CLINICAL CASES
IN TROPICAL MEDICINE

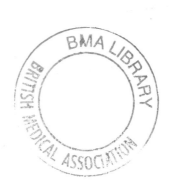

CLINICAL CASES IN TROPICAL MEDICINE

CAMILLA ROTHE MD DTM&H

Clinical Lecturer
Department of Medicine
Division of Tropical Medicine and Infectious Diseases
University of Hamburg School of Medicine
Hamburg, Germany

For additional online content visit ExpertConsult.com

ELSEVIER
SAUNDERS

ELSEVIER
SAUNDERS

Notices

ISBN: 9780702058240
Reprinted 2014, 2015

e-book ISBN: 9780702058264
Printed in China
Last digit is the print number: 9   8   7   6   5   4   3

Content Strategist: Belinda Kuhn
Content Development Specialist: Poppy Garraway
Content Coordinator: Humayra Rahman Khan
Project Manager: Caroline Jones
Design: Miles Hitchen
Marketing Manager: Katie Alexo

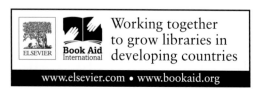

Working together to grow libraries in developing countries

www.elsevier.com • www.bookaid.org

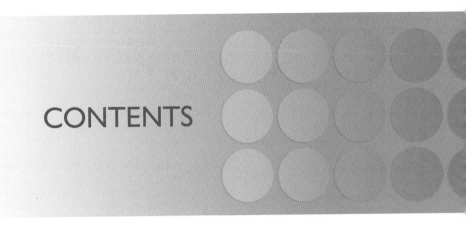

CONTENTS

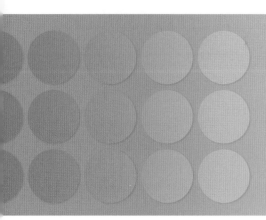

FOREWORD

Peter Hotez MD PhD FAAP FASTMH*

Information from the recently published Global Burden of Disease Study 2010 indicates that the world's major tropical infections, including malaria and the 17 major neglected tropical diseases (NTDs) identified by the World Health Organization, exert a horrific toll on human life[1,2]. Together these diseases kill more than one million people annually,[1] while causing chronic and disabling effects measured in DALYs (disability-adjusted life years) that exceed almost any other cause of illness.[2] Tuberculosis and HIV/AIDS are also devastating infections that disproportionately occur in tropical developing countries.

Even beyond their adverse health impact, the leading tropical diseases are significant causes of economic underdevelopment – indeed they are the most common diseases of poor people and have been shown to thwart economic productivity through their negative effects on child health and the productivity of agricultural workers.[3] These diseases also disproportionately devastate girls and women through their ability to damage the female urogenital tract or cause disfigurement and stigma.[4] Tropical diseases are the secret scourge of girls and women.

Despite their enormous global importance, there is a surprising lack of knowledge about tropical diseases among health care professionals including physicians. For example, recent studies from the United States Centers for Disease Control and Prevention indicate that very few US medical doctors know how to recognize and diagnose Chagas disease (American trypanosomiasis) even though it is now an important cause of heart disease in the US.[5,6] As a result, thousands of Chagas disease cases may go undiagnosed every year and patients inadvertently denied access to essential trypanocidal medicines. This finding emphasizes an emerging concept in tropical medicine that many parasitic and related infections occur outside of the poorest countries, with high levels of transmission also occurring in generally wealthy countries such as in the US or Eastern and Southern Europe.[7,8] The term 'blue marble health' has been coined to account for the finding that many of the world's neglected tropical diseases are found predominantly among the extreme poor living amidst wealth.[9] In other words, poverty has emerged as the overriding social determinant of neglected tropical diseases.

Clinical Cases in Tropical Medicine ('*Clinical Cases*') is a key companion volume to the recently published 23rd Edition of Manson's Tropical Diseases, but it will also be useful alongside other complete tropical medicine textbooks. An important role for *Clinical Cases* is to provide important practical applications and illustrative case reports in order to reinforce the material in these comprehensive texts. Comprised of 76 detailed clinical cases from as many tropical medicine physicians across the world, *Clinical Cases* provides an excellent learning opportunity to reinforce concepts on practical approaches to the diagnosis, management, and treatment of the major tropical diseases endemic to Africa, Asia and the Americas. The book should be useful for trainees and practitioners working in disease-endemic developing countries, as well as those working in clinical settings that see immigrants or travelers from affected regions and now people living in poverty in North America and Europe who also suffer from these afflictions. *Clinical Cases* should serve as a powerful learning tool for years to come!

Peter Hotez is Texas Children's Hospital Endowed Chair of Tropical Pediatrics, Professor of Pediatrics and Molecular Virology and Microbiology, and Dean of the National School of Tropical Medicine at Baylor College of Medicine in Houston, Texas.

References Cited

1. Lozano R, Naghavi M, Foreman K, et al. Global and regional mortality from 235 causes of death for 20 age groups in 1990 and 2010: a systematic analysis for the Global Burden of Disease Study 2010. Lancet 2012;380:2095–128.

2. Murray CJ, Vos T, Lozano R, et al. Disability-adjusted life years (DALYs) for 291 diseases and injuries in 21 regions, 1990-2010: a systematic analysis for the Global Burden of Disease Study 2010. Lancet 2012;380:2197–223.

3. Hotez PJ, Fenwick A, Savioli L, et al. Rescuing the bottom billion through control of neglected tropical diseases. Lancet 2009;373:1570–5.

4. Hotez PJ, Whitham M. Helminth infections: a new global women's health agenda. Obst Gynecol 2014;in press.

5. Stimpert KK, Montgomery SP. Physician awareness of Chagas disease, USA. Emerg Infect Dis 2010;16:871–2.

6. Verani JR, Montgomery SP, Schulkin J, et al. Am J Trop Med Hyg 2010;83:891–5.

7. Hotez PJ. Neglected infections of poverty in the United States of America. PLOS Negl Trop Dis 2008;2:e256.

8. Hotez PJ, Gurwith M. Europe's neglected infections of poverty. Int J Infect Dis 2011;15:e611–19.

9. Hotez PJ. NTDs V.2.0: 'Blue marble health' – neglected tropical disease control and elimination in a shifting health policy landscape. PLOS Negl Trop Dis 2013;7:e2570.

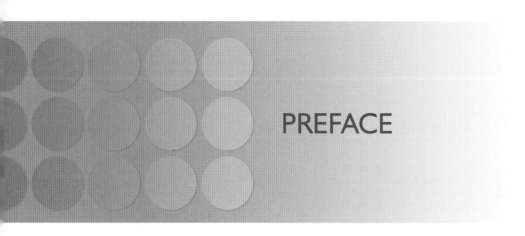

PREFACE

Do you speak any Latin? No? – You may have spent quite a few years of your life studying an ancient language, but you still would not be able to survive in a place like ancient Rome if a time machine took you there since you were never trained to converse in that language. Reading medical textbooks may be a similar experience: you may acquire a considerable amount of theoretical knowledge, but still struggle to apply it when suddenly confronted with a patient. This is why this book has been written – to enable you to effortlessly put your knowledge of tropical medicine into practice.

This book contains 76 real cases from all over the tropical world. It has no claim to be a comprehensive textbook of tropical medicine, however, all cases are real and their authors have extensive experience working in the tropics. Apart from confronting you with a challenging clinical problem the authors will share with you the daily realities at their workplacein the tropics – few available investigations, patchy test results, conflicting cultural beliefs, stock-outs of essential drugs and other challenges that you may only read between the lines of a conventional textbook.

The book equally covers tropical medicine and medicine in the tropics, infectious diseases and travel medicine, since for the practising clinician working in the tropics the division into subspecialties is of little use. Also, the same tropical disease may present in a very different manner in a returning traveller compared to a patient born in an endemic country.

Clinical Cases in Tropical Medicine has been written for doctors and senior medical students who already have some background knowledge in tropical medicine which they wish to put into practice. It shall help the reader prepare for an occupational stay in a tropical country and equally be useful to prepare for examinations, like the Diploma in Tropical Medicine and Hygiene (DTM&H) or a specialist examination. It can also just be used by anyone who takes pleasure in puzzling cases in tropical medicine for the mere fun of it.

This book has been developed as a companion book to *Manson's Tropical Diseases* 23rd edition, however, it can be read alongside any other textbook of tropical medicine. It can also be used on its own since every case presentation closes with a 'summary box' providing a brief synopsis of the clinical problem discussed.

LIST OF CONTRIBUTORS

Charlotte Adamczick, MD DTM&H MScIH
General Paediatrician, Private Practice,
St Gallen, Switzerland, Guest Lecturer,
Tropical Institute, Berlin, Germany

Andrew Bastawrous, MB ChB BSc (Hons)
FHEA MRCOphth
Clinical Research Fellow in International Eye
Health, International Centre for Eye Health,
Clinical Research Department, London
School of Hygiene & Tropical Medicine,
London, UK

Sudhir Babji, MD
Assistant Professor, The Wellcome Trust
Research Laboratory, Division of
Gastrointestinal Sciences, Christian
Medical College, Vellore, India

M. Jane Bates, BSc MB ChB MPhil
(Pall Med)
Clinical Lecturer, Department of Medicine,
College of Medicine, Blantyre, Malawi

Daniel G. Bausch, MD MPH&TM
Associate Professor, Department of Tropical
Medicine, Tulane School of Public Health
and Tropical Medicine, Clinical Associate
Professor, Department of Medicine, Section
of Adult Infectious Diseases, Tulane Medical
Center, New Orleans, LA, USA

Nicholas A.V. Beare, MA MBChB
FRCOphth MD
Consultant Ophthalmologist, St Paul's Eye
Unit, Royal Liverpool University Hospital,
Liverpool, UK

Marleen Boelaert, MD PhD
Professor, Department of Public Health,
Institute of Tropical Medicine, Antwerp,
Belgium

Gerd-Dieter Burchard, MD
Professor, ifi-Institut for Interdisciplinary
Medicine, Hamburg, Germany

Beatriz Bustamante, MD
Head of the Mycology Laboratory and
Associate Researcher, Instituto de Medicina
Tropical Alexander con Humboldt,
Universidad Peruana Cayetano Heredia,
Lima, Peru, Assistant Physician, Department
of Transmissible and Dermatological
Diseases, Hospital Nacional Cayetano
Heredia, Lima, Peru

Fátima Concha, MD
Medical doctor, Instituto de Medicina Tropical
Alexander von Humbolt, Universidad
Peruana Cayetano Heredia, Lima, Peru

Bart Currie, FRACP
Professor in Medicine and Head of Infectious
Diseases, Infectious Diseases Department
and Global and Tropical Health Division,
Royal Darwin Hospital and Menzies School
of Health Research, Darwin, NT, Australia

David Dance, MB ChB MSc FRCPath
Clinical Research Microbiologist, Lao–Oxford–
Mahosot Hospital–Wellcome Trust Research
Unit, Microbiology Laboratory, Mahosot
Hospital, Vientiane, Lao PDR and Centre
for Tropical Medicine, University of Oxford,
Oxford, UK

Sebastian Dieckmann, MD
Senior Clinical Consultant, Institute of Tropical
Medicine and International Health, Charité
– Universitätsmedizin Berlin, Berlin,
Germany

Viravong Douangnoulak, MD
Head, Department of Otorhinolaryngology, Mahosot Hospital, Vientiane, Laos PDR

Ivy Ekem, MB ChB FWACP FGCP
Senior Lecturer and Consultant Haematologist, Department of Haematology, University of Ghana Medical School and Korle-Bu Teaching Hospital, Accra, Ghana

Nadia El-Dib, PhD
Professor of Parasitology, Head of the Permanent Scientific Committee of Parasitology in Egyptian Universities, Department of Medical Parasitology, Faculty of Medicine, Cairo University, Cairo, Egypt

Jeremy Farrar, FRCP DPhil
Professor of Tropical Medicine, Oxford University Clinical Research Unit, Hospital for Tropical Diseases, Ho Chi Minh City, Vietnam

Facundo M. Fernández, PhD
Associate Professor, School of Chemistry and Biochemistry, Georgia Institute of Technology, Atlanta, GA, USA

Arthur M. Friedlander, MD
Senior Scientist, US Army Medical Research Institute of Infectious Diseases, Frederick, MD, USA, Adjunct Professor of Medicine, Uniformed Services University of the Health Sciences, Bethesda, MD, USA

Eduardo Gotuzzo, MD FACP FIDSA
Principal Professor of Medicine, Universidad Peruana Cayetano Heredia, Director, Instituto de Medicina Tropical Alexander von Humboldt, Lima, Peru

Michael D. Green, PhD
Research Chemist, Division of Parasitic Diseases and Malaria, US Centers for Disease Control and Prevention, Atlanta, GA, USA

Anthony D. Harries, OBE MA MD FRCP DTM&H
Senior Advisor, Department of Research, International Union Against Tuberculosis and Lung Disease, Paris, France

William P. Howlett, FRCPI PhD
Physician/Neurologist, Department of Internal Medicine, Kilimanjaro Christian Medical Centre, Moshi, Tanzania

Ralf Ignatius, MD
Head of Diagnostic Laboratory, Institute of Tropical Medicine and International Health, Charité – Universitätsmedizin Berlin, Berlin, Germany

Saythong Inthalad, MD
Luang Nam Tha Provincial Health Department, Luang Nam Tha Province, Lao PDR

Kentaro Ishida, MD DTM&H
Obstetrics and Gynecology Resident, Department of Obstetrics and Gynecology, Tokyo Metropolitan Bokutoh Hospital, Tokyo, Japan

Frederique Jacquerioz, MD DTM&H MPH
Visiting Clinical Research Fellow, Instituto de Medicina Tropical Alexander von Humboldt, Universidad Peruana Cayetano Heredia, Lima, Peru, Assistant Clinical Professor, Department of Tropical Medicine, Tulane School of Public Health and Tropical Medicine, New Orleans, LA, USA

Benjamin Jeffs, MRCP
Consultant in Infectious Diseases, Bradford Royal Infirmary, Yorkshire, UK

Sabine Jordan, MD DTM&H (LSTM)
Senior Physician, Division of Tropical Medicine and Infectious Diseases, University of Hamburg School of Medicine, Hamburg, Germany

Gagandeep Kang, MD PhD FRCPath
Professor and Head, Division of Gastrointestinal Sciences, Christian Medical College, Vellore, India

Juri Katchanov, MD DTMH (BKK)
Specialist in Neurology, Auguste-Viktoria Klinikum, Department of Infectious Diseases and Gastroenterology, Berlin, Germany

Valy Keoluangkhot, MD MSc
Chief of Adult Infectious and Tropical Diseases Center, Senior Clinical Research, Mahosot Hospital, Ministry of Health, Vientiane, Lao PDR, Clinical Coordinator, Institut Francophone pour la Medicine Tropicale Vientiane, Lao PDR

Guido Kluxen, MD, Professor Dr. med.
Senior Clinical Research Fellow,
    Ophthalmological Regional Community
    Consulting, and, Clinic Wermelskirchen–
    Solingen–Remscheid, Wermelskirchen,
    Germany

Vatthanaphone Latthaphasavang, MD
Senior Clinical Research Fellow, Adult
    Infectious Disease Ward, Mahosot Hospital,
    Vientiane, Lao PDR

Alejandro Llanos-Cuentas, MD MSc PhD
Full Professor, School of Public Health,
    Universidad Peruana Cayetano Heredia,
    Lima, Peru

David Mabey, DM FRCP
Professor of Communicable Diseases, Faculty
    of Infectious and Tropical Diseases, London
    School of Hygiene & Tropical Medicine,
    London, UK

Ciro Maguiña, MD
Principal Professor of Medicine, Instituto de
    Medicina Tropical, Alexander van Humboldt,
    Universidad Peruana Cayetano Heredia,
    Lima, Peru

Dalila Martínez, MD MSPH
Associated Investigator, Instituto de Medicina
    Tropical Alexander von Humboldt,
    Universidad Peruana Cayetano Heredia,
    Lima, Peru

Haruhiko Maruyama, MD
Professor, Department of Infectious Diseases,
    University of Miyazaki, Faculty of Medicine,
    Miyazaki, Japan

Mayfong Mayxay, MD PhD (Clin Trop Med)
Associate Professor of Tropical Medicine and
    Infectious Diseases, University of Health
    Sciences and Lao-Oxford-Mahosot
    Hospital-Wellcome Trust Research Unit,
    Mahosot Hospital, Vientiane, Lao PDR

James McCarthy, FRACP
Professor of Tropical Medicine and Infectious
    Diseases, Infectious Diseases Program,
    QIMR Berghofer Medical Research Institute
    and Department of Infectious Diseases,
    Royal Brisbane and Women's Hospital,
    Brisbane, QLD, Australia

Fernando Mejía Cordero, MD
Associated Clinical Research Fellow, Instituto
    de Medicina Tropical Alexander Von
    Humboldt, Universidad Peruana Cayetano
    Heredia, Lima, Peru

Robert F. Miller, MB BS FRCP FSB
Reader in Clinical Infection, Research
    Department of Infection and Population
    Health, University College London, London,
    UK

Elizabeth M. Molyneux, OBE MB BS
DObsRCOG FRCPCH FRCP FCEM
Hon Professor of Paediatrics, Paediatric
    Department, College of Medicine, Blantyre,
    Malawi

Andreas J. Morguet, MD
Senior Cardiology Attending and Lecturer,
    Department of Cardiology and Pulmology,
    Campus Benjamin Franklin, Charité –
    Universitätsmedizin Berlin, Berlin, Germany

Yukifumi Nawa, MD PhD
Consultant/Invited Professor, Research Affairs,
    Faculty of Medicine, Khon Kaen University,
    Khon Kaen, Thailand

Paul N. Newton, BM BCh, D.Phil, MRCP,
DTM&H
Hon Professor, Lao–Oxford–Mahosot
    Hospital–Wellcome Trust Research Unit,
    Mahosot Hospital, Vientiane, Lao PDR and
    Centre for Tropical Medicine, Nuffield
    Department of Medicine, Churchill
    Hospital, University of Oxford, Oxford, UK

Caoimhe Nic Fhogartaigh, MBBS MRCP
FRCPath DTM&H
Infectious Diseases and Microbiology Registrar,
    Lao-Oxford-Mahosot Hospital-Wellcome
    Trust Research Unit, Mahosot Hospital,
    Vientiane, Lao PDR

Buachan Norindr, MD
Deputy, Department of Otorhinolaryngology,
    Mahosot Hospital, Vientiane, Lao PDR

Joep J. van Oosterhout, MD PhD
Medical and Research Director, Dignitas
    International, Zomba, Malawi

Gregor Pollach, Dr Med FCAI (Hon)
MA(pol sc) DTM&P
Head of Department, Associate Professor,
   Department of Anaesthesiology and
   Intensive Care, University of Malawi,
   College of Medicine Blantyre, Malawi

Douglas G. Postels, MD
Associate Professor of Pediatric Neurology,
   Department of Neurology and
   Ophthalmology, Michigan State University,
   East Lansing, MI, USA

Ranjan Premaratna, MD
Professor in Medicine, Department of
   Medicine, Faculty of Medicine, University of
   Kelaniya, Ragama, Sri Lanka

Sayaphet Rattanavong, MD
Research Clinician, Lao Oxford Mahosot
   Hospital Wellcome Trust Research Unit,
   Microbiology Laboratory, Mahosot Hospital,
   Vientiane, Lao PDR

Koert Ritmeijer, PhD
Lead Neglected Tropical Diseases, Public
   Health Department, Médecins Sans
   Frontières, Amsterdam, The Netherlands

Hillary K. Rono, MBChB MMed
(Ophthalomology) FEACO Msc
Ophthalmologist, Kitale District Hospital,
   Ministry of Health, Kenya, Kitale, Kenya

Karen Roodnat, MD MRCP MSc DTM&H
Medical Doctor in Tropical Medicine and
   International Health, Medecins Sans
   Frontières, Amsterdam, The Netherlands

Camilla Rothe, MD DTM&H
Clinical Lecturer, Department of Medicine,
   Division of Tropical Medicine and Infectious
   Diseases, University of Hamburg School of
   Medicine, Hamburg, Germany

Carlos Seas, MD
Associate Professor of Medicine, Instituto de
   Medicina Tropical Alexander von Humboldt,
   Universidad Peruana Cayetano Heredia,
   Lima, Peru

Fredericka Sey, MB ChB
Principal Medical Officer, Sickle Cell Clinic,
   Ghana Institute of Clinical Genetics, Korle
   Bu, Accra, Ghana.

Thomas Schneider, Univ. Prof. PhD MD
Head of Infectious Diseases, Charite –
   Universitätsmedizin Berlin, Berlin, Germany

Markus Schulze Schwering, MD FEBO
Lecturer; Consultant Ophthalmologist,
   Department of Ophthalmology within the
   Department of Surgery, College of Medicine
   and Department für Augenheilkunde,
   Blantyre, Malawi and, Tübingen, Germany

Omar Siddiqi, MD
Clinical Instructor, Department of Neurology,
   Beth Israel Deaconess Medical Center,
   Harvard Medical School, Boston, MA, USA,
   Honorary Lecturer, Department of Internal
   Medicine, University of Zambia School of
   Medicine, Lusaka, Zambia

Eberhard Siebert, MD
Staff Neuroradiologist, Department of
   Neuroradiology, Charité –
   Universitätsmedizin Berlin, Berlin, Germany

Siho Sisouphonh, MD
Senior Infectious Disease Clinician, Adult
   Infectious Disease Ward, Mahosot Hospital,
   Vientiane, Lao PDR

Günther Slesak, Dr.med., DTM&H
Consultant for Tropical Medicine, Department
   for Tropical Medicine, Hospital for Tropical
   Diseases Paul-Lechler-Krankenhaus,
   Tübingen, Germany

Douangdao Soukaloun, MD
Professor, Department of Pediatrics, Mahosot
   Hospital, Vientiane, Lao PDR

M. Leila Srour, MD MPH DTM&H
Professional Development Coordinator,
   Pediatrics, Health Frontiers, Muang Sing,
   Laos

Hartmut Stocker, MD
Consultant, Auguste-Viktoria Klinikum,
   Department of Infectious Diseases and
   Gastroenterology, Berlin, Germany

Marija Stojkovic, MD DTM&H
General Practitioner, Section Clinical Tropical
   Medicine, University Hospital Heidelberg,
   Heidelberg, Germany

Masaki Tomita, MD
Associate professor, Department of Surgery II,
University of Miyazaki, Miyazaki, Japan

Kristien Verdonck, MD PhD
Research Fellow, Department of Public Health,
Institute of Tropical Medicine, Antwerp,
Belgium

Moritz Vogel, Pediatrician DTM&H
Clinical Investigator, Section Clinical Tropical
Medicine, Department of Infectious
Diseases, Heidelberg University Hospital,
Heidelberg, Germany

Emma C. Wall, MRCP DTM&H MRes
Wellcome Trust Clinical PhD Student, Clinical
Research Group, Liverpool School of
Tropical Medicine and the, Malawi–
Liverpool–Wellcome Trust Clinical Research
Programme, Malawi, Africa

Thomas Weitzel, MD DTMP
Consultant in Tropical and Travel Medicine,
Travel Medicine Program, Clínica Alemana,
Universidad del Desarrollo, Santiago, Chile

Christopher J.M. Whitty, FRCP DTM&H
Professor of International Health, London
School of Hygiene & Tropical Medicine,
London, UK

Yohannes W. Woldeamanuel, MD
Postdoctoral Scholar, Department of Neurology
and Neurological Sciences, Stanford
University, School of Medicine, Stanford,
California, Department of Neurology, Addis
Ababa University School of Medicine, Addis
Ababa, Ethiopia

Katherine L. Woods, MBBS DTMH MSc
MRCP FRCPath
Infectious Diseases/ Microbiology Registrar,
Infectious Diseases Department, Royal Free
Hospital NHS Trust, London, UK

Mary E. Wright, MD MPH
Division of Clinical Research, National
Institute of Allergy and Infectious Diseases,
National Institutes of Health, Bethesda, MD,
USA

Sophie Yacoub, MRCP MSc DTM&H
Clinical Research Fellow, Centre for Tropical
Medicine, Oxford University Clinical
Research Unit, Wellcome Trust Major
Overseas Programme, Hanoi, Vietnam,
Department of Medicine, Imperial College,
London, UK

ACKNOWLEDGEMENTS

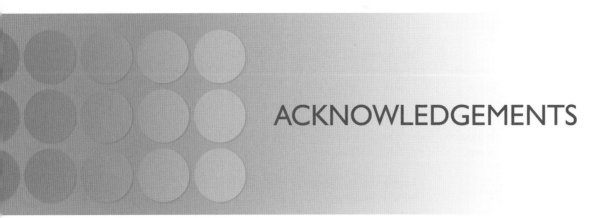

I would like to thank the whole editorial team at Elsevier's for their great and completely uncomplicated cooperation. In particular I would like to thank Poppy Garraway, Belinda Kuhn and Caroline Jones.

I am very grateful to all authors for their spontaneous enthusiasm and their willingness to share their cases.

Special thanks go to Chris Whitty for his continous support, advice and encouragement, and to Anthony D. Harries, who's own wonderful case book is sadly out of print but was the key inspiration to edit this book. I'd also like to thank David Lalloo and Malcolm Molyneux for their encouragement and support.

Finally I'd like to thank Juri Katchanov for his patience and for being an inexhaustable source of inspiration.

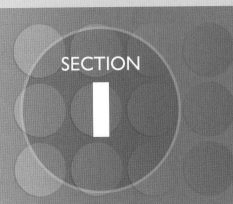

CASE 1

A 20-Year-Old Woman from Sudan With Fever, Haemorrhage and Shock

Daniel G. Bausch

History

A 20-year-old housewife presents to a hospital in northern Uganda with a two-day history of fever, severe asthenia, chest and abdominal pain, nausea, vomiting, diarrhoea and slight non-productive cough. The patient is a Sudanese refugee living in a camp in the region. She denies any contact with sick people.

Clinical Findings

The patient was prostrate and semi-conscious on admission. Vital signs were: temperature 39.6°C, blood pressure 90/60 mmHg, pulse 90 bpm, respiratory rate 24 breath cycles per minute. Physical examination revealed abdominal tenderness, especially in the right upper quadrant, hepatosplenomegaly and bleeding from the gums. The lungs were clear. No rash or lymphadenopathy was noted.

Questions

1. Is the patient's history and clinical presentation consistent with a haemorrhagic fever (HF) syndrome?
2. What degree of nursing precautions need to be implemented?

CASE 2

A 7-Year-Old Girl from Peru With a Chronic Skin Ulcer

Dalila Martínez / Kristien Verdonck / Marleen Boelaert / Alejandro Llanos-Cuentas

History

A 7-year-old girl who lives in Lima, the Peruvian capital, is brought to your clinic with a lesion on the nose as the main complaint. The lesion appeared four months ago as a small nodule and slowly turned into an ulcer. It is a bit itchy but not painful. There is no history of trauma. The girl is otherwise healthy. Six months ago she travelled to a valley on the western slopes of the Andes.

Clinical Findings

The lesion is a localized ulcer on the nose (Figure 2-1, p 49). The borders of the ulcer are indurated and there is plaque-like infiltration of the surrounding skin. The diameter of the whole lesion is about 2 cm. There are no palpable lymph nodes. Body temperature is 37°C. The rest of the physical examination is normal.

1. What are your differential diagnoses?
2. How would you approach the diagnosis of this patient?

CASE 3

A 26-Year-Old Woman from Malawi With Headache, Confusion and Unilateral Ptosis

Juri Katchanov

History

A 26-year-old Malawian woman is brought to the emergency department of a local central hospital by two relatives. She has been unwell for at least one week. She complained of a headache of insidious onset and has been confused for two days. One day before presentation the guardians noticed an eyelid drooping on the left side.

The guardians say her past medical history is unremarkable. The patient lives in an urban high-density area. She works as a businesswoman, selling vegetables. She has three healthy children, but another four of her children have died as toddlers. Her husband died a year ago of 'high fever'.

Clinical Findings

On examination she looks seriously unwell. Glasgow Coma Scale 14/15, temperature 38.4°C, blood pressure 115/75 mmHg, heart rate 86 bpm, respiratory rate 18 breath cycles per minute. There is no neck stiffness. The chest is clear. Figure 3-1 (p 53) shows the examination of her eyes. The remainder of her neurological examination is normal.

Laboratory Results

Her blood results are shown in Table 3-1 (p 53). A lumbar puncture was done. The opening pressure was markedly raised, at 32 cmH$_2$O (12–20 cmH$_2$O). The available CSF results are shown in Table 3-2 (p 53).

1. What is the clinical syndrome and what is the differential diagnosis?
2. How would you manage this patient?

CASE 4

A 4-Year-Old Girl from Uganda in Coma

Douglas G. Postels

History

It is the rainy season in rural eastern Uganda. A 4-year-old girl, previously healthy, is carried into the Accident and Emergency (A&E) Department. Her father reports that she was well until yesterday. She had a bad headache in the early afternoon but later in the evening developed shaking chills. Believing this was yet another episode of malaria, a common problem in their village, the family planned to take her to the Health Centre in the morning. The child slept restlessly. At 5 a.m. today the family woke to find the girl was in the midst of a seizure which lasted about ten minutes. It has taken four hours for the family to reach A&E and the little girl has not awoken. The child has not had any recent head trauma and the family knows of no other reason that the child might be ill.

Clinical Findings

Her temperature is 38.7°C, pulse 150 bpm, respiratory rate 36 breath cycles per minute. Her blood pressure 98/40 mmHg. She has no neck stiffness or jaundice. Capillary refill is normal. There is nasal flaring with respirations. Blantyre Coma Score is 1/5. Pupils are 2 mm and reactive, and extraocular movements are normal by oculocephalic manoeuvres. She has no papilloedema on direct ophthalmoscopy. With stimulation there is decerebrate posturing that resolves spontaneously. On cardiac examination she has a gallop rhythm. Her liver is palpable 2 cm below the right costal margin and her spleen is 4 cm below the left costal margin. A rapid test for glucose is normal.

Laboratory Results

Laboratory results are given in Table 4-1 (p 57).

Questions

1. What is the differential diagnosis?
2. What additional work-up should be performed?

CASE 5

A 4-Year-Old Boy from Laos With a Lesion of the Lip and Cheek

M. Leila Srour

History

You are sent a picture of a 4-year-old boy taken by a visitor at a remote district hospital in Laos (Figure 5-1, p 60). You receive a limited history and physical exam. Three days ago the family noticed a dark sore on the child's cheek. The child's breath smells bad, he is not eating and appears listless. The lesion progressed quickly from a sore to eat through the child's cheek. The child, who is unimmunized, had a fever and rash about two months ago and recovered. The family is very poor. The local doctors do not recognize this disease.

Clinical Findings

The 4-year-old child appears small and quiet. His mouth has a gangrenous lesion that has destroyed part of his upper and lower lips and cheek, exposing his teeth. The child appears stunted and thin.

Questions

1. What is your differential diagnosis?
2. What should you recommend to help this child?

CASE 6

A 36-Year-Old Male Traveller Returning from Botswana With a Creeping Eruption

Emma C. Wall

History

A 36-year-old male restaurant owner presents to a travel clinic in Europe with a mobile itchy mass under his skin. Three weeks ago he noted the mass in his groin for four days after which it subsided. He then noted an itchy, serpiginous rash tracking from his groin to his chest which moved over the course of several days, disappeared and then he noted the mass reappearing on his right shoulder, at which point he was referred for assessment. There is no history of fever or systemic illness.

Five weeks ago he returned from a fishing holiday with four friends to the Okavango Delta in Botswana. He took malaria chemoprophylaxis (atovaquone/proguanil), slept on the boat under a mosquito net and swam in fresh river water. He ate freshwater fish from the river.

He is married with a child and denies sexual contact on the trip. Of the four friends who accompanied him, two also have the same complaint.

Clinical Findings

The patient is afebrile and organ system examination is normal. On his right upper deltoid is a firm mass with clear margins 3 × 8 cm in size. On further questioning this mass has recently migrated across his upper chest wall and a serpiginous tract is visible (Figure 6-1, p 62). There is no additional rash and no lymphadenopathy.

Laboratory Results

Total white cell count 8.9×10^9/L (reference range: 4–10), eosinophil count 0.9×10^9/L (reference value: <0.5), liver function tests, creatinine and electrolytes are normal. HIV antibodies are negative.

Questions

1. What is the likely diagnosis and what are your differentials?
2. What is the risk of this condition if untreated?

CASE 7

A 28-Year-Old Male Fisherman from Malawi With Shortness of Breath
Camilla Rothe

History

A 28-year-old Malawian man presents to a local hospital with progressive shortness of breath for the past five days. He reports orthopnoea and paroxysmal nocturnal dyspnoea, but there is no cough and no fever. He has also developed bilateral flank pain in the past days, which he describes as continuous and dull in nature, and he has been feeling constantly nauseated. However, there is no diarrhoea and no jaundice.

According to his health passport book, the patient was diagnosed with arterial hypertension two years earlier. He was prescribed some antihypertensive drugs which he never took. No investigations were done at that time.

His past medical history and family history are otherwise unremarkable. A recent HIV test was negative. The patient comes from a town on the Southern shore of Lake Malawi. He is a fisherman by profession. He is married and has two healthy children.

Clinical Findings

The patient is a 28-year-old man with an athletic build, who is not chronically ill looking, but is in respiratory distress. His conjunctivae are notably pale. His blood pressure is 200/130 mmHg, pulse 66 bpm, temperature 36.8°C and respiratory rate 32 breath cycles per minute.

His apex beat is slightly displaced, but his heart sounds are clear and regular, and the jugular venous pressure is not raised. On auscultation of the lungs there are bilateral fine crackles over the lung bases. The abdomen is flat and non-tender. There is bilateral renal angle tenderness and the kidneys are ballottable. There is no peripheral oedema.

Laboratory Results

His laboratory results on admission are shown in Table 7-1 (p 65).

Imaging

His chest radiograph on admission is shown in Figure 7-1 (p 66).

Questions

1. What is your clinical impression?
2. What further investigations would you like to do to establish the diagnosis?

CASE 8

A 26-Year-Old Female Traveller Returning from Ghana With a Boil on the Leg

Camilla Rothe

History

A 26-year-old German student presents to your clinic because of a localized swelling on her right leg. She has just returned from a six-week trip to Ghana.

The swelling has developed slowly over the past three weeks. It is itchy, but not painful. There is no history of fever; no history of arthropod bites. The patient is otherwise fine.

Clinical Findings

There is localized swelling on the right leg, about 1.5 cm in diameter (Figure 8-1, p 70). The skin surrounding the swelling is slightly hyperaemic. At the centre of the boil a dark scab can be seen. There is no lymphadenopathy. The patient is afebrile while the rest of the physical examination is normal.

Questions

1. What are your most important differential diagnoses?
2. How would you approach this patient?

CASE 9

A 16-Year-Old Girl from Vietnam With Fever, Headache and Myalgias

Sophie Yacoub / Jeremy Farrar

History

A 16-year-old girl presents to the outpatient department of an urban hospital in Vietnam having had fevers of 39–40°C, headache, lethargy and muscle aches for five days. Today she has vomited three times and is complaining of abdominal pain. She also noticed some bleeding from her gums after brushing her teeth this morning. She is normally fit and well and has not travelled outside the city.

Clinical Findings

On examination, the patient looks lethargic but has a GCS of 15/15. Her temperature is 37.5°C, blood pressure is 94/68 mmHg, pulse 88 bpm and the respiratory rate is 20 breath cycles per minute. There is a maculopapular rash on the chest, abdomen and extremities that is fading (Figure 9-1, p 73). Cardiovascular and respiratory examination is normal. There is mild abdominal tenderness and the liver edge is palpable, bowel sounds are normal. The spleen is not enlarged and there is no palpable lymphadenopathy.

Laboratory Findings

The laboratory results are shown in Table 9-1 (p 73).

Questions

1. What is your differential diagnosis?
2. What further investigations would you request?

CASE 10

A 55-Year-Old Indigenous Woman from Australia With a Widespread Exfoliating Rash and Sepsis

Bart Currie / James McCarthy

History

You are working in a remote indigenous community in tropical northern Australia, and the community health worker asks you to visit a house to assess an elderly woman who has been living in the crowded back room. Her family are worried that she has become increasingly withdrawn and hasn't been getting out of the house much at all.

Clinical Findings

The patient is a 55-year-old indigenous Australian woman with a widespread exfoliative rash involving all limbs and especially the armpits, buttocks and thighs (Figure 10-1, p 76). Many flakes of skin cover the mattress she is lying on. In addition, she has fissures over her wrists and knees. She also looks pale and is clammy and poorly responsive. You take her observations and her temperature is 39.5°C, heart rate 110 bpm, respiratory rate 28 breath cycles per minute and blood pressure 85 mmHg systolic to radial pulsation. Oxygen saturation by pulse oximetry is 92% on room air.

Laboratory Results

You take blood cultures, full blood count, CRP and biochemistry. Samples are sent into the regional laboratory, with results expected the next day. You also take skin scrapings, which you can look at yourself using the community clinic microscope.

Questions

1. What is your provisional diagnosis?
2. What is your initial management?

CASE 11

A 45-Year-Old Male Security Guard from Malawi With Difficulties in Walking and Back Pain

Juri Katchanov

History

A 45-year-old security guard from Malawi is brought to the admission ward of a local tertiary hospital by two relatives because of back pain and progressive difficulties in walking.

His troubles started one year earlier with back pain and he presented to a local health centre. He was given paracetamol and sent home. The pain did not improve and over the following weeks he also developed difficulties in walking and 'pins and needles' sensations in his legs.

Three months after the first visit he presented again to the same health centre. His temperature was documented as slightly elevated (37.5°C). He was given antimalarials, a single dose of praziquantel and paracetamol. He consulted a local traditional healer who applied tattoos to his chest and his back (Figure 11-1A, p 79). Over the following six months his condition further deteriorated and he finally became bedridden.

The patient denies fever, night sweats and weight loss, and there is no chronic cough. There is neither haematuria nor diarrhoea and he is continent for stool and urine. There is no history of trauma or past tuberculosis. He has never been tested for HIV.

He is a non-smoker, but drinks two paper cartons (about one litre) of chibuku, a locally brewed beer, per day. He is married with three children, who are all well. He resides in an urban area and used to work as a security guard but has been unemployed for the last six months due to his illness.

Clinical Findings

He looks well and is afebrile with normal vital signs. There is tenderness over the lower thoracic spine and severe spasticity of both legs (Figure 11-1B, p 79). The power in his legs is 1/5 (visible muscle flicker). Deep tendon reflexes of the lower limbs are exaggerated. The plantar reflexes are upgoing (Figure 11-1C, p 79). There is a sensory level for pain and temperature sensation between T9 and T 11 (Figure 11-1D, p 79), with diminished joint sense in his big toes bilaterally. The examination of his cranial nerves and the upper limbs is normal.

Laboratory Results

Full blood count results are: WBC 4.3×10^9/L (reference range: 4–10), haemoglobin 14.8 g/dL (13–15), platelets 391×10^9/L (150–400).

Questions

1. What is the neuroanatomical syndrome and what is your differential diagnosis?
2. What further management should be carried out?

CASE 12

A 29-Year-Old Man from The Gambia With Genital Ulceration

David Mabey

History

A 29-year-old man comes to your clinic in The Gambia complaining of painful sores involving his private parts for seven days. He has been previously well. He admits to having had sex with a commercial sex worker two weeks ago, when he had not used a condom.

Clinical Findings

He is in considerable pain and is only able to walk with difficulty because of this. He is afebrile and well nourished. General examination is unremarkable. The only abnormality is the presence of numerous painful ulcers on his penis, scrotum and inner thigh (Figure 12-1, p 84). The ulcers are tender, soft and bleed on contact. There is no inguinal lymphadenopathy.

Questions

1. What are the most important differential diagnoses?
2. How would you manage this patient?

CASE 13

A 16-Year-Old Girl from Malawi With Fever and Abdominal Pain

Camilla Rothe

History

A 16-year-old girl presents to the emergency room of a hospital in Malawi because of fever, generalized abdominal pain and frontal headache for the past five days. There is no history of diarrhoea.

She delivered a baby five months ago. A HIV test done in the antenatal clinic was negative. Her further past medical history is unremarkable.

She lives with her parents, her three siblings and her baby in an urban high-density area. There is no running water and no electricity in the house. They fetch water from a community tap. She went to primary school but recently dropped out during her pregnancy.

Clinical Findings

The patient is a 16-year-old girl in a fair nutritional state. Temperature 38.1°C, blood pressure 110/60 mmHg, pulse 78 bpm, respiratory rate 20 breath cycles per minute, Glasgow Coma Scale 15/15. There is mild scleral jaundice, no neck stiffness. The examination of the abdomen shows diffuse tenderness but no guarding. The liver is not enlarged, the spleen is palpable at 2 cm below the left costal margin. The chest is clear and there is no lymphadenopathy. Pelvic examination is unremarkable and there is no vaginal discharge.

Investigations

Her laboratory results on admission are shown in Table 13-1 (p 85). Thick smear for malaria parasites is positive. Liver function tests are not available since reagents are out of stock.

1. What are your most important differential diagnoses?
2. How would you approach this patient?

CASE 14

A 22-Year-Old Woman from Bangladesh With Profuse Watery Diarrhoea

Gagandeep Kang / Sudhir Babji

History

A 22-year-old woman from a village near Dhaka, Bangladesh, is brought to the district hospital emergency room with a history of passing 12–15 large-volume stools which resemble diluted milk or rice water with white flakes in the past day. Her husband reports that she became unresponsive about an hour previously and he hired a rickshaw to bring her to the hospital. He says that she had not complained of pain and did not have fever.

The patient has recently returned from her village after attending a religious festival, where water was supplied in large metal containers. Her husband reports that there were five or six people who had attended the same event and who were also ill with diarrhoea, although none as severely affected as his wife.

Clinical Findings

A thin young woman, who is stuporous, and responds minimally to a painful stimulus (Glasgow Coma Scale 9/15). She is afebrile, with sunken eyes, dry mouth and eyes, and a scaphoid abdomen. A skin pinch returns very slowly. Her pulse rate is 110 bpm, low volume, and her blood pressure is 90/50 mm Hg. The remainder of her systemic examination is normal.

Laboratory Results

The results of her blood tests on admission are shown in Table 14-1 (p 88).

Stool Examination

Macroscopic: Liquid stool, rice-water appearance with no faecal matter.

Hanging drop preparation shows small slender curved bacilli with darting motility. Motility is completely inhibited by using *Vibrio cholerae* antiserum O1.

Stool culture grows *V. cholerae* (Figure 14-1, p 89) and the organism was typed as *V. cholerae* O1, Serotype Ogawa, biotype El Tor. The organism was susceptible to tetracycline, furazolidone and quinolone groups of antibiotics.

1. How was the infection most likely acquired? Is there an outbreak?
2. How is dehydration assessed and managed?

CASE 15

A 3-Year-Old Boy from Laos With Right Suppurative Parotitis

Sayaphet Rattanavong / Viravong Douangnoulak / Buachan Norindr / Paul N. Newton / Caoimhe Nic Fhogartaigh

History

A 3-year-old rural Lao boy, whose parents are rice farmers, presents to the ENT clinic with a ten-day history of gradual, painful swelling of the right cheek with associated fever and poor appetite. Three days previously his mother noticed a purulent discharge from the ear. He has no cough, vomiting or diarrhoea. There is no history of previous ear infection or dental problems, and no known history of trauma. The child is developing normally and is up to date with vaccinations.

Clinical Findings

The child looks unwell, with a fever of 39.5°C. There is a localized, fluctuant, hot, tender swelling below and anterior to the right ear, 6–8 cm in diameter, extending from the lower cheek to the sub-mandibular region, consistent with a parotid mass (Figure 15-1, p 92). Ear examination reveals purulent discharge in the auditory canal and a suspicion of a small fistula from which the pus is arising, with a right lower motor neuron facial nerve palsy. The oral cavity and throat are unremarkable. There is no lymphadenopathy and no hepatosplenomegaly. Heart sounds are normal and the chest is clear.

Questions

1. What are your differential diagnoses?
2. What investigations would you perform?

CASE 16

A 25-Year-Old Female School Teacher from Malawi With Abrupt Onset of a Febrile Confusional State

Emma C. Wall

History

A 25-year-old Malawian primary school teacher presents to a local central hospital. She was reported to be well at 8 a.m., confused by 10 a.m. and drowsy with a high fever and convulsions on admission at 11 a.m.

She is HIV-reactive and has been on antiretroviral therapy (ART) with tenofovir, lamivudine and efavirenz for six months with good adherence. Her CD4 count starting ART was 320 cells/μL. She completed treatment for pulmonary tuberculosis two months ago.

Clinical Findings

The patient is restless and agitated; Glasgow Coma Scale 10/15. Pupils are equal and reactive with photophobia, the neck is stiff and there is no rash. Plantar responses are down-going, Kernig's sign is positive. Chest and abdominal examinations are unremarkable.

Observations: temperature 40°C, pulse 125 bpm, blood pressure 125/68 mmHg, oxygen saturation 93% on room air. During the physical examination she suffers renewed seizure.

Laboratory Results

Her blood results are shown in Table 16-1 (p 95). A spinal tap is done. The CSF appears hazy; CSF results are shown in Table 16-2 (p 95). Rapid antigen test for *Plasmodium falciparum* is negative.

Questions

1. What are your treatment priorities for this woman?
2. What adjunctive interventions should be used in this setting?

CASE 17

A 34-Year-Old Man from Thailand With Fever and a Papular Rash

Juri Katchanov / Hartmut Stocker

History

A 34-year-old man from Phuket, Thailand, presents to a European hospital with a two-week history of fever. He has also noticed a papular rash affecting his whole body, particularly his face and trunk. When asked, he reports having lost 7 kg in the last three months.

He lives in Thailand and has arrived in Europe only three days previously to visit friends.

Clinical Findings

On examination, the patient is febrile with a temperature of 38.2°C. His conjunctivae are pale. He is very wasted, with a body mass index of 14 kg/m².

The patient has a generalized non-pruritic rash, predominantly on his face and trunk, which consists of small umbilicated papules (Figure 17-1, p 98). There is generalized lymphadenopathy with visibly swollen lymph nodes in the left supraclavicular region (Figure 17-2, p 98); his inguinal and axillary lymph nodes are also enlarged. On abdominal examination, the spleen is palpable two fingers below the left costal margin. The liver span was 15 cm in the midclavicular line.

Laboratory Results

Full blood count: WBC 2.1 × 10⁹/L (reference range 4–10), haemoglobin 9.8 g/dL (13–16), platelets 110 × 10⁹/L (150–350). C-reactive protein 150 mg/L (<5).

Questions

1. What is the single most important test to be done in this patient?
2. What is your differential diagnosis?

CASE 18

A 43-Year-Old Male Traveller With Fever and Eosinophilia

Gerd-Dieter Burchard

History

A 43-year-old German man presents to a local travel clinic on 21 May because of fever. He had been in Mozambique from 16 April to 30 April, afterwards in Chile from 30 April to 17 May. He did not take any malaria chemoprophylaxis in Mozambique and reports self-treatment for malaria with atovaquone/proguanil because of fever (27 April to 29 April). He is now complaining of renewed fever for the past three days. The day prior to presentation his temperature was as high as 39.8°C. He also has some headache and diarrhoea.

He reports freshwater contact in a small lake near Maputo. His past medical history is unremarkable.

Clinical Findings

The patient is a 43-year-old man, febrile, with a temperature of 39.2°C. The rest of the physical examination is normal and there is no rash, no hepatomegaly, no splenomegaly and no lymphadenopathy.

Laboratory Results

The relevant laboratory results on admission are shown in Table 18-1 (p 101).

Further Investigations

Electrocardiogram is normal. Chest radiography reveals some nodular lesions ranging in size from 2 mm to 5 mm in the periphery of the lower lung zones bilaterally (Figure 18-1, p 102); this finding is confirmed by a CT scan of his chest.

Questions

1. What are your differential diagnoses and which investigations would you like to do?
2. What is the significance of eosinophilia in returning travellers?

CASE 19

A 40-Year-Old Man from Togo With Subcutaneous Nodules and Corneal Changes

Guido Kluxen

History

A 40-year-old man from Togo presents to a local clinic. He has noticed changes in both of his eyes over the past four years. There are no visual disturbances, but he is worried. In his village there are adults in each family who have turned completely blind after their eyes had shown features very similar to the changes he has noticed in his own eyes.

He has also observed some painless bumps under his skin which have developed over the past two decades. The patient also complains of suffering from intense itching of his skin that keeps him awake at night.

The patient has always lived in a village in the savannah near a fast-flowing river. He reports that small biting flies are common near the river.

Clinical Findings

Opacities are noticeable in the cornea of both eyes. The patient's left eye is shown in Figure 19-1 (p 104).

The skin shows evidence of atrophy in some areas (thinning with loss of elasticity), and there are multiple scratch marks. Subcutaneous nodules are palpable in various regions of his body, especially over bony prominences like the ribs (Figure 19-2, p 104), iliac crest, femoral trochanters and on the head. The nodules are firm, non-tender and measure 1–3 cm in diameter.

Questions

1. What is your most important differential diagnosis?
2. What investigations would you like to carry out?

CASE 20

A 56-Year-Old Man Returning from a Trip to Thailand With Eosinophilia

Sebastian Dieckmann / Ralf Ignatius

History

A 56-year-old European man is referred to a local specialist clinic for further work-up of peripheral eosinophilia. Clinically, he suffers from fatigue and back pain. The patient returned from a three-week round trip to Thailand four months ago.

He is known to have mild hypertension and suffered a transient ischaemic attack (TIA) five years ago. He has never experienced any allergic reactions. The patient has taken aspirin since suffering the TIA and an angiotensin receptor blocker (sartan) for one year.

Clinical Findings

The vital signs are normal, he is afebrile. His physical examination does not reveal any pathological findings.

Laboratory Results

The patient's full blood count is shown in Table 20-1 (p 107).

Questions

1. How is eosinophilia defined and what is the differential diagnosis?
2. How do you narrow down your differential diagnosis in a traveller with eosinophilia?

CASE 21

A 35-Year-Old American Man With Fatigue and a Neck Lesion

Mary E. Wright / Arthur M. Friedlander

History

A 35-year-old Caucasian male presents to a clinic in the United States with fatigue and a rash on his neck that started as a papule two days earlier. The lesion is non-pruritic, but it is associated with significant swelling and a pressure sensation in the neck. There is no history of fever, but the patient reports at least one episode of diaphoresis with mild confusion and headache.

The patient recalls a break in the skin at the site of the lesion three days before while shaving, and is sure that he has not been bitten by an insect. He has had no contact with animals or foreign travel within the previous year.

He had come into the clinic 24 hours earlier with similar symptoms. After blood cultures were obtained he was given one dose of a first-generation cephalosporin and discharged on a ten-day oral course. He returns because of worsening malaise and neck swelling associated with mild difficulty breathing.

The past medical history is unremarkable. The patient is a postal worker by profession.

Clinical Findings

Examination reveals a 2 cm irregularly shaped, indurated non-tender patch on the left anterior neck with mild overlying erythema and several 2–3 mm vesicles. The main lesion has a 6 mm shallow ulceration. There is massive neck oedema making lymph nodes difficult to assess (see Figure 21-1, p 110). His neck circumference had increased from 57 cm at baseline to a peak of 81 cm. Temperature is 36.9°C, pulse 118 bpm, blood pressure 138/90 mmHg and respiratory rate 20 breath cycles per minute. The remainder of the initial physical examination is normal.

Investigations

Full blood count, Na+, K+, Cl⁻ HCO_3, BUN, creatinine and random glucose are normal except for a mildly elevated haemoglobin at 18.7 g/dL (reference range: 13.0–18.0 g/dL).

Questions

1. What are the distinguishing features of this lesion that help narrow down your differential diagnosis?
2. What investigations need to be performed to establish early diagnosis and appropriate treatment?

CASE 22

A 32-Year-Old Woman from Nigeria With Jaundice and Confusion

Christopher J.M. Whitty

History

A 32-year-old, previously fit woman of African ethnicity but born in Europe travelled to rural Jos in Nigeria to visit relatives. According to her husband, 18 days after her return to Europe she developed a fever, and three days later became very unwell with abnormal behaviour.

Clinical Findings

On examination she has a temperature of 37.5°C, is mildly jaundiced and confused, Glasgow Coma Scale 14/15. She has no rash or palpable lymph nodes, and throat and sclerae are not injected. She has some fine crepitations at the lung bases.

Laboratory Results

The laboratory refuses to undertake tests because of recent rural exposure in an area known to have viral haemorrhagic fever (Lassa).

1. What is the differential diagnosis?
2. Is viral hemorrhagic fever (VHF) a real risk, and which single test is the most important?

CASE 23

A 31-Year-Old HIV-Positive Man With Extensive Travel History, With Cough and Night Sweats

Katherine Woods / Robert F. Miller

History

You are on-call in a London hospital and are referred a 31-year-old HIV-positive man from Accident and Emergency. He has a six-week history of drenching night sweats, dry cough and increasing short-ness of breath on exertion. He also reports general fatigue and a loss of about 10 kg in weight over the past five months.

He works in the retail industry and travels extensively for business. In the past six months he has had work trips to Europe, China, Korea, Japan, Singapore and the United States. He lives with his male partner, denies any recreational drug use and has never smoked tobacco. He was diagnosed with HIV six years ago. He says that one month ago his CD4 was 280/μL. He is not yet on antiretroviral therapy (ART), or any other regular medications. There is no other significant past medical history.

Clinical Findings

On examination, he is alert, short of breath at rest but able to complete full sentences. He has a tem-perature of 39.2°C. Respiratory rate is 26 breath cycles per minute, oxygen saturation is 87% on air, 97% on 15 L O_2 via reservoir bag. Pulse 100 bpm, blood pressure 120/70 mmHg. Chest is clear on auscultation. The rest of the physical examination is unremarkable.

Laboratory Results

His arterial blood gases on air are shown in Table 23-1 (p 116), the full blood count and blood chem-istry results are given in Table 23-2 (p 117).

Chest Radiography

His chest radiograph is shown in Figure 23-1 (p 117).

1. What further investigations would you perform in order to confirm the diagnosis?
2. What is your immediate management of the patient?

CASE 24

A 14-Year-Old Boy from Rural Tanzania With Difficulties in Walking

William P. Howlett

History

A 14-year-old boy presents to his local hospital in rural Tanzania with a history of difficulty in walking. He had been well up until just over two years earlier when his illness suddenly started. He describes that he was walking home from school when he first noticed that his legs began to feel heavy and started to tremble, which caused him difficulty in walking, with a tendency to fall over. He slowly completed the journey home and since that day has been unable to stand or walk unaided. He now stands on his toes and drags his legs around with the aid of a stick (Figure 24-1, p 120). He denies any history of fever, pain, sensory, bladder or bowel symptoms or disease progression.

His past history is otherwise unremarkable. He lives in a village in northern Tanzania in a rural area with limited agricultural suitability where the main staple food crop is cassava. His diet for the two months before the illness was almost exclusively cassava. He has three other siblings, one of whom is similarly affected, whereas their parents remained fine. He mentions that identical cases had occurred in his own and neighbouring villages at around the same time.

Clinical Examination

Clinically he is well nourished with normal vital signs. General examination is unremarkable. On neurological examination he is fully orientated and higher mental function appears normal. Cranial nerves are normal but bilateral optic pallor was noted on fundoscopy. Limbs reveal signs of spastic paraparesis with flexion contractures at both ankles and knees. Power in the legs is graded 3–4/5 (= just overcoming gravity) with the knee extensors and foot dorsiflexors involved to the greatest extent (Figure 24-1, p 120). There is bilateral hypertonia, hyperreflexia and sustained ankle clonus with extensor plantar responses. The arms are normal apart from generalized hyperreflexia. There is no impairment or loss of sensation. A lumbar lordosis with thoracic kyphoscoliosis is noticeable only on standing.

Investigations

Full blood count, erythrocyte sedimentation rate, blood glucose and creatinine are normal. Urine analysis is normal. Microscopy of urine and stool specimens does not show any ova of *Schistosoma* spp. HIV serology and VDRL are negative. Lumbar puncture is normal. Radiographs of the chest and thoracolumbar spine are normal.

Questions

1. What is the clinical diagnosis and the likely cause in this patient?
2. How do you plan to manage this patient?

CASE 25

A 72-Year-Old Male Farmer from Laos With Extensive Skin Lesions on the Lower Leg

Günther Slesak / Saythong Inthalad / Paul N. Newton

History

A 72-year-old male farmer is admitted to a provincial hospital in northern Laos with extensive, painful verrucous skin lesions on his left foot and lower leg.

Ten years prior he had a leech bite on the dorsum of his left foot. One week later a small painless red nodule developed at the site of the bite. Over the following years the lesion slowly increased in size; further lesions developed and spread up to his knee. Three days before admission his ankle became painful and swollen.

Clinical Findings

Vital signs are normal and the patient is afebrile. His left lower leg and foot are grossly swollen (Figure 25-1, p 123); the skin is hyperaemic and feels hot. There are several cauliflower-like masses and oval plaque-like lesions on his left lower leg and foot. The lesions are partly erythematous, partly fungating and purulent, oozing a bad odour.

Investigations

Radiography of the left leg and foot showed no bone involvement.

Questions

1. What are the important differential diagnoses?
2. Which diagnostic tests should be done?

CASE 26

A 14-Year-Old Boy from Malawi Who Has Been Bitten by a Snake

Gregor Pollach

History

A 14-year-old Malawian boy presents to a local hospital because of an extensive necrotic wound on his right foot.

Three weeks earlier he was playing with his friends on a path leading through rocky grassland to the maize field of his family when he stepped on a snake. The snake was brown with V-shaped black bands on its back, and it was approximately one metre long. His friends told his mother later that the snake had hissed loudly but did not move away before biting him – which the boy did not even realize, being busy chasing a football. Shortly after the bite, haemorrhagic bullae formed on the right leg. His gums started to bleed and he vomited extensively. He was taken to a local traditional healer for treatment. His bleeding and vomiting settled, however, he developed intense pain and swelling at the site of the bite.

Clinical Findings

The patient is a 14-year old boy, who appears weak and is in respiratory distress. His vital signs are: temperature 39.4°C, pulse 126 bpm, blood pressure 85/60 mmHg, respiratory rate 30 breath cycles per minute. There is an extensive foul-smelling necrosis affecting his right foot and ankle where the tendons are exposed (Figure 26-1, p 126). The right lower leg is swollen and he is unable to bend the ankle of his right foot. The inguinal lymph nodes are enlarged on the right side.

The urine is clear, rectal exam does not show any signs of bleeding and upon provoked coughing there is no haemoptysis. Fundoscopy is normal.

Investigations

The 20 minute whole blood clotting test is normal. The results of the other blood tests are shown in Table 26-1 (p 127).

Questions

1. Which snake was most probably responsible for the bite?
2. What first-aid measures should have been taken?

CASE 27

A 16-Year-Old Boy from Sri Lanka With Fever, Jaundice and Renal Failure

Ranjan Premaratna

History

A 16-year-old Sri Lankan boy presents to a local hospital with fever, frontal headache and severe body aches for two days. He has vomited two to three times during the illness and has not passed any urine for the previous 12 hours. He does not have a cough, coryza or shortness of breath. He has been attending school until his illness. He had been fishing in an urban water stream five days prior to falling ill.

Clinical Examination

The boy looks ill and drowsy. He is jaundiced and has subconjunctival haemorrhages (Figure 27-1, p 130). There is no neck stiffness, however there is severe muscle tenderness, mainly involving the abdominal wall and in the calves so that the patient finds it difficult to walk. There is no lymphadenopathy. The liver is palpable at 4 cm below the right costal margin and is tender. The spleen is not palpable. There is mild bilateral renal angle tenderness. Body temperature is 38.3°C. The pulse rate is 100 bpm and is low in volume. The blood pressure is 90/60 mmHg. The cardiac apex is not shifted. Examination of the lungs and the CNS are normal.

Further Investigations

The laboratory findings are summarized in Table 27-1 (p 131). The urine microscopy shows 20 red blood cells per high-power field, proteins '+' and granular casts '+'. A chest radiograph is normal. An ECG shows sinus tachycardia.

Questions

1. What is the most likely diagnosis and what are your differentials?
2. What tests are indicated to confirm the diagnosis?

CASE 28

A 67-Year-Old Female Expatriate Living in Cameroon With Eosinophilia and Pericarditis

Sebastian Dieckmann / Ralf Ignatius

History

A 67-year-old German woman who has lived as an expatriate in Cameroon for the past four years presents with palpitations at a tropical medicine clinic in Germany. She also reports transient subcutaneous swellings for the past year. There is no history of fever or constitutional symptoms and the past medical history is otherwise unremarkable.

A 24 hour ECG was done elsewhere, which showed paroxysmal supraventricular extrasystoles. Echocardiography revealed a minimal pericardial effusion.

Clinical Findings

Vital signs are normal and the patient is afebrile. There are no visible subcutaneous swellings. Heart sounds are clear and regular and there are no murmurs. No pathological findings are noted on physical examination.

Laboratory Results

Full blood count results are shown in Table 28-1 (p 133).

Further Investigations

The chest radiograph does not show any abnormalities.

Questions

1. What are the key findings?
2. What are your differential diagnoses?

CASE 29

A 35-Year-Old Woman from Malawi With Fever and Progressive Weakness

Camilla Rothe

History

A 35-year-old Malawian woman presents to a local hospital because of fever and weakness.

The fever started three days earlier, but the weakness has progressed over the past several months. There is no cough and no night sweats but she reports some weight loss. There is no diarrhoea, no dysuria and no history of abnormal bleeds.

Two months earlier she presented to a local health centre because of her weakness. She was found to be clinically pale and was prescribed iron tablets, which she took. Nevertheless, the weakness progressed. Otherwise, the patient does not report any abnormalities.

She is divorced, with three children (17, 15 and 12 years old), who are all well. She works as a small-scale farmer and sells vegetables on the local market. The family can afford three meals a day and occasionally meat or fish.

Clinical Findings

A 35-year-old woman, wasted, body mass index 17 kg/m². Blood pressure 90/60 mmHg (difficult to measure on the wasted arm), pulse 110 bpm, temperature 37.8°C, respiratory rate 25 breath cycles per minute, oxygen saturation 97% on ambient air, Glasgow Coma Scale 15/15.

Her conjunctivae are very pale, but there is no jaundice. The examination of her mouth is normal, there is no oral thrush, no Kaposi's sarcoma lesions and no oral hairy leukoplakia. The chest is clear. The abdomen is soft, with slight diffuse tenderness, but no guarding. The spleen is palpable 3 cm below the left costal margin. The rectal examination is normal.

Investigations

The malaria rapid diagnostic test is negative. The HIV serology comes back reactive.

The results of her full blood count are shown in Table 29-1 (p 136).

Questions

1. What is the suspected diagnosis?
2. How would you manage this patient?

CASE 30

A 12-Year-Old Boy from Rural Kenya With Painful Eyes

Hillary K. Rono / Andrew Bastawrous / Nicholas A.V. Beare

History

A 12-year-old boy is brought to a health centre in rural north-west Kenya. He reports a two-month history of pain, watering and redness of both eyes. The watering of his eyes is worse in the sun and he is struggling to keep his eyes open.

Six months previously he was treated at a dispensary for similar, but less severe symptoms. He was given a course of tetracycline ointment but his symptoms did not improve. Following this, he went to a traditional healer who applied some herbal medication made from juice extracts from the ecucuka plant (*Aloe vera* species). After instillation he experienced severe eye pain and discharge, both eyes became red and his vision was reduced.

The boy lives with his parents in the hot, dusty and dry area of Loima in Turkana County. They keep large herds of cows and sheep and the boy helps with herding and watering the animals. They fetch water for domestic use from a dried river bed about 6 kilometres from their home.

Clinical Findings

A 12-year-old boy who appears systemically fit and well. Visual acuity is markedly reduced in both eyes. He can only perceive hand movements in the right eye and the vision is 6/60 in the left eye. The findings on inspection of his eyes are shown in Table 30-1 (p 139) and Figures 30-1, 30-2 (p 140).

Questions

1. What are your differential diagnoses?
2. What features fit the criteria for trachoma?

CASE 31

A 6-Year-Old Boy from Malawi With Fever, Cough and Impaired Consciousness

Charlotte Adamczick

History

You review a 6-year-old boy in the paediatric high dependency unit of a Malawian Central Hospital. The boy was admitted the night before because of a high fever, dyspnoea and a dry cough which started three days before. On admission he was started on antibiotics and presumptive antimalaria treatment; the results of the malaria smear are pending.

The boy is known to be HIV-reactive. Antiretroviral therapy (ART) was deferred on his last visit to the clinic six months ago when his CD4 count was high and he was clinically not deemed eligible for ART (WHO clinical stage 2).

Clinical Findings

Examination reveals a sick child with a temperature of 39.8°C and laboured breathing. The Blantyre coma score is 3/5. The boy has coryza and a bilateral conjunctivitis. Behind both ears and on the forehead you notice a fine maculopapular rash (see Figure 31-1, p 142) that has not been described before. There is bilateral axillary lymphadenopathy.

Questions

1. What is your most important differential diagnosis?
2. What complications should you expect and how do you manage the patient?

CASE 32

A 44-Year-Old Male Farmer from Laos With Diabetes and a Back Abscess

Sayaphet Rattanavong / Valy Keoluangkhot / Siho Sisouphonh / Vatthanaphone Latthaphasavang / David Dance / Caoimhe Nic Fhogartaigh

History

A 44-year-old male rice farmer presents to a provincial hospital in Southern Laos in the rainy season with a one-month history of fever, headache, generalized myalgia and arthralgia, and a painful swelling over the left scapula. The swelling has gradually increased in size, without any history of preceding trauma. He has not noticed any lesions elsewhere. He was diagnosed with type 2 diabetes four years previously, but was not compliant with oral antidiabetic drugs or follow-up. The lesion on his back was incised and drained at a local health centre the previous week, since when he has been taking cloxacillin 1 g four times daily. However, there has been no improvement and during the two days prior to admission he has deteriorated, with high fever, chills and severe malaise.

Clinical Findings

The patient appears septic, with a fever of 40°C, a heart rate of 136 bpm, blood pressure of 140/80 mmHg and a respiratory rate of 30 breath cycles per minute. He is pale and jaundiced. In the left scapular region there is an erythematous swelling of 2.5 × 4 cm with pus discharging from a central wound (Figure 32-1, p 145). There is no regional lymphadenopathy. On chest auscultation there are bilateral crepitations and reduced breath sounds at both lung bases. Heart sounds are normal. The abdomen is soft, without any palpable organomegaly.

Laboratory Results

The laboratory results are shown in Table 32-1 (p 146).

Questions

1. What are your differential diagnoses?
2. What additional investigations would you like to do?

CASE 33

A 53-Year-Old Man from Malawi With a Chronic Cough

Camilla Rothe

History

A 53-year-old Malawian man presents to a local hospital because of a productive cough for three months. He also reports night sweats and that he has lost some weight, but he is unable to quantify this.

Two months earlier he presented to a health centre with the same complaints. He was given presumptive antimalarials and amoxicillin for five days, but to no avail. The patient is not aware of any tuberculosis (TB) contacts. He is currently not on any medication and his past medical history is unremarkable. He is a farmer. He has never worked in a mine or in the construction industry. He is a non-smoker. He is married with five children; all are well.

Clinical Findings

The patient is a 53-year-old man, slightly wasted. Temperature 38.8°C, blood pressure 100/80 mmHg, pulse 88 bpm, oxygen saturation 97% in ambient air. He appears mildly anaemic. On inspection of his mouth there is no oral thrush, no Kaposi's sarcoma and no oral hairy leukoplakia. His chest is clear and there are normal heart sounds without any murmurs. There is no lymphadenopathy; liver and spleen are not enlarged.

Investigations

The patient is sent for HIV voluntary counselling and testing. The HIV test result is reactive. His further laboratory results are shown in Table 33-1 (p 149).

Chest Radiography

His chest radiograph on admission shows prominent hili bilaterally but is otherwise normal (Figure 33-1, p 150).

Questions

1. What is your suspected diagnosis?
2. How would you approach this patient?

CASE 34

A 35-Year-Old Male Farmer from Peru With a Chronic Ulcer and Multiple Nodular Lesions on the Arm

Fernando Mejía Cordero / Beatriz Bustamante / Eduardo Gotuzzo

History

A 35-year-old farmer from the Peruvian highlands presents to a reference hospital in the capital, Lima, with a two-month history of a slowly growing ulcer and multiple painless nodules on his left arm.

Two months prior to presentation the patient suffered a scratch on his left hand from a tree branch while working in the fields. After a few days he noticed a small painless erythematous papule that later developed into a pustule. He took antibiotics without improvement. Over the following weeks new pustules appeared and the lesion started to ulcerate and increased in size, despite continued antibiotics and topical traditional medicines. Four weeks after the initial papule the patient noticed painless firm nodules on his left forearm. The patient was seen at a regional hospital and treated empirically for cutaneous leishmaniasis with a 20-day course of pentavalent antimonials but showed no improvement. He was then referred for further diagnosis and treatment. The patient was previously healthy. He denied recent contact with animals or travel.

Clinical Findings

The patient appears generally well. His vital signs are normal and he is afebrile.

On his left hand there is a single ulcerative lesion (20 × 30 mm) with irregular elevated borders (Figure 34-1, p 153) and multiple subcutaneous erythematous nodules (10 × 10 mm) along the lymphatic tract of the left arm (Figure 34-2, p 154). The rest of the physical examination is normal.

Laboratory Results

The WBC is 4.5×10^9/L (reference range $4–10 \times 10^9$/L) with normal differential count; haemoglobin is 11.3 g/dL (12–16 g/dL). The remainder of the full blood count is normal.

Questions

1. What are your differential diagnoses?
2. How would you approach this patient?

CASE 35

A 32-Year-Old Woman from Malawi With Headache and Blurred Vision

Camilla Rothe

History

A 32-year-old Malawian woman presents to a local hospital with a three-week history of headache and blurred vision. The headache has been gradual in onset and does not respond to over-the-counter painkillers. There is no fever and no history of convulsions or of head trauma.

The patient presented to a local health centre where she received presumptive antimalarial treatment (artemether/lumefantrine) and a course of antibiotics (amoxicillin 500 mg tds for five days), which was of no benefit.

Clinical Findings

The patient appears wasted and slightly anaemic. All vital signs are normal and she is afebrile. The GCS is 15/15. There is no neck stiffness. The visual acuity is normal on both sides. On left lateral gaze there is an abduction deficit of the left eye with 'blurring of vision' reported by the patient (Figure 35-1, p 156). The rest of the examination is normal.

Laboratory Results

See Table 35-1 (p 157).

Questions

1. What are your differential diagnoses?
2. What investigations would you like to do?

CASE 36

A 25-Year-Old Buddhist Monk from Myanmar With Unilateral Scrotal Swelling

Kentaro Ishida / Camilla Rothe

History

A 25-year-old Buddhist monk presents to a district hospital in Myanmar with a three-year history of left-sided scrotal swelling. The swelling is non-tender and has gradually increased in size. There is no history of fever. He has attempted to treat the swelling with traditional herbal medicine, but to no avail.

The patient comes from the central part of Myanmar. He reports that scrotal swelling is not an uncommon problem in his home region.

Clinical Findings

The patient is a 25-year-old man in fair general condition. His vital signs are normal and he is afebrile. There is left-sided scrotal swelling, which cannot be reduced (Figure 36-1, p 159). There are no palpable inguinal lymph nodes.

Questions

1. What is the differential diagnosis?
2. What investigations would you like to do?

CASE 37

A 29-Year-Old Woman from Malawi With Confusion, Diarrhoea and a Skin Rash

Camilla Rothe

History

A 29-year-old woman is brought to a hospital in Malawi by her relatives. She has been confused, restless and irritable for the past month. She also has watery diarrhoea, which started one week ago. She does not have a fever. It is January, which is the rainy season in that country.

Her past medical history has been uneventful. There have been no psychiatric disorders in the past. Her HIV status is unknown. She is not taking any medication. There are no known intoxications, no use of alcohol or recreational drugs.

The patient is married with four children. She is a housewife. Her husband works as a farmhand on a local chicken farm. The family come from a village where they live in a grass-thatched mud-hut and collect their water from a borehole. There is no electricity at home. They eat two meals a day, mainly maize porridge with a few vegetables. Only rarely can the family afford fish or meat.

Clinical Findings

The patient is slim but not wasted. Glasgow Coma Scale 14/15 (confusion), the remaining vital signs are normal and she is afebrile. There is no neck stiffness. The patient's conjunctivae are pale. There is a noticeable skin rash around the patient's neck (Figure 37-1, p 162), on her forearms, hands and feet (Figure 37-2, p 162), where the skin appears hyperpigmented and dry. The skin changes are clearly demarcated. The rest of the physical examination is unremarkable. When asked, her relatives report that the rash had been present for the past two months.

Questions

1. What is the suspected diagnosis and what are your differential diagnoses?
2. How would you manage this patient?

CASE 38

A 24-Year-Old Female Globetrotter from The Netherlands With Strange Sensations in the Right Side of Her Body

Juri Katchanov / Eberhard Siebert

History

A 24-year-old Dutch yoga instructor presents to an emergency room in Berlin, Germany, with one episode of strange sensations in the right side of her body. This started in the right side of her face, marched to her right arm and then continued, to involve her right leg. She describes the feeling as 'pins and needles' lasting for about two minutes. She had a similar episode several months ago. At that time she did not consult a doctor.

Four years prior to this presentation, after finishing school she had left her home town in The Netherlands to go backpacking for two years. She travelled extensively through South America (Ecuador, Peru, Argentina) and South-east Asia (Thailand, Laos, Cambodia), staying in hostels or private accommodations. She describes herself as an 'eco-traveller', visiting the countryside and staying with local people. She has been a strict vegan for the past eight years. She would eat food from local vendors but never any animal products. Her main diet during her travelling consisted of fruits, vegetables, nuts and rice.

Clinical Findings

On examination she looks well. Her body temperature is 36.7°C. Her neurological examination is completely unremarkable. The rest of her physical examination is also normal.

Laboratory Results

Her routine blood investigations, including C-reactive protein, are completely unremarkable. Her differential blood count and CSF examination are normal.

Imaging

The MR imaging of her brain shows multiple cortical and subcortical cystic lesions in both hemispheres with gadolinium enhancement (Figure 38-1, p 166).

(Figure 38-1, p 166)

Questions

1. What is the clinical syndrome the patient presents with and what is the most likely diagnosis in the light of the imaging findings and the patient's travel history?
2. How would you treat this patient?

CASE 39

A 30-Year-Old Male Trader from China With Persistent Fever

Paul N. Newton / Valy Keoluangkhot / Mayfong Mayxay / Michael D. Green / Facundo M. Fernández

History

A 30-year-old, male, Chinese, itinerant trader presents in Vientiane, Laos, with a seven-day history of fever, chills, headache and a dry cough. He developed slide-positive falciparum malaria whilst living in southern Laos and was treated with intravenous infusions and intramuscular artemether 80 mg for five days, which he had brought from China as standby therapy, but he did not improve. The fever persisted, jaundice developed and he was therefore transferred to Mahosot Hospital, Vientiane.

Clinical Findings

On admission he was febrile (39.5°C), with normal blood pressure and Glasgow Coma Scale (GCS) score, but had nausea, dry cough, moderate dehydration, chest pain and abdominal tenderness. His chest was clear and no hepatosplenomegaly was detected.

Investigations

Giemsa-smear was negative for malaria parasites but a rapid diagnostic test (HRP-2) was positive for Plasmodium falciparum, consistent with recent falciparum malaria. Serum creatinine and glucose were normal. His further laboratory results are shown in Table 39-1 (p 168).

Questions

1. What are your most important differential diagnoses?
2. How would you approach this patient?

CASE 40

A 62-Year-Old Woman from Ethiopia With Difficulty Eating

Christopher J.M. Whitty

History

A 62-year-old woman from rural Ethiopia had flown to Europe to visit her daughter and meet her new grandchild. She was normally fit and well and very physically active, as she worked on her smallholding in Ethiopia. Three days after arrival she began to find it difficult to chew, with what she described through her daughter as 'stiffness of the mouth'. This had never happened before.

Clinical Findings

No abnormal findings are discovered on examination. Her pulse, blood pressure and respiratory rate are within normal limits.

1. What are the important differential diagnoses and what would help to establish the diagnosis?
2. What is the immediate management?

CASE 41

A 7-Year-Old Girl from West Africa With Two Skin Ulcers and a Contracture of Her Right Wrist

Moritz Vogel

History

A grandmother presents her 7-year-old granddaughter to a district hospital in the tropical region of a West African country. She reports that following an insect bite approximately three months ago the girl had noticed an itchy papule on the back of her right hand, which increased in size over time. When the child complained of pain, a traditional healer was consulted who prescribed local herbal remedies. After some weeks the lesion ulcerated with increasing pain. Diclofenac and dexamethasone were prescribed at the local health post.

When a second lesion appeared on her right wrist, oral oxacillin was given. However, there was no improvement and the girl became increasingly unable to extend her wrist or to use her right hand. There is no history of major trauma or any systemic symptoms.

Clinical Findings

A 7-year-old, anxious girl in good general condition holds her right wrist in a 45° flexion and 20° abduction position. Vital signs: pulse 108 bpm (normal 70–110), blood pressure 100/70 mmHg, temperature 37.9°C.

There are two skin ulcers: one is on the back of the right hand, measuring 3 × 3 cm, the second ulcer is on the medial side of her right wrist (0.5 × 1 cm). The larger ulcer is filled with necrotic tissue (Figure 41-1, p 173). The skin around the lesions shows hypo- and hyperpigmentation, lichenification and desquamation. On palpation there is an ill-defined induration surrounding the ulcers measuring 12 × 8 cm, which is itself encompassed by an oedema extending from the lower arm to the fingers. There is a 0.5 × 0.5 cm nodule above the medial right elbow. The flexion of the wrist is actively and passively limited to 45° ± 10°.

1. What is the most likely diagnosis and what is the differential diagnosis?
2. What is the appropriate clinical approach in the given context?

CASE 42

A 41-Year-Old Male Traveller Returning from Australia With Itchy Eruptions on Both Upper Thighs

Camilla Rothe

History

A 41-year-old male yoga teacher presents to a travel clinic in Europe because of itchy skin eruptions on both upper thighs for the past week.

He has just returned from a ten-day trip to northern Australia where he attended a yoga seminar. On his way to Australia he had stopped over on a Thai island for a three-day beach holiday. Just after his arrival in Australia he developed three intensely itchy skin eruptions on both upper thighs. The itch is so intense that at times it keeps him awake at night.

There has been no fever, no cough or wheeze and he is otherwise completely well.

Clinical Findings

On both upper thighs there are a total of three reddish, serpiginous tracks, about 2 mm in width (Figure 42-1, p 176). The inguinal lymph nodes are not enlarged. The chest is clear. The rest of the examination is unremarkable.

Questions

1. What is the clinical syndrome and what is the differential diagnosis?
2. What management would you recommend?

CASE 43

A 35-Year-Old Woman from Malawi With a Painful Ocular Tumour

Markus Schulze Schwering

History

A 35-year-old woman presents to the outpatient department of a Malawian tertiary hospital. She has been referred by an ophthalmic clinical officer from a district hospital for exenteration of the left eye because of an ocular tumour.

The first symptoms started eight months ago when she noticed a whitish lesion growing on the conjunctiva of her left eye. She presented to a health centre and was prescribed nonspecified eye drops. However, over the following months the lesion grew bigger and turned reddish. She went to a traditional healer who prescribed herbal eye drops, which did not help either. The lesion grew constantly bigger and she finally lost her eyesight in the affected eye. Pain also increased, which made her present at her local district hospital.

The patient is known to be HIV-reactive. She has been on antiretroviral treatment for the past three years. The CD4-count is unknown.

Clinical Findings

There is localized swelling of the left eyeball and orbit; lid closure is incomplete (Figure 43-1, p 179). The visual acuity in her right eye is 6/6, whereas the left eye has no light perception. Her left preauricular lymph nodes are swollen. She is afebrile and the rest of her physical examination is unremarkable.

Questions

1. What is the suspected diagnosis?
2. How would you manage the patient?

CASE 44

A 7-Year-Old Girl from South Sudan With Undulating Fever

Karen Roodnat / Koert Ritmeijer

History

A 7-year-old girl presents to a clinic in South Sudan with a four-week history of undulating fever. The fever occurs mainly in the afternoon hours accompanied by chills and sometimes convulsions. In between the febrile episodes she was initially fine and played normally. However, over time she has developed progressive anorexia, dry cough, chest pain, joint and back pain.

She has never been admitted to hospital but she has presented at another clinic recently where she received some unspecified tablets that did not bring any improvement.

Clinical Findings

The girl is alert, pale, but not jaundiced. She is severely malnourished (Z-score <3). Her vital signs are: temperature 39.6°C, pulse 96 bpm, blood pressure 100/60 mmHg. Her chest sounds clear; normal antituberculous therapy, vitamin B6, antiretrovirals and co-trimoxazole prophylaxis, all of which she is currently taking.

The patient works as a street vendor selling mobile phone vouchers. Despite her left-sided weakness she is still able to work sitting on a plastic chair and managing her vouchers and money with her right hand. She is divorced and does not have any children. She lives in an urban high-density area.

Clinical Findings

She is afebrile and her vital signs and general examination are normal apart from slightly pale conjunctivae. On fundoscopy her fundi are normal without any signs of papilloedema or retinitis.

The neurological examination reveals a spastic hemiparesis on the left with hyperreflexia. The power in the left leg is 2/5 (active movement with gravity eliminated) and in her left arm 3/5 (active movement against gravity). There is a pronator drift on the left (Figure 51-1, p 205) indicating proximal weakness. Sensation of pain is reduced in her left leg and hand. The examination of her cranial nerves is normal.

Laboratory Results

Full blood count: WBC 3.8×10^9/L (reference range: 4–10), haemoglobin 9.9 g/dL (12–14), platelets 140×10^9/L (150–350).

Questions

1. What is your differential diagnosis?
2. What is your diagnostic approach in the resource-limited setting?

CASE 52

A 56-Year-Old Man from Peru With Prolonged Fever and Severe Anaemia

Ciro Maguiña / Carlos Seas / Frederique Jacquerioz

History

A 56-year-old male Peruvian is admitted to a hospital in the capital, Lima, with a two-week history of fever, jaundice and confusion.

Daily fever started three months after leaving a rural area in the highlands of Northern Peru (altitude of 2400 m), where the patient spent three weeks on vacations. In the second week of illness the patient noticed dark urine and jaundice, and few days before admission his wife noticed confusion and somnolence. While in the rural area, the patient and his wife were bitten at night by tiny mosquitoes; no personal protection was used. Otherwise there has been no animal contact. The past medical history is unremarkable.

Clinical Findings

His blood pressure is 90/60 mmHg, pulse 110 bpm and regular, temperature 39.2°C, respiratory rate 22 breath cycles per minute. The patient appears confused and disorientated without any focal neurological findings or meningeal signs (GCS 14/15). Skin and conjunctivae are markedly pale and there is scleral jaundice. Cardiovascular and pulmonary examination are normal. The liver is slightly enlarged but there is no splenomegaly.

Laboratory Results

Creatinine, electrolytes and alkaline phosphatase are normal. His further routine laboratory results are shown in Table 52-1 (p 209). Coomb's test is negative. The CSF results are within normal range.

Further Investigations

A CT of the brain is normal. Abdominal ultrasound reveals hepatomegaly, but no focal lesions.

Questions

1. What are your differential diagnoses?
2. How would you approach this patient?

CASE 53

A 24-Year-Old Woman from Uganda With Fever and Shock

Benjamin Jeffs

History

A 24-year-old woman presents to a small hospital in rural Uganda because of a five-day history of a febrile illness. Apart from fever, the illness started with a sore throat and aching all over. She also developed some abdominal pain and diarrhoea. The patient has become increasingly unwell over the course of the past days. She is very weak and needs help to stand.

Her husband died of a severe febrile illness six days before she herself became ill. He had worked in a local gold mine and had previously been in good health. He had fallen ill about a week before his death. His wife had looked after him during his final illness and he had died at home.

Clinical Findings

The patient looks very unwell. Her blood pressure is 85/65 mmHg, pulse rate 105 bpm, temperature 38°C. She has bilateral conjunctivitis. There is no rash and no lymphadenopathy. The heart sounds are normal and her chest is clear. Her abdominal examination is normal.

Questions

1. What are your differential diagnoses?
2. How would you approach the patient and what tests would you do?

CASE 54

A 52-Year-Old Male Safari Tourist Returning from South Africa With Fever and a Skin Lesion

Camilla Rothe

History

A 52-year-old man presents to a tropical medicine clinic in Germany with fever for the past two days. He is also complaining of night sweats and a frontal headache. There are no joint pains and he has not noticed a rash.

Ten days ago he returned from a two-week holiday trip to South Africa. He visited Cape Town and travelled the Garden Route and through KwaZulu–Natal. He went on safari in Kruger Park and several other game reserves. He did not take any antimalarial chemoprophylaxis. His past medical history is unremarkable.

Clinical Findings

Fair general condition. Tympanic temperature 37.5°C (after taking 1 g of paracetamol), pulse 80 bpm, blood pressure 130/70 mmHg.

No jaundice; neck supple. Enlarged lymph nodes in the left groin. You notice a small sticking plaster on the left upper thigh of the patient. He tells you that he has noted a skin lesion that he meant to show to a medical practitioner for advice. You ask the patient to take off the plaster (see Figure 54-1, p 215).

Questions

1. What is the diagnosis?
2. How would you manage this patient?

CASE 55

A 40-Year-Old Male Farmer from Peru With Chronic Cough and Weight Loss

Frederique Jacquerioz / Carlos Seas

History

A 40-year-old farmer from the Peruvian Amazon is referred to a hospital in the capital, Lima, with a four-month history of chronic productive cough and chest pain. The patient reports dyspnoea on exertion and weight loss of about 20 kg. He denies diarrhoea, fever or night sweats.

Three and half months earlier, the patient was hospitalized at a regional hospital in the Peruvian Amazon for similar complaints. During the hospitalization, three sputum smears for acid-fast bacilli (AFB) were reported negative. No tuberculin skin test was performed. The chest radiograph was described as abnormal but no report is available and the patient does not have the film. A diagnosis of pulmonary tuberculosis (TB) was made based on clinical presentation and abnormal chest radiographic findings. The patient received first line TB therapy consisting of isoniazid, rifampicin, pyrazinamide and ethambutol.

In the following months, despite adherence to treatment, he showed no clinical improvement and reported persistence of productive cough with streaking of blood in the sputum. He was then referred to Lima with a suspected diagnosis of multi-drug resistant TB (MDR TB) for further work-up.

The patient had been found to be HTLV-1-positive ten years previously. A recent HIV ELISA test was negative. The patient denies recent travels.

Clinical Findings

A 40-year-old man appears fatigued and cachectic. Temperature 37.2°C, blood pressure 120/75 mmHg, pulse 70 bpm regular, respiratory rate 15 breaths per minute. On inspection, few cervical and retro-auricular lymph nodes are palpable, which are small, mobile, soft and non-tender. Lungs: crackles and rhonchi bilaterally. No hepatosplenomegaly. The rest of the physical examination is normal.

Laboratory Results

Platelets: 1093×10^9/L (reference range: 150-450); the rest of the full blood count is within normal limits.

Questions

1. What are your differential diagnoses?
2. How would you approach this patient?

CASE 56

A 21-Year-Old Pregnant Woman from The Gambia With a Rash

David Mabey

History

A 21-year-old woman comes to your clinic in The Gambia complaining of a generalized, non-itchy rash that she has had for five days. She is otherwise well, and has no significant past medical history. She is 32 weeks pregnant. This is her first pregnancy.

Clinical Findings

She has a generalized rash (Figure 56-1, p 222). Her mouth is normal, and there is no lymphadenopathy. She is not anaemic or jaundiced, and general examination is unremarkable.

Questions

1. What is the most likely diagnosis, and how might this affect the outcome of her pregnancy?
2. How would you manage the patient?

CASE 57

A 37-Year-Old Woman from Southern Malawi With Haematemesis

Camilla Rothe

History

A 37-year-old woman from the Lower Shire Valley in Southern Malawi is referred from a clinic on one of the local sugar plantations to the district hospital. She has vomited blood three times over the past 24 hours. The blood is bright red in colour. There is no epigastric pain and no previous history of vomiting. There is no history of fever and abnormal bleeding and her stool has been normal in colour. Before the onset of symptoms she was fine. She has not taken any regular painkillers and does not drink any alcohol.

Her past medical history is unremarkable. She lives and works on a large sugar plantation in the area. She is married with three children, all are well. An HIV test done three months previously was negative.

Clinical Findings

The patient is a 37-year-old woman who is slim but not wasted. Conjunctivae are slightly pale, but there are no subconjunctival effusions and she is not jaundiced. Her blood pressure is 90/60 mmHg, pulse 110 bpm, temperature 36.8°C, respiratory rate 28 breath cycles per minute.

On examination of the abdomen there is no abdominal tenderness. The spleen is palpable at 10 cm below the left costal margin. The liver is slightly enlarged but there are no stigmata of chronic liver disease. There is no shifting dullness and no peripheral oedema. Her lymph nodes are not enlarged. The rest of the physical examination is normal.

Laboratory Results

Her laboratory results on admission are shown in Table 57-1 (p 225).

Questions

1. What is the most likely cause of her haematemesis?
2. What further investigations would you like to do to establish the diagnosis?

CASE 58

A 25-Year-Old Woman from Egypt With Severe Chronic Diarrhoea and Malabsorption

Thomas Weitzel / Nadia El-Dib

History

A 25-year-old woman from Bani Suwaif in Upper Egypt (115 km south of Cairo) presents to a hospital in Cairo complaining of severe diarrhoea for two months accompanied by weight loss of about 15 kg and amenorrhoea. The symptoms started with stomach rumbles and colicky abdominal pain; later on she suffered anorexia and vomiting. The diarrhoea is voluminous, not related to meals, and occurs both during the day and at night (five to ten times in 24 hours).

She received various antibiotics, including metronidazole, as well as antidiarrhoeal drugs, without any improvement. During the last month she has developed lower limb swelling and severe prostration.

Clinical Findings

The patient appears generally unwell; she is pale and has angular stomatitis. Her temperature is 36.6°C, heart rate 100 bpm, blood pressure 100/60 mmHg, scaphoid abdomen with borborygmi, pitting oedema of the lower limbs, and decreased skin turgor.

Laboratory Results

Laboratory results are summarized in Table 58-1 (p 228). D-xylose test shows evidence of malabsorption. On stool microscopy, numerous helminth ova are detected (Figure 58-1, p 228).

Clinical Findings

He is thin and slightly breathless in the supine position. His pulse is regular at 130 bpm with pronounced pulsus paradoxus measured at 15 mmHg. Blood pressure in the supine position is 90/60 mmHg. The jugular venous pulse is difficult to visualize but is judged to be elevated. The apex beat is impalpable. The heart sounds are quiet but audible; no triple rhythm and no heart murmurs are heard. Auscultation of the chest is normal. There is an enlarged tender palpable liver measured at 8 cm below the right costal junction and evidence of mild peripheral oedema of the legs and sacral area.

Investigations

Haemoglobin 10.5 g/dL ; WBC 9.8×10^9/L (reference range: 4–10). Chest radiography (see Figure 66-1, p 253) shows an enlarged globular heart with clear lung fields.

Questions

1. Based on the clinical history and examination and investigations done, what is the most likely pathology to explain this man's illness and what would be the most frequent cause of the problem?
2. What other investigations should be carried out? Outline the immediate and long-term management of his condition.

CASE 67

A 24-Year-Old Woman from the Peruvian Andes With Fever and Abdominal Pain

Fátima Rosario Concha Velasco / Eduardo Gotuzzo

History

A 24-year-old woman from the highlands of Peru is transferred to a hospital in the capital Lima with a two-month history of upper abdominal pain, weight loss (5 kg), nausea and vomiting. She tried analgesics, which did not control the pain. She also reports intermittent fevers for the past two months.

Three days previously, she was seen at the emergency room of the same hospital for the above complaints. Abdominal ultrasound revealed multiple hypoechoic lesions. She was treated with ceftriaxone and metronidazole for suspected pyogenic liver abscesses but did not show any clinical improvement.

The patient reported that about 2–3 months ago she started taking over-the-counter medicines to lose weight and changed her diet to vegetarian food. She also reported the consumption of energetic hot drinks made from alfalfa and watercress. Prior to her current illness, she was healthy. She is single and has no children.

Clinical Findings

An ill-looking patient with pale mucous membranes but no jaundice. Her blood pressure is 95/60 mmHg, pulse 105 bpm and temperature 38.5°C. On palpation of the abdomen there is right upper quadrant tenderness and the liver is slightly enlarged with a liver span of 15 cm. The rest of the physical examination is within normal limits.

Laboratory Results

Table 67-1 (p 256) shows the patient's laboratory results, taken in the emergency room.

Imaging

A contrast-enhanced CT scan of her abdomen shows multiple hypodense, non-enhancing lesions in the liver (Figure 67-1, p 257).

Questions

1. What are your differential diagnoses?
2. What would be the most useful investigation to establish the diagnosis?

CASE 68

A 31-Year-Old Woman from Malawi With a Generalized Mucocutaneous Rash

Camilla Rothe

History

A 31-year-old woman presents to a hospital in Malawi with a generalized skin rash. The rash started three days previously on the trunk, and then spread to the extremities and the mucosal membranes involving lips, oral mucosa, conjunctivae and genital mucosa.

There is also productive cough with whitish sputum that started one day before the rash appeared and she also reports a sore throat and dysuria for the past two days.

The patient had been found to be HIV-positive two months earlier when she was hospitalized with cryptococcal meningitis. She was treated with high-dose oral fluconazole, since amphotericin B and flucytosine were unavailable. She improved and was discharged home on a maintenance dose of fluconazole. Antiretroviral treatment with stavudine (d4T), lamivudine (3TC) and nevirapine (NVP), as well as co-trimoxazole prophylaxis, were started one month previously.

The rest of the medical history is unremarkable and there are no known allergies.

Clinical Findings

Her temperature is 37.7°C, blood pressure 120/68 mmHg, pulse 90 bpm and respiratory rate 24 breath cycles per minute. There is a generalized, non-itchy maculopapular rash involving the skin and mucous membranes but sparing the palms and soles. There is bilateral conjunctivitis. The eyelids and lips are covered with haemorrhagic crusts (Figure 68-1, p 259). The lips are swollen and she can hardly open her mouth; talking and eating is difficult and painful. The chest is clear.

Questions

1. What is the most likely diagnosis and what is it caused by?
2. How would you approach the patient?

CASE 69

A 22-Year-Old Farmer from Rural Ethiopia With Difficulty Walking

Yohannes W. Woldeamanuel

History

A 22-year-old male farmer from rural northern Ethiopia presents to a hospital in the capital with difficulty walking.

His problem started 10 years ago, when he woke from sleep one morning and noticed a weakness in both legs. There was no history of trauma and no prodromal symptoms; he had been in excellent health before. The weakness in his legs rapidly progressed over 4–5 days, leading to him needing a cane for mobility. He had no back pain, sensory complaints, sphincter disturbance or upper limb symptoms.

The start of his illness coincided with a period of drought and famine, when his diet almost exclusively consisted of grasspeas (*Lathyrus sativus*, local name guaya), which is known to be drought-resistant (Figure 69-1, p 262). Despite the monotonous diet, he had been engaged in hard physical labour on his family farm where he acted as the main breadwinner, despite his young age. He lived with his mother and three sisters, who took care of household chores; they consumed a similar diet but of overall smaller amounts of guaya.

During that time, several similar cases of weakness among young male farmers occurred in his village. His walking difficulty finally meant that he could not return to farm work. At the age of 20, he moved to the capital city seeking an alternative job. He migrated along with another young male farmer from his village who had suffered a similar fate; he had weakness of both legs and arms, which he had developed during the same period of drought. There was no history of cassava exposure in the region.

Clinical Findings

An alert young man with a normal mental state. The gait is spastic ('scissor gait'), with foot-dragging and toe-scraping (Figure 69-2, p 263). There is mild bilateral lower limb spastic weakness of pyramidal pattern, with pathological brisk deep tendon reflexes and sustained foot clonus. Extensor plantar response is elicited on the right, while equivocal on the left. Cranial nerves and upper limbs are normal. There is no sensory or bladder dysfunction.

Laboratory Results

Full blood count, liver and renal function tests, cerebrospinal fluid, nerve conduction studies and electromyography are normal. His HIV-1 serology is non-reactive. HTLV-1 and -2 serology and MRI are not available.

Questions

1. What clinical syndrome can you apply for a diagnostic approach and how do you narrow down your differential diagnoses?
2. What management and disease prevention plans can be used?

CASE 70

A 58-Year-Old Woman from Sri Lanka With Fever, Deafness and Confusion

Ranjan Premaratna

History

A 58-year-old Sri Lankan woman who resides in a rural area presents to a local hospital with high-grade fever, chills, body aches, non-productive cough and progressive shortness of breath for ten days. Two days previously, she developed tinnitus and hearing loss. One day prior to admission she became increasingly confused.

Clinical Findings

On admission the patient is confused, with a Glasgow Coma Scale score of 13/15 (E4 V4 M5). Her hearing is severely impaired (WHO grade 3). Temperature 39.3°C, heart rate 120 bpm, blood pressure 90/60 mmHg. There are enlarged axillary lymph nodes on the right side. There is no rash and no neck stiffness; Kernig's and Brudzinski's signs are negative. Scattered crackles are audible on auscultation over the bases of both lungs. Her liver is enlarged to 5 cm below the right costal margin and the spleen is just palpable.

Laboratory Findings

Her basic laboratory results on admission are shown in Table 70-1 (p 265); her cerebrospinal fluid results are shown in Table 70-2 (p 265).

Her blood cultures grow no organisms; *Leptospira-* and *Salmonella*-serologies are negative. A thick film for malaria parasites is negative as well.

Further Investigations

Chest radiography does not show any pathological changes. Her ECG shows sinus tachycardia. The EEG reveals widespread slowing; the CT scan of the brain is normal.

Questions

1. What clinical sign will you be specifically looking for?
2. What antibiotic would you include in your empirical regimen?

CASE 71

A 71-Year-Old Man from Japan With Eosinophilia and a Nodular Lesion in the Lung

Yukifumi Nawa / Haruhiko Maruyama / Masaki Tomita

History

A 71-year-old Japanese man is referred to a local tertiary care hospital for further work-up of a nodular lesion in his right lung. He is clinically well and does not report any complaints.

The lesion was first detected two years earlier during a routine health check. Initially it was of linear shape. The patient has been regularly followed up since then. At his most recent follow-up visit it was found by chest radiography (Figure 71-1A, p 269) and CT scan (Figures 71-1B, 71-1C, p 269) that his linear lung shadow had turned into a nodular lesion of about 2 cm in diameter.

The patient was born in Kyushu district, southern Japan, where he is still living. He has no history of travelling overseas.

Clinical Findings

The vital signs were normal. The chest was clear. The remainder of the physical examination was also normal.

Investigations

His full blood count and total IgE are shown in Table 71-1 (p 270). Liver and renal function tests as well as electrolytes are normal. LDH and CRP are not raised.

Serologies

Cryptococcus Ag negative, *Aspergillus* Ag negative, ß-D-glucan 6.0 pg/mL (<20 pg/mL), Quantiferon-test (QFT-2G) negative.

Imaging

Fluorodeoxyglucose-positron emission tomography (FDG-PET-CT) shows increased FDG-uptake into the lesion in the right upper lobe (Figures 71.1D–F, p 269).

Questions

1. What kind of diseases should be considered in your differential diagnosis?
2. What further information should you obtain from the patient?

CASE 72

A 4-Year-Old Boy from Mozambique With Severe Oedema and Skin Lesions

Charlotte Adamczick

History

An oedematous 4-year-old boy from Mozambique with low serum albumin is seen in the paediatric department of a central hospital in Malawi.

On admission five days earlier, the suspected diagnosis had been nephrotic syndrome and the child was started on furosemide and prednisolone; however, his oedema did not settle.

Three weeks earlier the little boy had been treated for pneumonia at a health centre. The past medical history is otherwise reported as normal. The boy is accompanied by his mother, who is visiting her sister in Malawi. The rainy season has just started.

Clinical Findings

The patient is a miserable, apathetic boy with a puffy face and pitting oedema, most prominently on the back of his feet. The hair of the child is brittle, sparse and fair in colour. The skin is dry and hyperpigmented; it is peeling off like 'flaky paint' to reveal hypopigmented skin underneath (Figure 72-1, p 273). There are ulcerative skin lesions, most prominently in the groins (Figure 72-2, p 273). The child is refusing to eat.

Laboratory Results

Albumin 2.2 g/dL (reference range 3.0–5.2 g/dL), haemoglobin 7 g/dL (reference range 12–14 g/dL).

Questions

1. What is the likely diagnosis and how can it be distinguished from nephrotic syndrome?
2. How should the child be treated and what is the prognosis?

CASE 73

A 38-Year-Old Woman from Malawi With Chronic Anaemia and Splenomegaly

Camilla Rothe

History

A 38-year-old woman presents to a local hospital in Malawi because of general body weakness and left-sided abdominal discomfort. The symptoms have been there 'for quite some time'. There is no history of fever, night sweats or weight loss.

Her file reveals that she has presented with similar complaints many times in the past seven years. The attending clinicians repeatedly noticed a massively enlarged spleen and clinical anaemia. The patient was prescribed iron and folic acid several times.

She is a farmer residing in the lower Shire Valley in southern Malawi.

Clinical Findings

The patient is in fair general condition. She is afebrile, with normal vital signs. She has pale conjunctivae. The spleen is visibly enlarged; on palpation it is felt about 15 cm below the left costal margin. The liver is moderately enlarged (about 4 cm below the right costal margin) with a smooth margin. There is no clinical ascites and no lymphadenopathy.

Laboratory Results

The full blood count results are: WBC 2.4×10^9/L (reference: 4–10); haemoglobin 7.2 g/dL (reference: 12–14); MVC 88 fL (reference: 80–98); platelets 115×10^9/L (reference: 150–350).

Ultrasound Abdomen

Spleen $22 \times 12 \times 7$ cm, homogeneous pattern. No abdominal lymphadenopathy. Liver 17 cm in diameter, normal echopattern.

Questions

1. What are the most important differential diagnoses in this patient?
2. How would you manage the patient?

CASE 74

A 28-Year-Old Woman from Sierra Leone With Fever and Conjunctivitis

Benjamin Jeffs

History

A 28-year-old woman presents to a small rural hospital in Eastern Sierra Leone with a six-day history of fever, weakness, sore throat and retrosternal chest pain. She has had loose stools twice a day for the past two days. She was seen in a local health post the day before admission and given a course of artemether with amodiaquine and amoxicillin but she had continued to get worse on this. Her examination was unremarkable except some mild pharyngitis. On arrival in hospital she was treated with IV ceftriaxone and she completed the course of her antimalarial medications. Her malaria slide was negative.

She remained on this treatment for two days but continued to get worse. On the second day after admission she develops conjunctivitis. By this stage she is very unwell and is unable to walk unaided. She has developed a cough and breathlessness.

Physical Examination

Axillary temperature 38.2°C, blood pressure 80/55 mmHg, pulse rate 100 bpm. On chest auscultation she has bilateral fine crepitations.

Investigations

Her chest radiograph reveals diffuse bilateral infiltrates. Blood chemistry shows mild renal impairment and raised transaminases (aspartate transaminase 514 U/L (<50 U/L)).

Questions

1. What is the differential diagnosis?
2. What tests would you do and how would you manage the patient?

CASE 75

A 25-Year-Old Woman from Zambia With a New Onset Seizure

Omar Siddiqi

History

A 23-year-old HIV-reactive Zambian woman is referred from a health centre to a local teaching hospital in Lusaka after suffering her first ever seizure. The seizure occurred out of sleep. Her son walked into her bedroom after hearing a noise and found his mother on the floor unresponsive and shaking all four limbs. This continued for 5–10 minutes.

The patient had been diagnosed with HIV infection one month earlier. She is not yet on antiretroviral therapy (ART) but has been taking co-trimoxazole prophylaxis for seven days. She was successfully treated for pulmonary tuberculosis four years ago.

The patient is unmarried with three children. She works in the hospital cafeteria. She does not drink alcohol or use any recreational drugs.

Clinical Findings

On examination she looks well, her GCS score is 15/15, her vital signs are normal and she is afebrile. There is no meningism. The chest is clear. The neurological examination is unremarkable.

Laboratory Results

The malaria rapid diagnostic test is negative. Further blood results are shown in Table 75-1 (p 282).

A lumbar puncture is done. The opening pressure is normal. The cerebrospinal fluid (CSF) is clear. CSF results are shown in Table 75-2 (p 283).

Imaging and EEG Results

A CT scan of her brain shows frontal and parietal hypodense lesions in the white matter of the right hemisphere (Figure 75-1, p 283). No contrast enhancement is present. Electroencephalography (EEG) demonstrates focal slowing in the right hemisphere (Figure 75-2, p 283).

Questions

1. How would you manage this patient?
2. What is your general approach to a patient presenting with new onset seizures in sub-Saharan Africa?

CASE 76

A 55-Year-Old Woman from Turkey With Fever of Unknown Origin

Andreas J. Morguet / Thomas Schneider

History

A 55-year-old Turkish woman presents to a hospital in Germany with remittent fever up to 39.5°C, night sweats, chest pain and abnormal fatigue. The patient had visited her relatives in Turkey several weeks before. There is a history of rheumatic fever in her childhood and mechanical mitral and aortic valve replacement at the age of 37 and 53, respectively (St Jude Medical prostheses).

Clinical Findings

The patient's blood pressure and heart rate were within normal limits. There were unremarkable prosthetic heart sounds and a systolic grade 1 murmur over the aortic area without radiation. Liver and spleen were not enlarged. No lymph nodes were palpable. No haemorrhages or petechiae were detectable.

Laboratory Results

On admission, there was slight anaemia (Hb 11.5 g/dL [reference >12 g/dL]). White blood cell count, lymphocyte–neutrophil ratio and platelet count were within normal limits. The C-reactive protein was 15 mg/dL (reference <0.5 mg/dL). Serum creatinine and transaminases were not elevated. Blood cultures were negative. Urinary cultures yielded enterobacteriaceae.

Further Investigations

Chest radiography showed no infiltrates. Transthoracic echocardiography demonstrated competent prosthetic valves.

The patient was diagnosed with a urinary tract infection and treated with co-trimoxazole. Body temperature dropped to normal values and the patient's condition improved, but not completely. She complained of increasing dyspnoea and eventually went into congestive heart failure.

Questions

1. What are further differential diagnoses in this patient after deterioration?
2. What are the most promising next diagnostic steps?

CLINICAL CASES –
DISCUSSION AND ANSWERS

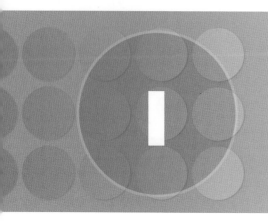

A 20-YEAR-OLD WOMAN FROM SUDAN WITH FEVER, HAEMORRHAGE AND SHOCK

Daniel G. Bausch

Clinical Presentation

HISTORY

A 20-year-old housewife presents to a hospital in northern Uganda with a two-day history of fever, severe asthenia, chest and abdominal pain, nausea, vomiting, diarrhoea and slight non-productive cough. The patient is a Sudanese refugee living in a camp in the region. She denies any contact with sick people.

CLINICAL FINDINGS

The patient was prostrate and semi-conscious on admission. Vital signs were: temperature 39.6°C, blood pressure 90/60 mmHg, pulse 90 bpm, respiratory rate 24 cycles per minute. Physical examination revealed abdominal tenderness, especially in the right upper quadrant, hepatosplenomegaly and bleeding from the gums. The lungs were clear. No rash or lymphadenopathy was noted.

QUESTIONS

1. Is the patient's history and clinical presentation consistent with a haemorrhagic fever (HF) syndrome?
2. What degree of nursing precautions need to be implemented?

Discussion

This patient was seen during an outbreak of Ebola HF in northern Uganda in 2000–2001, so the diagnosis was strongly suspected. She was admitted to the isolation ward that had been established as part of the international outbreak response. No clinical laboratory data were available because, for biosafety reasons, such testing is often suspended during HF virus outbreaks. While it is a reasonable precaution, the suspension of routine testing often causes difficulty in ruling out the many other febrile syndromes in the differential diagnosis. Fortunately, many clinical laboratory tests can now be safely performed with point-of-care instruments, often brought into a specialized laboratory in the isolation ward, as long as the laboratory personnel are properly trained and equipped.

ANSWER TO QUESTION I

Is the Patient's History and Clinical Presentation Consistent with an HF Syndrome?

The clinical presentation is indeed one of classic viral HF. However, most times the diagnosis is not so easy. Although some patients, such as this one, do progress to the classic syndrome with haemorrhage, multi-organ system failure and shock, haemorrhage is not invariably seen (and may even be noted in only a minority of cases with some virus species), and severe and fatal disease may still occur in its absence. The clinical presentation of viral HF is often very non-specific. Furthermore, haemorrhage may be seen in numerous other syndromes, such as complicated malaria, typhoid fever, bacterial

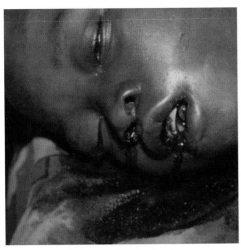

FIGURE 1-1 Oral bleeding in Ebola HF. *(From Bausch DG. Viral hemorrhagic fevers. In: Schlossberg D, editor. Clinical Infectious Disease. New York: Cambridge University Press; 2008. Used with permission. Photo by D. Bausch)*

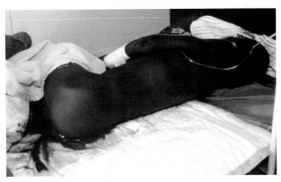

FIGURE 1-2 Rectal bleeding in Ebola HF. *(From Bausch DG. Viral hemorrhagic fevers. In: Schlossberg D, editor. Clinical Infectious Disease. New York: Cambridge University Press; 2008. Used with permission. Photo by D. Bausch)*

gastroenteritis and leptospirosis, which are the primary differential diagnoses, depending upon the region.

ANSWER TO QUESTION 2

What Degree of Nursing Precautions Need to be Implemented?

The spread of Ebola virus between humans is through direct contact with blood or bodily fluids. Secondary attack rates are generally 15–20% during outbreaks in Africa, and much lower if proper universal precautions are maintained. Specialized viral HF precautions and personal protective equipment (surgical mask, double gloves, gown, protective apron, face shield and shoe covers) are warranted when there is a confirmed case or high index of suspicion, such as in this case.

THE CASE CONTINUED ...

Intravenous fluids, broad-spectrum antibiotics and analgesics were begun on admission. Nevertheless, the patient's condition rapidly worsened, with subconjunctival haemorrhage, copious bleeding from the mouth, nose and rectum (Figures 1-1 and 1-2), dyspnoea and hypothermic shock (temperature 36.0°C, blood pressure = unreadable, pulse 150 bpm, respiratory rate 36 cycles per minute). She became comatose and died approximately 24 hours after admission. Laboratory testing at a specialized laboratory established as part of the outbreak response showed positive ELISA antigen and PCR tests for Ebola virus and a negative result for ELISA IgG antibody, confirming the diagnosis of Ebola HF.

SUMMARY BOX

Filoviral Diseases

Ebola HF and Marburg HF are the two conditions caused by filoviruses.[1] Microvascular instability with capillary leak and impaired haemostasis, often including disseminated intravascular coagulation, are the pathogenic hallmarks. There are six known pathogenic species of Ebola and one of Marburg virus, with relatively consistent case fatality ratios associated with each, ranging from 25% to 85%. Ebola and Marburg HF are generally indistinguishable, both with nonspecific presentations typically including fever, headache, asthenia, myalgias, abdominal pain (especially over the liver), nausea, vomiting and diarrhoea. Conjunctival infection is common. A fleeting maculopapular rash is occasionally seen. Typical laboratory findings include mild lymphopenia and thrombocytopenia, and elevated hepatic transaminases, with AST>ALT. Leucocytosis may be seen in late stages. The differential diagnosis is extremely broad, including almost all febrile diseases common in the tropics.

Ebola and Marburg HF are endemic in sub-Saharan Africa, with Ebola HF typically found in tropical rainforest in the western part of the continent and Marburg HF in the drier forest or savannah in the east. Recent evidence strongly implicates fruit bats as the filovirus reservoir, with human infection likely occurring from inadvertent exposure to infected bat excreta or saliva. Miners,

Continued on following page

spelunkers, forestry workers and others with exposure in environments typically inhabited by bats are at risk, especially for Marburg HF. Non-human primates, especially gorillas and chimpanzees, and other wild animals may serve as intermediate hosts that transmit filoviruses to humans through contact with their blood and bodily fluids, usually associated with hunting and butchering. These wild animals are presumably also infected by exposure to bats and usually develop severe and fatal disease similar to human viral HF. Most outbreaks are thought to result from a single or very few human introductions from a zoonotic source followed by nosocomial amplification through person-to-person transmission in a setting of inadequate universal precautions, usually in rural areas of countries where civil unrest has decimated the healthcare infrastructure, as was the case in northern Uganda where the government has been battling against the Lord's Resistance Army rebel group for decades.

Since symptoms are generally nonspecific and laboratory testing is not widely available, viral HF outbreaks are usually recognized only if a cluster of cases occurs, especially when healthcare workers are involved. Having been into caves or mines, and direct or indirect contact with wild animals or people with suspected viral HF, are key diagnostic clues, but these are not uniformly present. Outside consultation with experts in the field and testing of suspected cases should be rapidly undertaken and public health authorities must be alerted.

Treatment is supportive, following the guidelines for septic shock.[2] Antimalarials and broad-spectrum antibiotics should be given until the diagnosis of viral HF is confirmed. There are presently no approved vaccines. Contact tracing should be undertaken to identify all persons with direct unprotected exposure with the case patient, with surveillance of contacts for fever for 21 days (the maximum incubation period for Ebola and Marburg HFs). Any contact developing fever or showing other signs of viral HF should immediately be isolated and tested.[3]

Further Reading

1. Blumberg L, Enria D, Bausch DG. Viral haemorrhagic fevers. In: Farrar J, editor. Manson's Tropical Diseases. 23rd ed. London: Elsevier; 2013 [chapter 16].
2. Dellinger RP, Levy MM, Rhodes A, et al. Surviving Sepsis Campaign Guidelines Committee including The Pediatric Subgroup. Surviving Sepsis Campaign: international guidelines for management of severe sepsis and septic shock, 2012. Intensive Care Med 2013;39(2):165–228.
3. WHO. Interim Infection Control Guidelines for Care of Patients with Suspected or Confirmed Filovirus (Ebola, Marburg) Haemorrhagic Fever. Geneva: WHO; 2008.

A 7-YEAR-OLD GIRL FROM PERU WITH A CHRONIC SKIN ULCER

2

Dalila Martínez / Kristien Verdonck / Marleen Boelaert / Alejandro Llanos-Cuentas

Clinical Presentation

HISTORY

A 7-year-old girl who lives in Lima, the Peruvian capital, is brought to your clinic with a lesion on the nose as the main complaint. The lesion appeared four months ago as a small nodule and slowly turned into an ulcer. It is a bit itchy but not painful. There is no history of trauma. The girl is otherwise healthy. Six months ago she travelled to a valley on the western slopes of the Andes.

CLINICAL FINDINGS

The lesion is a localized ulcer on the nose (Figure 2-1). The borders of the ulcer are indurated and there is plaque-like infiltration of the surrounding skin. The diameter of the whole lesion is about 2 cm. There are no palpable lymph nodes. Body temperature is 37°C. The rest of the physical examination is normal.

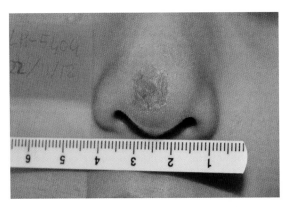

FIGURE 2-1 Lesion at first consultation.

QUESTIONS

1. What are your differential diagnoses?
2. How would you approach the diagnosis of this patient?

Discussion

A 7-year-old Peruvian girl presents with an ulcerative skin lesion on her nose, which has been present for the past four months. There are no systemic symptoms.

ANSWER TO QUESTION 1

What are Your Differential Diagnoses?

Infectious diseases that can cause similar lesions in the face are cutaneous leishmaniasis, sporotrichosis, cutaneous tuberculosis and infection by *Balamuthia mandrillaris*, a free-living amoeba.

Although common bacterial infections of the skin that are partially treated or masked as a consequence of traditional remedies (e.g. chemical burns) are another possibility, this is less likely in our case given the chronic nature of the lesion. Cutaneous anthrax and tularaemia could be considered in the differential diagnosis of lesions located on the extremities, but the latter is endemic in the Northern hemisphere only.

Cutaneous leishmaniasis is a common, vector-borne, parasitic disease that affects people living in or travelling to endemic areas. It typically begins as a small papule on air-exposed parts of the skin, progresses to a nodule or plaque and then turns into an ulcer with raised borders. The ulcer is painless unless there is bacterial co-infection. Patients may have several lesions.

Sporotrichosis is caused by *Sporothrix schenckii*, a dimorphic fungus that is found in soil and on plants. It enters the skin through direct inoculation (e.g. thorny plants or animal scratch). The disease usually starts with a papule that turns into a tender ulcer. Lesions can spread along draining lymphatic vessels. Sporotrichosis occurs throughout the world as a sporadic disease of farmers and gardeners. This disease is hyper-endemic in parts of the Peruvian Andes, where it often affects children and typically produces facial lesions. However, our patient did not travel to such a hyper-endemic place.

Cutaneous tuberculosis is an uncommon manifestation of tuberculosis. It occurs by direct inoculation of mycobacteria into the skin of non-sensitized individuals (e.g. children) or as a result of reactivation in persons with previous immunity against mycobacteria. As our patient lives in a poor neighbourhood with a high incidence of tuberculosis, we cannot rule out this diagnosis. Not only *Mycobacterium tuberculosis*, but also environmental mycobacteria and *M. leprae* can cause ulcerating skin lesions.

Balamuthia mandrillaris is a free-living amoeba that causes an uncommon, highly fatal disease. It usually starts as a painless plaque, often after local trauma. *Balamuthia* lesions are characterized by reddish or purplish infiltrations; ulceration is uncommon. The most frequent location of the initial lesion is the central face, over the nose. In a few months, it can progress to the brain (granulomatous amoebic encephalitis). If this occurs, the survival time is usually less than eight weeks.

The most likely diagnosis in our case is cutaneous leishmaniasis, due to the frequency of leishmaniasis in the valley our patient had travelled to and the characteristic presentation (localized painless ulcer with raised edges).

ANSWER TO QUESTION 2

How Would You Approach This Patient?

Gently clean the lesion with water, remove the scab and take a closer look at the process underneath. A definitive diagnosis of cutaneous leishmaniasis requires the demonstration of the parasite through microscopic examination, culture, or molecular techniques.

The simplest approach is to scrape with a lancet under the edges of the lesion, and use the obtained material for a smear examination with Giemsa staining, looking for *Leishmania* amastigotes. The sensitivity of this technique is about 70%, decreasing as the duration of the lesion increases. The specificity is 100%.

Culture can be done on samples obtained by fine-needle aspiration or biopsy. In reference centres, polymerase chain reaction (PCR) is used to confirm the presence of *Leishmania* and to identify the species.

The Montenegro or leishmanin skin test detects delayed immune response against *Leishmania* antigens and is sometimes used as a diagnostic aid. It can be negative in early stages of the disease and cannot distinguish current from past infection.

If leishmaniasis is ruled out, the following tests can be useful for the diagnosis of alternative causes of our patient's lesion: smear microscopy and culture in Sabouraud's medium (for sporotrichosis), a PPD skin test (for tuberculosis) and, if necessary, a histopathological examination of a biopsy specimen.

THE CASE CONTINUED ...

The scab was removed revealing an ulcer with cobblestone-patterned bottom and raised edges, typical of cutaneous leishmaniasis. The microscopic examination of a sample obtained by scraping was negative. The leishmanin skin test was positive. PCR was also positive; and the infecting species was identified as *Leishmania Viannia peruviana*.

With a definitive diagnosis of cutaneous leishmaniasis, treatment was started with intravenous sodium stibogluconate (SSG, 20 mg/kg/day for 20 days) which is the first-line treatment of choice

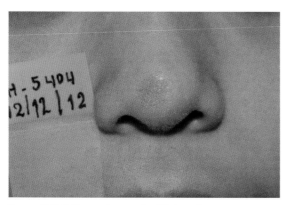

FIGURE 2-2 Follow-up image after 20 days of treatment.

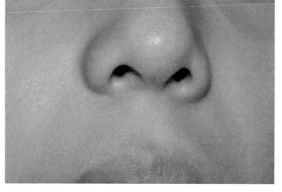

FIGURE 2-3 Follow-up image of the scar 3 months after the end of treatment.

for cutaneous leishmaniasis caused by *L. (V.) braziliensis* or *L. (V.) peruviana* in Peru. In addition, the girl received topical imiquimod therapy, which was administered every other day for 20 days. In our centre we we use imiquimod, an immune-modulating drug, as part of the therapy for facial lesions and relapses.

In our patient, response after 20 days of treatment was good (Figure 2-2).

Treatment failure occurs in almost 24% of patients after a first course of SSG monotherapy in Peruvian series, usually within three months. Follow-up is therefore recommended. Factors linked to treatment failure include young age and short stay in endemic area (as in this case) as well as recent onset of disease (≤5 weeks), multiple lesions, and *L. (V.) braziliensis* infection (not present in this case). At the third month of follow-up, our patient did not have any signs of relapse (Figure 2-3).

The treatment of cutaneous leishmaniasis is challenging because SSG has a high failure rate and several side-effects, including myalgia, arthralgia, loss of appetite, nausea, fever, increased levels of liver and pancreatic enzymes, reactivation of varicella zoster virus and cardiotoxicity, which can lead to prolongation of QT-segment, severe arrhythmias and death. Information about the safety of this drug in children is limited. It is also unclear from the literature if there are safe and effective alternatives to SSG in children with *L. (V.) peruviana* infection. This is particularly relevant since, in endemic areas, cutaneous leishmaniasis often affects children.

SUMMARY BOX

Cutaneous Leishmaniasis

Cutaneous leishmaniasis (CL) is caused by protozoa of the genus *Leishmania*.[1] Some twenty *Leishmania* species are associated with human disease. Cutaneous leishmaniasis can be anthroponotic or zoonotic (reservoir: small mammals). The parasite is transmitted by sand flies of the genus *Lutzomyia* (New World) and *Phlebotomus* (Old World). Ninety per cent of the estimated 1.5 million annual cases occur in Afghanistan, Algeria, Brazil, Colombia, Iran, Pakistan, Peru, Saudi Arabia and Syria.[2]

The incubation period between sand fly bite and appearance of skin lesions ranges from weeks to months. Clinical manifestations depend on characteristics of the parasite and the host immune response. Localized cutaneous leishmaniasis is the most common form. Some species of the *Leishmania Viannia*-complex can produce mucosal lesions resulting in disfiguring disease.

The lesions can heal spontaneously; this is more common in Old World (>50%) than in New World leishmaniasis (<20%). The aim of treatment is to accelerate healing, reduce scarring and decrease the risk of metastasis and recurrence. Topical therapy is recommended for Old World CL and for New World CL caused by species not belonging to the *Leishmania Viannia*-complex. This topical approach consists of intralesional pentavalent antimony, paramomycin cream and/or cryo- or thermotherapy. Systemic therapy is indicated for CL caused by species of the *Leishmania Viannia*-complex, when lesions are extensive, or when topical treatment fails. Pentavalent antimonials are the first-line systemic treatment of choice for all New World forms except *L. guyanensis*, for which pentamidine is recommended. Miltefosine and azoles are alternatives. Amphotericin B deoxycholate and liposomal amphotericin B are second-line drugs.[3,4]

Further Reading

1. Boelaert M, Sundar S. Leishmaniasis. In: Farrar J, editor. Manson's Tropical Diseases. 23rd ed. London: Elsevier; 2013 [chapter 47].
2. WHO. Control of the Leishmaniases. WHO TEchnical Report Series 949. Geneva: World Health Organization; 2010.
3. Llanos-Cuentas A, Tulliano G, Araujo-Castillo R, et al. Clinical and parasite species risk factors for pentavalent antimonial treatment failure in cutaneous leishmaniasis in Peru. Clin Infect Dis 2008;46(2):223–31.
4. Reveiz L, Maia-Elkhoury AN, Nicholls RS, et al. Interventions for American cutaneous and mucocutaneous leishmaniasis: a systematic review update. PLoS ONE 2013;8(4):e61843.

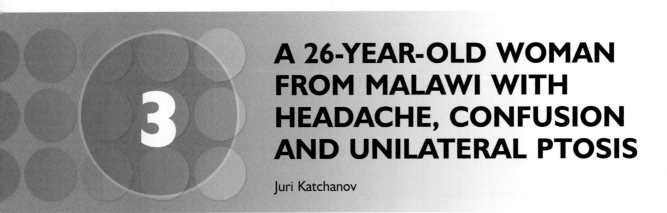

A 26-YEAR-OLD WOMAN FROM MALAWI WITH HEADACHE, CONFUSION AND UNILATERAL PTOSIS

Juri Katchanov

Clinical Presentation

HISTORY

A 26-year-old Malawian woman is brought to the emergency department of a local central hospital by two relatives. She has been unwell for at least one week. She complained of a headache of insidious onset and has been confused for two days. One day before presentation the guardians noticed an eyelid drooping on the left side.

The guardians say her past medical history is unremarkable. The patient lives in an urban high-density area. She works as a businesswoman, selling vegetables. She has three healthy children, but another four of her children have died as toddlers. Her husband died a year ago of 'high fever'.

CLINICAL FINDINGS

On examination she looks seriously unwell. Glasgow Coma Scale 14/15, temperature 38.4°C, blood pressure 115/75 mmHg, heart rate 86 bpm, respiratory rate 18 breath cycles per minute. There is no neck stiffness. The chest is clear. Figure 3-1 shows the examination of her eyes. The remainder of her neurological examination is normal.

LABORATORY RESULTS

Her blood results are shown in Table 3-1. A lumbar puncture was done. The opening pressure was markedly raised, at 32 cmH$_2$O (12–20 cmH$_2$O). The available CSF results are shown in Table 3-2.

QUESTIONS

1. What is the clinical syndrome and what is the differential diagnosis?
2. How would you manage this patient?

Discussion

A young Malawian widow presents with headache and confusion. She is febrile and has a unilateral third nerve palsy. The CSF examination reveals an inflammatory picture with a low glucose.

ANSWER TO QUESTION I

What is the Clinical Syndrome and What is the Differential Diagnosis?

The clinical syndrome is that of infectious meningitis. Infectious encephalitis should also be considered, however, the cranial nerve involvement makes this diagnosis less likely. Moreover, the main causes of infectious encephalitis are viral or protozoan and the CSF findings of very high protein and very low glucose are not consistent with a viral or protozoan CNS infection.

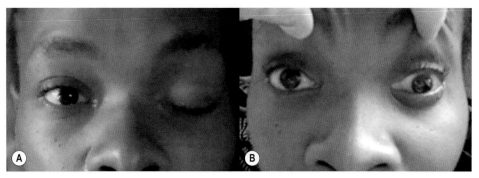

FIGURE 3-1   (A) There is a complete ptosis on the left. (B) On primary gaze, the left eye is in a 'down and out' position.

TABLE 3-1 Blood Results on Admission

Parameter	Patient	Reference
WBC (×10⁹/L)	3.2	4–10
Hb (g/dL)	10.2	12–14
Platelets (×10⁹/L)	155	150–350
Serum glucose (mmol/L)	4.0	3.9–11.1
Thick film for malaria	Negative	Negative

TABLE 3-2 CSF Results on Admission

Parameter	Patient	Reference
White cell count (/μL)	54	0–5
CSF protein (g/L)	3.0	0.25–0.55
CSF glucose (mmol/L)	1.3	2.0–2.64*

*½ to ⅔ of paired serum glucose sample.

The differential diagnosis comprises bacterial, tuberculous and cryptococcal meningitis (Table 3-3). Neither the patient's clinical presentation nor her CSF results can help differentiate reliably between the three. Furthermore, onset and duration of symptoms and signs may have to be interpreted with caution in many cultures, particularly when the history cannot be taken from the patients themselves.

ANSWER TO QUESTION 2

How Would You Manage This Patient?

The patient has a suspected CNS infection and is seriously ill with confusion, cranial nerve palsy and a high fever. Immediate action should be taken and treatment should not be delayed whilst further test results are being awaited. Pragmatic treatment should cover bacterial, cryptococcal as well as tuberculous meningitis.

Gram-stain and bacterial culture should be done from the CSF. A Ziehl–Neelsen stain should be ordered, although the sensitivity of this technique is low in many settings. India Ink stain and fungal culture should be done for detection of *Cryptococcus neoformans*.

An HIV-serology is crucial as cryptococcal meningitis is associated with immunosuppression. Also tuberculous meningitis is more common in HIV-reactive than in uninfected persons.

THE CASE CONTINUED ...

The patient was started on ceftriaxone 2 g bid, fluconazole 1200 mg od (local protocol for cryptococcal meningitis in the absence of amphotericin B and flucytosin) and on treatment for presumptive TB-meningitis.

The HIV test came back reactive. India Ink stain, cryptococcal and bacterial culture were reported negative, but acid-fast bacilli were detected in the CSF (Figure 3-2).

The diagnosis of tuberculous meningitis was established. A few days into treatment the patient slipped into a coma. An MRI scan of her brain revealed bilateral basal ganglia infarctions. She died in hospital.

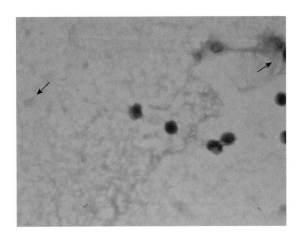

FIGURE 3-2 Ziehl–Neelsen stain of CSF sample showing acid-fast bacilli (arrows). *Courtesy Dr Jeremy Day.*

TABLE 3-3 Clinical and CSF Features of Acute Bacterial, Tuberculous and Cryptococcal Meningitis

	Bacterial Pathogen	Clinical Features	CSF Features
Acute Bacterial Meningitis	*Streptococcus pneumoniae*, *Neisseria meningitides*, *Streptococcus suis* (Asia)	Often very rapid onset with high fever and meningism, cranial nerve involvement less common	Often cloudy, high leukocyte cell count, predominance of polymorphs, low glucose
Tuberculous Meningitis	*Mycobacterium tuberculosis*	Often a history of several days of illness, onset less abrupt, cranial nerve involvement common	Often clear, high CSF protein, low CSF glucose
Cryptococcal Meningitis	*Cryptococcus neoformans*	Often subacute onset, severe headache common, cranial nerve involvement common	CSF can be normal in at least 25% of cases

TABLE 3-4 Four Pillars of Clinical Diagnosis of Tuberculous Meningitis

Clinical Criteria	Symptom duration >5 days
	Systemic symptoms suggestive of tuberculosis (one or more of the following): weight loss (or poor weight gain in children), night sweats, or persistent cough for more than two weeks
	History of close contact with an individual with pulmonary tuberculosis or a positive tuberculin skin test within the past year
	Focal neurological deficit
	Cranial nerve palsy
	Altered consciousness
CSF Criteria	Clear appearance
	Leukocytes: 10–500/μL
	Lymphocytic predominance (>50%)
	Protein concentration >1 g/L
	CSF to plasma-glucose ratio <50% or absolute CSF glucose concentration <2.2 mmol/L
Neuroimaging Criteria	Hydrocephalus
	Basal meningeal enhancement
	Tuberculoma
	Infarct
	Pre-contrast basal hyperdensity
Evidence of TB Elsewhere	Chest radiography suggestive of active TB
	Evidence for TB outside the CNS on CT, MRI or ultrasound
	AFB identified or *M. tuberculosis* cultured from another source (sputum, lymph node, gastric washing, urine, blood culture)
	Positive commercial *M. tuberculosis*-PCR from extra-neural specimen

Source: After Marais et al.[2]

SUMMARY BOX

Tuberculous Meningitis

Tuberculous meningitis is the most dramatic form of tuberculosis. After the release of bacilli and granulomatous material into the subarachnoid space, a florid gelatinous exudate forms, which may impair CSF circulation and cause hydrocephalus, cranial nerve palsies and vasculitis.[1] Vasculitis is the most serious complication of tuberculous meningitis and may lead to cerebrovascular accidents.

A definitive diagnosis of TB-meningitis is established when acid-fast bacilli are seen in the CSF, or *Mycobacterium tuberculosis* is cultured from the CSF or detected by a reliable molecular method such as PCR. However, these diagnostic tools are either time-consuming or lack sensitivity. Therefore, clinical diagnosis is crucial (Table 3-4).

TB-meningitis is an emergency. Treatment should be started without delay once the diagnosis is considered.[3] WHO recommends treatment with the same regimen as any form of tuberculosis starting with isoniazid, rifampicin, ethambutol and pyrazinamide, but some national guidelines include streptomycin. Usually, treatment is for 9–12 months. Corticosteroids seem to improve clinical outcome and are currently recommended; however, their effect may vary in different clinical settings.

Further Reading

1. Thwaites G. Tuberculosis. In: Farrar J, editor. Manson's Tropical Diseases. 23rd ed. London: Elsevier; 2013 [chapter 40].
2. Marais S, Thwaites G, Schoeman JF, et al. Tuberculous meningitis: a uniform case definition for use in clinical research. Lancet Infect Dis 2010;10:803–12.
3. Thwaites G. Advances in the diagnosis and treatment of tuberculous meningitis. Curr Opin Neurol 2013;26:295–300.

4

A 4-YEAR-OLD GIRL FROM UGANDA IN COMA

Douglas G. Postels

Clinical Presentation

HISTORY

It is the rainy season in rural eastern Uganda. A 4-year-old girl, previously healthy, is carried into the Accident and Emergency (A&E) Department. Her father reports that she was well until yesterday. She had a bad headache in the early afternoon but later in the evening developed shaking chills. Believing this was yet another episode of malaria, a common problem in their village, the family planned to take her to the Health Centre in the morning. The child slept restlessly. At 5 a.m. today the family woke to find the girl was in the midst of a seizure which lasted about ten minutes. It has taken four hours for the family to reach A&E and the little girl has not awoken. The child has not had any recent head trauma and the family knows of no other reason that the child might be ill.

CLINICAL FINDINGS

Her temperature is 38.7°C, pulse 150 bpm, respiratory rate 36 breath cycles per minute. Her blood pressure 98/40 mmHg. She has no neck stiffness or jaundice. Capillary refill is normal. There is nasal flaring with respirations. Blantyre Coma Score is 1/5. Pupils are 2 mm and reactive, and extraocular movements are normal by oculocephalic manoeuvres. She has no papilloedema on direct ophthalmoscopy. With stimulation there is decerebrate posturing that resolves spontaneously. On cardiac examination she has a gallop rhythm. Her liver is palpable 2 cm below the right costal margin and her spleen is 4 cm below the left costal margin. A rapid test for glucose is normal.

LABORATORY RESULTS

Laboratory results are given in Table 4-1.

QUESTIONS

1. What is the differential diagnosis?
2. What additional work-up should be performed?

Discussion

A 4-year-old Ugandan girl is brought to hospital unconscious with no neurological localizing signs, a supple neck, hepatosplenomegaly and a positive malaria rapid diagnostic test. Early laboratory testing reveals anaemia and thrombocytopenia.

ANSWER TO QUESTION I

What is the Differential Diagnosis?

The most important underlying aetiologies of coma to consider are cerebral malaria, acute bacterial meningitis, viral encephalitis and intoxication (particularly organophosphates). Metabolic

TABLE 4-1 Laboratory Results on Admission

Parameter	Patient	Reference Range
Haematocrit (%)	17.6	≥30
Platelet count (×10⁹/L)	28	150–450
Malaria RDT	Positive	Negative

abnormalities (hypoglycaemia, or renal or hepatic failure) and non-convulsive *status epilepticus* may be primary causes of coma or complicate these infectious and toxic aetiologies. Although there is no neck stiffness, she is deeply comatose, making this clinical finding less reliable; the absence of neck stiffness should not lower the clinician's suspicion of meningitis. Rapid testing shows that hypoglycaemia is not the cause of the child's abnormal mental status and it has been four hours since her last clinical seizure, making a post-ictal state unlikely.

The World Health Organization (WHO) defines cerebral malaria as an 'otherwise unexplained coma in a patient with malaria parasitaemia'. This clinical diagnosis is highly sensitive but has low specificity due to high rates of asymptomatic parasitaemia in those geographic areas where malaria is most common. People living in an area of high malaria transmission (such as rural Uganda in the rainy season) may be frequently bitten by infectious mosquitoes. Initially this produces clinical illness (either uncomplicated or complicated malaria), but with repeated infectious challenges a state of asymptomatic parasitaemia may be attained. Therefore, in comatose African children, a positive malaria RDT does not rule out an underlying non-malarial aetiology of acute illness.

In parasitaemic comatose African children, direct or indirect ophthalmoscopy may be useful in differentiating malarial from non-malarial aetiologies of coma (see Summary Box).

ANSWER TO QUESTION 2

What Additional Work-Up Should be Performed?

Although the child has a positive RDT, a lumbar puncture should be performed to rule out bacterial meningitis. If available, an EEG may be useful to rule out non-convulsive *status epilepticus* as either a primary coma aetiology or a contributor to illness. More sophisticated laboratory evaluations (creatinine, electrolytes, bilirubin) may be useful but are seldom available in the geographic contexts where malaria is most prevalent.

An ophthalmoscopic examination to evaluate for malarial retinopathy may be helpful. The presence of one or more retinal findings (retinal whitening, haemorrhages, or orange–white vessels with or without papilloedema) would lend support to a malarial aetiology of acute illness (Figure 4-1). Children with retinopathy-negative cerebral malaria may be more likely to have a non-malarial aetiology for their coma. As both retinopathy-negative and retinopathy-positive cerebral malaria may be complicated by bacteraemia, bacterial meningitis, seizures, and/or metabolic abnormalities, a complete work-up for non-malarial coma aetiologies (including non-convulsive *status epilepticus*) is indicated in all patients presenting with WHO clinically defined cerebral malaria.

THE CASE CONTINUED ...

A lumbar puncture was performed. The CSF was clear and acellular and opening pressure was normal. Blood cultures were taken and mydriatic drops instilled to perform ophthalmoscopy. This revealed white-centred haemorrhages in both eyes. A diagnosis of retinopathy-positive cerebral malaria was made.

After administration of artesunate 2.4 mg/kg IV in A&E, the child was admitted to the high dependency section of the hospital's paediatric unit for frequent monitoring of vital signs and serum glucose. Artesunate was repeated at 12 and 24 hours and then once daily. An EEG showed diffuse slowing but no epileptiform activity. Twelve hours after admission the child had one short (1 minute) generalized seizure that spontaneously resolved and did not recur. Forty hours after admission her Blantyre Coma Score was 4/5. The child was discharged home on hospital day five, with a follow-up appointment in the Neurology Clinic scheduled after four weeks.

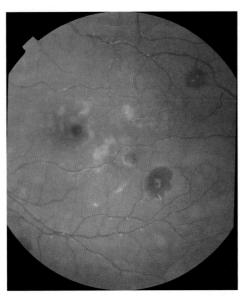

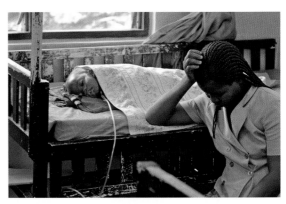

FIGURE 4-2 Infant with cerebral malaria hospitalized at Queen Elizabeth Central Hospital, Blantyre, Malawi *(courtesy of Mr James Peck)*

FIGURE 4-1 White-centred haemorrhages and retinal whitening, both features of malaria retinopathy *(courtesy of Dr Nicholas Beare)*

SUMMARY BOX

Cerebral Malaria and Malarial Retinopathy

Cerebral malaria is defined as an otherwise unexplained coma in a patient with *Plasmodium falciparum* parasitaemia.[1] Malaria kills approximately 600 000 people per year, the vast majority of them children less than 6 years old living in sub-Saharan Africa. Many of these children have cerebral malaria (Figure 4-2).

In parasitaemic comatose African children, direct or indirect ophthalmoscopy may be useful in differentiating malarial from non-malarial aetiologies of coma.[2] In autopsy studies, identification of malarial retinopathy during life was 95% sensitive and 100% specific for the post-mortem identification of sequestered parasitized erythrocytes in cerebral vasculature.[3] Sequestered parasitized erythrocytes in the central nervous system are a pathological hallmark of cerebral malaria and likely indicate that acute malarial infection was responsible for the patient's illness and death. In these autopsy studies, children who fulfilled WHO clinical criteria for cerebral malaria but lacked malarial retinopathy (i.e. they had retinopathy-negative cerebral malaria) had other non-malarial aetiologies of death on autopsy, including systemic infections (pneumonia) and Reye syndrome.

The mainstay of therapy is antimalarials, intensive supportive care, and diagnosis and treatment of non-malarial infectious and non-infectious contributors to illness. Even in specialized centres, the mortality rate for cerebral malaria is 15–25%. One-third of survivors are left with neurological sequelae, including epilepsy, cognitive impairment, attention problems and behavioural disorders.[4]

Further Reading

1. White NJ. Malaria. In: Farrar J, editor. Manson's Tropical Diseases. 23rd ed. London: Elsevier; 2013 [chapter 43].
2. Beare NA, Taylor TE, Harding SP, et al. Malarial retinopathy: a newly established diagnostic sign in severe malaria. Am J Trop Med Hyg 2006;75(5):790–7.
3. Taylor TE, Fu WJ, Carr RA, et al. Differentiating the pathologies of cerebral malaria by postmortem parasite counts. Nat Med 2004;10(2):143–5.
4. Birbeck GL, Molyneux ME, Kaplan PW, et al. Blantyre Malaria Project Epilepsy Study (BMPES) of neurological outcomes in retinopathy-positive paediatric cerebral malaria survivors: a prospective cohort study. Lancet Neurol 2010;9(12): 1173–81.

A 4-YEAR-OLD BOY FROM LAOS WITH A LESION OF THE LIP AND CHEEK

M. Leila Srour

5

Case Presentation

HISTORY

You are sent a picture of a 4-year-old boy taken by a visitor at a remote district hospital in Laos (Figure 5-1). You receive a limited history and physical exam. Three days ago the family noticed a dark sore on the child's cheek. The child's breath smells bad, he is not eating and appears listless. The lesion progressed quickly from a sore to eat through the child's cheek. The child, who is unimmunized, had a fever and rash about two months ago and recovered. The family is very poor. The local doctors do not recognize this disease.

CLINICAL FINDINGS

The 4-year-old child appears small and quiet. His mouth has a gangrenous lesion that has destroyed part of his upper and lower lips and cheek, exposing his teeth. The child appears stunted and thin.

QUESTIONS

1. What is your differential diagnosis?
2. What should you recommend to help this child?

Discussion

This chronically malnourished child, living in a remote village of a poor developing country, has a rapidly advancing gangrenous lesion of the face.

ANSWER TO QUESTION 1

What is Your Differential Diagnosis?

A few days earlier, when the child had a sore on the face and bad breath, you may have suspected a tooth abscess and cellulitis. The rapid destruction of tissue is typical of noma, an opportunistic infection that affects poor children whose immune system is compromised by malnutrition and often other infections, commonly measles or malaria. Other ulcerating facial lesions such as oral cancer, leishmaniasis, syphilis and yaws are unlikely in a young child. There are no diagnostic laboratory tests as the diagnosis is made clinically.

ANSWER TO QUESTION 2

What Should You Recommend to Help This Child?

You recommend treating the child with penicillin and metronidazole to cover the suspected aerobic and anaerobic oropharyngeal bacteria. You emphasize the need for nutritional support, which can be challenging with a mouth lesion. Local foods including eggs, milk, soy products and peanuts can be liquefied

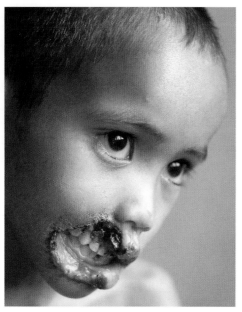

FIGURE 5-1 A 4-year-old Lao boy with a necrotizing lesion on the right cheek.

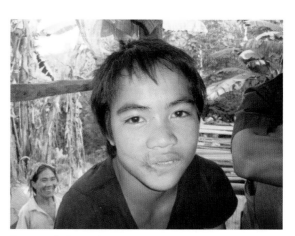

FIGURE 5-2 At age 9 after two surgeries correcting facial contractures and salivary incontinence.

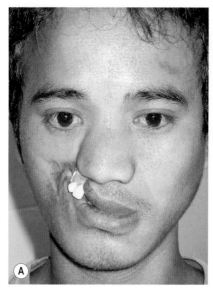

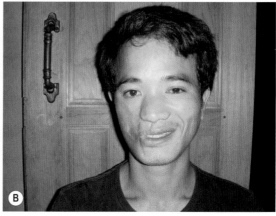

FIGURE 5-3 Young adult survivor of noma that occurred when he was 3 years old, before (A) and after surgery (B).

and fed orally or enterally. Other diseases such as malaria, intestinal parasites, tuberculosis and vitamin deficiencies should be looked for and treated. Dead tissue can be removed. Physiotherapy will be needed to prevent contractures with healing. Reconstructive surgery should not be attempted for at least one year by an experienced surgical team. Improved nutrition before surgery may improve the outcome.

Survivors of noma suffer from disfigurement and functional problems with speech and eating. They may present as young adults seeking help. Their history reveals the illness as a child of less than 10 years of age.

THE CASE CONTINUED ...

The child was treated successfully with antibiotics and nutritional support. His face healed with contractures, resulting in disfigurement and salivary incontinence. At age 9 years, he was referred for surgery by a visiting international surgical team. After two surgeries, his appearance was improved and the salivary incontinence corrected (Figure 5-2).

Another adult noma survivor had had noma at the age of 3. Aged 20 he presented asking for possibilities to improve his appearance (Figure 5-3A). He had surgery by a visiting international surgical team (Figure 5-3B), after which he got married and now has a family.

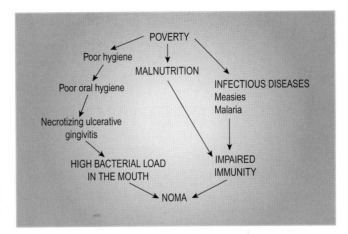

FIGURE 5-4 The pathogenesis of Noma. *(Reproduced with permission from Marck KW. 2003. Noma: the face of poverty. Hanover: MIT-Verlag GmbH. p. 108.)*

SUMMARY BOX

Noma

Noma is an opportunistic infection, primarily affecting children aged 1–7, whose immunity is compromised by malnutrition and vitamin deficiencies. Risk factors include extreme poverty, malnutrition, poor oral hygiene, viral infections (especially measles and HIV), poor sanitation and living in close proximity to livestock. The true aetiology of noma is unknown. The pathogenesis appears to be a complex combination of factors illustrated in Figure 5-4 by Klaas Marck, a reconstructive surgeon working with noma patients who named the disease the 'face of poverty'.

Noma is a neglected and forgotten disease, because it primarily affects the poorest children living in remote areas of developing countries. Health workers throughout the world often do not recognize this disease, so it remains underreported and unknown. Untreated mortality is 70–90%. Treatment with antibiotics and nutritional support can prevent disease progression and save the child's life. Survivors suffer with disfigurement, functional impairment and psychosocial isolation.

Noma is an indicator of extreme poverty and inadequate public health systems. The elimination of extreme poverty, provision of prenatal care, promotion of exclusive breastfeeding, immunizations, food security and improved nutrition for the poorest children can lead to the eradication of this preventable childhood disease.[1–3]

Further Reading

1. Srour L, Wong V, Wyllie S. Noma, actinomycosis and nocardia. In: Farrar J, editor. Manson's Tropical Diseases. 23rd ed. London: Elsevier; 2013 [chapter 29].
2. Enwonwu CO, Falkler WA Jr, Phillips RS. Noma (cancrum oris). Lancet 2006;368(9530):147–56.
3. Bolivar I, Whiteson K, Stadelmann B, et al. Bacterial diversity in oral samples of children in niger with acute noma, acute necrotizing gingivitis, and healthy controls. PLoS Negl Trop Dis 2012;6(3):e1556.

6

A 36-YEAR-OLD MALE TRAVELLER RETURNING FROM BOTSWANA WITH A CREEPING ERUPTION

Emma C. Wall

Case Presentation

HISTORY

A 36-year-old male restaurant owner presents to a travel clinic in Europe with a mobile itchy mass under his skin. Three weeks ago he noted the mass in his groin for four days after which it subsided. He then noted an itchy, serpiginous rash tracking from his groin to his chest which moved over the course of several days, disappeared and then he noted the mass reappearing on his right shoulder, at which point he was referred for assessment. There is no history of fever or systemic illness.

Five weeks ago he returned from a fishing holiday with four friends to the Okavango Delta in Botswana. He took malaria chemoprophylaxis (atovaquone/proguanil), slept on the boat under a mosquito net and swam in fresh river water. He ate freshwater fish from the river.

He is married with a child and denies sexual contact on the trip. Of the four friends who accompanied him, two also have the same complaint.

CLINICAL FINDINGS

The patient is afebrile and organ system examination is normal. On his right upper deltoid is a firm mass with clear margins 3×8 cm in size. On further questioning this mass has recently migrated across his upper chest wall and a serpiginous tract is visible (Figure 6-1). There is no additional rash and no lymphadenopathy.

LABORATORY RESULTS

Total white cell count 8.9×10⁹/L (reference range: 4–10), eosinophil count 0.9×10⁹/L (reference value: <0.5), liver function tests, creatinine and electrolytes are normal. HIV antibodies are negative.

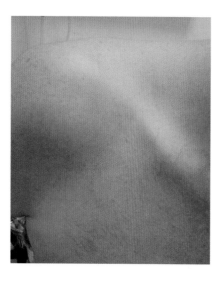

FIGURE 6-1 Itchy serpiginous rash tracking up the right shoulder.

1. What is the likely diagnosis and what are your differentials?
2. What is the risk of this condition if untreated?

Discussion

A 36-year-old European presents because of a mobile migratory mass he has been noticing for the past three weeks. There is some itch, but no fever and no further complaints. Five weeks ago he returned from a fishing trip to the Okavango Delta. Two of his travel companions have the same symptoms. Full blood count shows eosinophilia.

ANSWER TO QUESTION 1

What is the Likely Diagnosis and What Are Your Differentials?

This patient is systemically well, with a very unusual mobile itchy mass. The eosinophilia suggests a parasitic cause. The fact that two of his travel companions are experiencing similar symptoms indicates a common exposure factor.

The patient's presentation is classic for gnathostomiasis, even though his travel history appears uncommon. Gnathostomiasis is endemic in South-east Asia and Latin America, but only a few cases have been reported in Africa. It is a food-borne zoonotic nematode infection which classically presents with a mobile subcutaneous mass, intermittent creeping eruptions and eosinophilia. The infection is acquired by eating raw fish and other food items.

Intermittent migratory swellings are also typically seen in patients with *Loa loa* infection (calabar swelling), but *Loa loa* is not endemic in the Okavango Delta and the minimum incubation time is five months.

A very rare cause of migratory swellings and eosinophilia is sparganosis. It is caused by larvae ('spargana') of canine and feline tapeworms of the genus *Spirometra*. Sparganosis is acquired by drinking water containing infected copepods or by eating raw or undercooked intermediate hosts such as amphibians or reptiles. It mainly occurs in East and South-east Asia, but cases have also been reported in East Africa.

Several other infections acquired in the tropics can be migratory and are associated with an itchy track-like rash. Such creeping eruptions are commonly caused by larvae of animal hookworms or *Strongyloides stercoralis* but these present with fine, serpiginous tracks and not with a large mobile mass, as seen in this patient. Very rare causes of creeping eruption are ectopic fascioliasis and migratory myiasis.

ANSWER TO QUESTION 2

What is the Risk of This Condition If Untreated?

Deaths from gnathastomiasis have occurred when the parasite has entered the brain or spinal cord, causing severe neurological sequelae[1] (see Summary Box).

THE CASE CONTINUED ...

On further questioning, the patient admitted that on their trip they had made sushi from fresh fish caught in the river. A clinical diagnosis of cutaneous gnathostomiasis was made and the patient was started on albendazole 400 mg bid for 21 days and praziquantel 200 μg/kg as a stat dose. Serology for *Gnathastoma* was negative. Over the next six days, the serpiginous lesion migrated over his shoulder and neck, disappeared for 24 hours, then reappeared between his eyebrows, moved to his forehead and face (Figure 6-2), and then was felt inside his nose. On the sixth day of treatment he expressed a larva from his nostril, which was identified as *G. spinigerum*. His two friends were also seen at the same institution and were given similar treatment with full resolution of their symptoms.

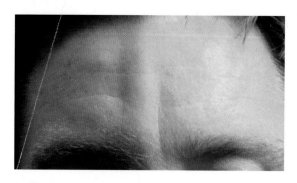

FIGURE 6-2 A picture taken after treatment of the mass tracking down the patient's forehead.

SUMMARY BOX

Gnathostomiasis

Gnathostomiasis is mostly caused by *Gnathostoma spinigerum*, a zoonotic nematode.[2] Humans are accidental hosts. Gnathostomiasis is endemic throughout areas where large amounts of raw or undercooked freshwater fish and crustaceans are consumed, most importantly in East and South-east Asia. It also occurs in Central and South America and case reports are emerging from Southern Africa.

Adult worms infect the gastrointestinal tract of felines and canines. When eggs excreted via the faeces get into water, first stage larvae hatch which then infect small freshwater crustaceans. A large variety of animals can act as a second intermediate host. Humans become infected by eating raw or undercooked meat of intermediate hosts, such as freshwater fish, crabs, shrimps, frogs, snakes, fowl and pork. Gnathostomiasis commonly occurs in outbreaks.

Larvae penetrate the human intestinal wall and wander around the body. Initial symptoms are nonspecific and may include fever, malaise, vomiting and diarrhoea lasting for 2–3 weeks. This is accompanied by marked eosinophilia. Within one month cutaneous infection may develop manifesting as non-pitting oedematous migratory swellings that may be pruritic or painful and mainly affect the trunk and the proximal limbs. Visceral disease occurs when the larvae migrate through the internal organs such as the lungs, gut, genitourinary tract, eye and CNS. CNS invasion may manifest as eosinophilic meningoencephalitis, subarachnoid haemorrhages cranial neuritis or painful radiculomyelitis due to invasion of the spinal cord.[1] Diagnosis is suggested by eosinophilia, migratory swellings and a history of geographic and food exposure. Gnathostomiasis is confirmed when demonstration of the parasite is made microscopically, radiologically or on a positive serology up to three months post presentation. Lumbar puncture and cranial imaging may be necessary in suspected CNS disease. Cerebrospinal fluid is often xanthochromic and may show eosinophilia. Imaging at times reveals larval tracks within the brain and cord parenchyma.[1] Treatment consists of albendazole 400 mg bid for 21 days or ivermectin 200 µg/kg on two consecutive days. For CNS infection, adjunctive corticosteroids are considered beneficial.[1,3]

Further Reading

1. Heckmann JE, Bhigjee AI. Tropical neurology. In: Farrar J, editor. Manson's Tropical Diseases. 23rd ed. London: Elsevier; 2013 [chapter 71].
2. Vega-Lopez F, Ritchie S. Dermatological problems. In: Farrar J, editor. Manson's Tropical Diseases. 23rd ed. London: Elsevier; 2013 [chapter 78].
3. Checkley AM, Chiodini PL, Dockrell DHm, et al. Eosinophilia in returning travellers and migrants from the tropics: UK recommendations for investigation and initial management. J Infect 2010;60(1):1–20.

A 28-YEAR-OLD MALE FISHERMAN FROM MALAWI WITH SHORTNESS OF BREATH

7

Camilla Rothe

Clinical Presentation

HISTORY

A 28-year-old Malawian man presents to a local hospital with progressive shortness of breath over the past five days. He reports orthopnoea and paroxysmal nocturnal dyspnoea, but there is no cough and no fever. He has also developed bilateral flank pain in the past days, which he describes as continuous and dull in nature, and he has been feeling constantly nauseated. However, there is no diarrhoea and no jaundice.

According to his health passport book, the patient was diagnosed with arterial hypertension two years earlier. He was prescribed some antihypertensive drugs which he never took. No investigations were done at that time.

His past medical history and family history are otherwise unremarkable. A recent HIV test was negative. The patient comes from a town on the Southern shore of Lake Malawi. He is a fisherman by profession. He is married and has two healthy children.

CLINICAL FINDINGS

The patient is a 28-year-old man with an athletic build, who is not chronically ill looking, but is in respiratory distress. His conjunctivae are notably pale. His blood pressure is 200/130 mmHg, pulse 66 bpm, temperature 36.8°C and respiratory rate 32 breath cycles per minute.

His apex beat is slightly displaced, but his heart sounds are clear and regular, and the jugular venous pressure is not raised. On auscultation of the lungs there are bilateral fine crackles over the lung bases. The abdomen is flat and non-tender. There is bilateral renal angle tenderness and the kidneys are ballottable. There is no peripheral oedema.

LABORATORY RESULTS

His laboratory results on admission are shown in Table 7-1.

TABLE 7-1 Laboratory Results on Admission		
Parameter	**Patient**	**Reference Range**
WBC (x10^9/L)	3.8	4–10
Haemoglobin (mg/dL)	6.0	13–15
MCV (fL)	92	80–99
Platelets (x10^9/L)	187	150–400
Creatinine (μmol/L)	1200	<120
BUN (mmol/L)	89.3	<17.9
K$^+$ (mmol/l)	7.2	3.5–5.2

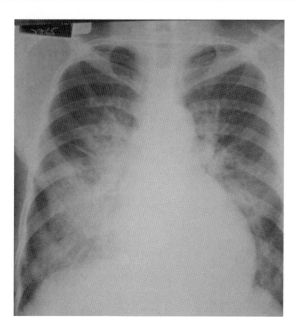

FIGURE 7-1 Chest radiograph on admission.

IMAGING

His chest radiograph on admission is shown in Figure 7-1.

QUESTIONS

1. What is your clinical impression?
2. What further investigations would you like to do to establish the diagnosis?

Discussion

A young Malawian fisherman presents to the hospital with signs and symptoms of left ventricular heart failure. He is hypertensive and severely anaemic. There is renal angle tenderness and his kidneys are palpable. His creatinine is very high and he is hyperkalaemic. His chest radiograph shows an enlarged cardiac silhouette and signs compatible with left-sided cardiac failure.

ANSWER TO QUESTION 1

What is Your Clinical Impression?

This young man presents with a combination of left-sided cardiac failure and renal failure. He has already been diagnosed with hypertension two years prior, but no further investigations were done, and it is unclear if his renal incompetence is a cause or the result of his raised blood pressure. On examination, however, his kidneys appear enlarged, which is against renal compromise secondary to hypertension, when you would expect the kidneys to shrink.

The reason for the enlargement of his kidneys could either be primary renal disease (e.g. polycystic kidneys) or postrenal obstruction with hydronephrosis.

The patient is a fisherman by profession. Since childhood he has been in regular contact with *Schistosoma haematobium*-infested water in Lake Malawi. Chronic schistosomiasis with hydronephrosis is one of the top differentials to suspect.

ANSWER TO QUESTION 2

What Further Investigations Would You Like to Do to Establish the Diagnosis?

The most useful investigation at this point is an ultrasound of the kidneys to differentiate between primary renal pathology and a postrenal problem. If there was hydronephrosis, obstruction at the level of the bladder seems most likely since both kidneys appear enlarged.

For a diagnosis of urogenital schistosomiasis in this man, the most useful investigation is a cystoscopy. Endoscopists can macroscopically establish the diagnosis, but ideally, biopsies should be taken to look for evidence of granulomatous inflammation and *S. haematobium* ova in the tissue and to rule out neoplasia. In chronic infection urine microscopy may be negative for ova of *S. haematobium*.

THE CASE CONTINUED ...

On admission the patient was given furosemide in view of his left ventricular failure. Yet, he only passed very small amounts of urine. Further doses of the diuretic were administered but the patient remained oliguric. Glucose and insulin were given for his hyperkalaemia.

Ultrasound of the kidneys showed bilateral grade IV hydronephrosis with massive dilatation of the renal pelvis and calyces. The remaining renal parenchyma was very thin in both kidneys.

The patient was sent for cystoscopy which revealed a hyperaemic mucosa with multiple 'sandy patches' suggestive of granulomatous lesions in the mucosa. No tumour was seen. An endoscopic diagnosis of urogenital schistosomiasis was made. Biopsies were not taken.

During the following day the patient deteriorated. He became drowsy and vomited repeatedly. He got progressively bradycardic, and on auscultation there was a new pericardial friction rub suggestive of uraemic pericarditis.

He was taken to theatre and a bilateral percutaneous nephrostomy was done; drainage catheters were inserted. The patient was taken to the intensive care unit and peritoneal dialysis (PD) was started, since haemodialysis was not available at that time.

The patient improved rapidly, vomiting and drowsiness ceased and his friction rub disappeared. He was discharged home on PD.

Two months later he was readmitted with fever and abdominal pain. He was treated for suspected bacterial peritonitis but sadly died three weeks later still in hospital.

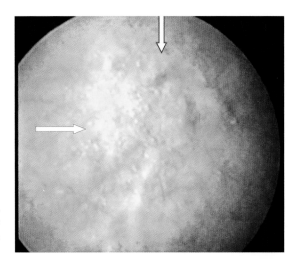

Figure 7-2 Cystoscopy findings of a patient with urogenital schistosomiasis. The white arrows show 'sandy patches' (*left*) and hyperaemia of the bladder mucosa (*top*). (*Courtesy of Iran Mendonça da Silva.*)

SUMMARY BOX

Genitourinary Schistosomiasis

Genitourinary schistosomiasis is caused by the trematode *Schistosoma haematobium*. It is endemic in large parts of Africa and in the Middle East.

In residents of endemic countries, recurrent infection during childhood leads to slow accumulation of worms. About 50% of *Schistosoma* eggs are shed via urine, the other half remain trapped in the tissue causing granulomatous inflammation. Egg excretion peaks between 12 and 15 years. Intensity of infection past adolescence is decreasing. It is as yet unclear if this is a result of developing immunity with immune-mediated destruction of invading cercariae, less intense water exposure in adults, or trapping of ova in the tissue leading to diminished sensitivity of egg testing.

An estimated 10% of people infected with schistosomiasis will progress to develop chronic late stage disease. Risk factors for disease progression are poorly understood. Apart from intensity and duration of infection, host genetic factors and parasite strain differences may play a role.

Continued on following page

Chronic infection with *S. haematobium* leads to granulomatous inflammation of the bladder wall and the ureteral mucosa resulting in obstructive uropathy, hydronephrosis, recurrent bacterial pyelonephritis and end-stage renal disease. As highlighted in the above case, these pathological changes can long go unnoticed. Chronic S. *haematobium* infection is also suspected to contribute to the development of squamous cell carcinoma of the bladder.[1]

Egg deposition in the female genital tract may result in dyspareunia, chronic lower abdominal pain, ectopic pregnancy and infertility. Female genital schistosomiasis has also been associated with an increased risk of HIV infection.[2] Men may present with scrotal swelling, orchitis and prostatitis, haemato- and oligospermia.

The advanced stages of schistosomiasis may be difficult to diagnose in the absence of biopsy results. The proof of *Schistosoma* eggs in the urine can be challenging since the adult flukes may have long died and egg production may have stopped. Serology is unhelpful in an endemic setting, as it can only detect past exposure without indicating the duration, activity or quantum of infection.

A plain abdominal radiograph may help show calcifications. Intravenous pyelography can be used to detect bladder and ureteral changes and obstructive uropathy. However, the investigation of choice is ultrasound, which has revolutionized the non-invasive diagnosis of schistosomiasis. Hydronephrosis and bladder wall abnormalities can easily be demonstrated.

On cystoscopy a characteristically hyperaemic mucosa with 'sandy patches' may be seen (Figure 7-2). Sandy patches are raised, yellowish mucosal irregularities associated with heavy egg deposition surrounded by fibrous tissue; they are pathognomonic for the disease.

Praziquantel may reverse the early stages of the infection, but it has little role to play in advanced hydronephrosis. A single dose of 40 mg/kg is usually still given to kill remaining adult flukes. Otherwise, late-stage urogenital schistosomiasis has to be managed symptomatically, which can be challenging in resource-limited settings where renal replacement therapy is usually not an option.

Further Reading

1. Bustinduy AL, King CH. Schistosomiasis. In: Farrar J, editor. Manson's Tropical Diseases. 23rd ed. London: Elsevier; 2013 [chapter 52].
2. Poggensee G, Feldmeier H. Female genital schistosomiasis: facts and hypotheses. Acta Trop 2001;79(3):193–210.

A 26-YEAR-OLD FEMALE TRAVELLER RETURNING FROM GHANA WITH A BOIL ON THE LEG

8

Camilla Rothe

Clinical Presentation

HISTORY

A 26-year-old German student presents to your clinic because of a localized swelling on her right leg. She has just returned from a six-week trip to Ghana.

The swelling has developed slowly over the past three weeks. It is itchy, but not painful. There is no history of fever; no history of arthropod bites. The patient is otherwise fine.

CLINICAL FINDINGS

There is localized swelling on the right leg, about 1.5 cm in diameter (Figure 8-1). The skin surrounding the swelling is slightly hyperaemic. At the centre of the boil a dark scab can be seen. There is no lymphadenopathy. The patient is afebrile while the rest of the physical examination is normal.

QUESTIONS

1. What are your most important differential diagnoses?
2. How would you approach this patient?

Discussion

A young traveller presents with a localized swelling on her leg after backpacking in Ghana. The swelling has been growing slowly and there are no systemic signs or symptoms.

ANSWER TO QUESTION I

What Are Your Most Important Differential Diagnoses?

There is a localized swelling with a central scab. This lesion may look similar to an eschar seen in rickettsial disease or in cutaneous anthrax, yet the absence of systemic symptoms renders these differentials unlikely. The clinical presentation suggests a topical process.

Localized bacterial skin and soft-tissue infections such as folliculitides, furuncles, carbuncles or abscesses are very common amongst backpacking travellers. A hot and humid tropical climate combined with low standards of hygiene favour bacterial and fungal skin infections. Itchy mosquito bites may serve as a portal of entry. Bacterial spread often occurs via scratching or contaminated items such as towels and shavers.

Another important differential diagnosis in this case is an infestation with fly maggots (myiasis). The slow growth of the boil, the absence of lymphadenopathy and systemic symptoms as well as the localized itch make myiasis the most likely differential diagnosis.

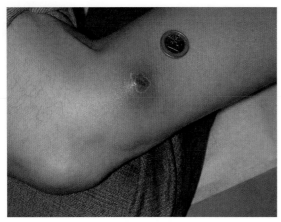

FIGURE 8-1 Boil on the right leg covered with a dark scab. *(Courtesy Dr Sebastian Dieckmann.)*

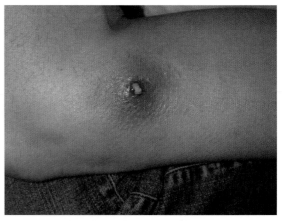

FIGURE 8-2 Skin lesion after removing the scab. *(Courtesy Dr Sebastian Dieckmann.)*

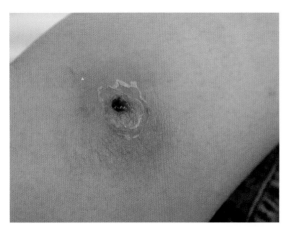

FIGURE 8-3 The residual lesion after removal of the maggot, looking clean. *(Courtesy Dr Sebastian Dieckmann.)*

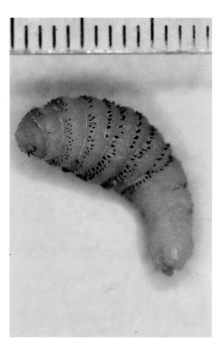

FIGURE 8-4 Larva of a botfly *(Dermatobia hominis)*. *(Courtesy Dr Sebastian Dieckmann.)*

ANSWER TO QUESTION 2

How Would You Approach This Patient?

Gently remove the scab and take a closer look at the lesion using a magnifying glass.

THE CASE CONTINUED ...

The scab was removed and a whitish matter was detected underneath (Figure 8-2). Using a magnifying glass one could see that the matter was not a pustular head but appeared to be pulsating and oozing transparent fluid. This appearance is typical of myiasis – the pulsating end of the larva seen contains the respiratory spiracles.

   The lesion was covered with white petroleum jelly and bandaged. The patient returned two days later for review. The maggot of a Tumbu fly was easily removed with a forceps. The remaining lesion looked clean (Figure 8-3) and no further treatment was required.

SUMMARY BOX

Myiasis

Myiasis is the infestation of live humans and vertebrate animals with larvae (maggots) of flies, which feed on the host's dead or living tissue, liquid body-substance or ingested food.[1,2] Cutaneous myiasis is one of the most common travel-associated skin disorders.

In sub-Saharan Africa, myiasis is usually caused by the larvae of *Cordylobia anthropophaga*, also known as Tumbu fly or Mango fly. Adult female flies deposit their eggs on sandy ground, or on damp laundry spread out on the ground or hung on a clothesline to dry. Normal hosts are dogs and rodents. Humans become infected when lying on the ground or wearing contaminated clothes without prior hot ironing. Larvae hatch and burrow into the skin. Over the following 2–3 weeks the developing larvae cause an itchy and at times painful 'blind boil'. Lesions are usually sterile since the larva oozes fluids with antibacterial properties.

Treatment aims to deprive the larva of oxygen which prompts it to extrude from the skin. This can be achieved by applying white petroleum jelly or liquid paraffin on the lesion to block its respiratory spiracles. Immature larvae are best left to develop for a while as they are difficult to retrieve and maceration of the larva can lead to a severe inflammatory reaction. Even untreated, cutaneous myiasis is self-limiting since the mature larva has to leave the host and pupate elsewhere.

In Central and South America, myiasis is caused by *Dermatobia hominis*, the human botfly (Figure 8-4). Unlike the Tumbu fly, this species lays its eggs directly on exposed skin. Furthermore it deposits its ova on blood-sucking insects such as mosquitoes, flies or ticks which afterwards convey it to the human host, a technique called 'hitch-hiking'.

Removal of botfly larvae can be slightly challenging due to their shape, and the process may require local anaesthesia and cruciate incision.

Further forms of myiasis exist whereby larvae may invade various body cavities such as nasal sinuses, ears, mouth, eye, vagina or anus (body cavity myiasis). Wounds can be infested as well.

Further Reading

1. Mumcuoglu KY. Other ectoparasites: leeches, myiasis and sand fleas. In: Farrar J, editor. Manson's Tropical Diseases. 23rd ed. London: Elsevier; 2013 [chapter 60].
2. Francesconi F, Lupi O. Myiasis. Clin Microbiol Rev 2012;25(1):79–105.

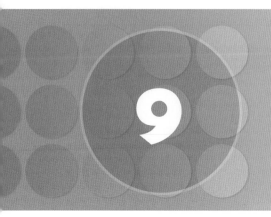

9

A 16-YEAR-OLD GIRL FROM VIETNAM WITH FEVER, HEADACHE AND MYALGIAS

Sophie Yacoub / Jeremy Farrar

Clinical Presentation

HISTORY

A 16-year-old girl presents to the outpatient department of an urban hospital in Vietnam having had fevers of 39–40°C, headache, lethargy and muscle aches for five days. Today she has vomited three times and is complaining of abdominal pain. She also noticed some bleeding from her gums after brushing her teeth this morning. She is normally fit and well and has not travelled outside the city.

CLINICAL FINDINGS

On examination, the patient looks lethargic but has a GCS of 15/15. Her temperature is 37.5°C, blood pressure is 94/68 mmHg, pulse 88 bpm and the respiratory rate is 20 breath cycles per minute. There is a maculopapular rash on the chest, abdomen and extremities that is fading (Figure 9-1). Cardio-vascular and respiratory examination is normal. There is mild abdominal tenderness and the liver edge is palpable, bowel sounds are normal. The spleen is not enlarged and there is no palpable lymphadenopathy.

LABORATORY FINDINGS

The laboratory results are shown in Table 9-1.

QUESTIONS

1. What is your differential diagnosis?
2. What further investigations would you request?

Discussion

This 16-year-old girl from urban Vietnam presents with a five-day history of a febrile illness with headache and myalgias. On examination she has a low grade temperature, a fading rash, some mild abdominal tenderness but otherwise normal examination. She is thrombocytopenic and has a low white cell count.

ANSWER TO QUESTION 1

What is Your Differential Diagnosis?

The main differential diagnoses would be dengue, other viral illnesses including rubella and measles, plus chikungunya if she had travelled to an endemic area. HIV seroconversion, EBV, CMV and influenza should also be considered.

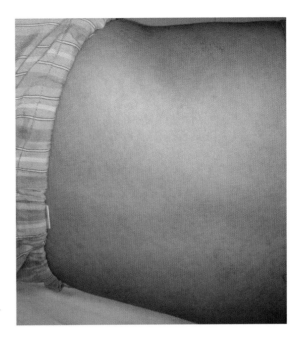

FIGURE 9-1 Maculopapular rash on the trunk of a 16-year-old Vietnamese girl.

TABLE 9-1 Laboratory Results on Admission		
Parameter	Patient	Reference Range
WCC (x10^9/L)	2.8	4–10
Haemoglobin (g/dL)	14.1	12–16
Haematocrit (%)	43.8	36.1–44.3
Platelets (x10^9/L)	38	150–300

Relevant bacterial infections include rickettsial diseases and leptospirosis. Malaria is a possibility if she has been in an endemic area of Vietnam, but since she has not left her city it is much less likely. Also, malaria does not present with a rash.

ANSWER TO QUESTION 2

What Further Investigations Would You Request?

This patient is presenting in a dengue-endemic area with a clinical syndrome that would fit very well with dengue. It is not essential to confirm the diagnosis of dengue immediately; more importantly the patient needs a thorough haemodynamic assessment and further tests for evidence of capillary leak and fluid accumulation. Classification by dengue clinical phase is also necessary, i.e. febrile, critical or recovery, to monitor for specific complications of that particular phase. Further investigations should include a biochemistry test to assess liver involvement and an ultrasound to look for pleural effusions, ascites or gallbladder wall thickening. Dengue diagnostics include NS1- (non-structural) antigen detection and viral isolation using real time PCR in the first 1–4 days of illness; after this time the sensitivity of these tests is reduced due to decreasing viraemia, so acute and convalescent serology for dengue IgM and IgG can be used. This patient already has some warning signs of more severe disease with persistent vomiting, gum bleeding, abdominal pain and low platelets with a borderline high haematocrit, so she needs to be admitted to hospital for careful monitoring.

THE CASE CONTINUED ...

The patient was admitted to hospital and a fluid balance chart was started. An ultrasound scan showed small bilateral pleural effusions, ascites and gallbladder wall thickening. Six hours later, on the ward, a repeat full blood count was performed and her haematocrit had risen to 46.4%. Her blood pressure was 90/75 mmHg, heart rate was 95 bpm and she had cool peripheries. A clinical diagnosis of severe dengue with compensated shock was made and she was fluid-resuscitated with 10 mL/kg of crystalloid over one hour. Her blood pressure improved to 100/70 mmHg and her heart rate was 86 bpm, her fluids were then reduced to 5 mL/kg over the next two hours and she was transferred to a high dependency ward.

Her haemodynamic status continued to improve, so hourly observations of pulse, blood pressure and urine output were made and 6-hourly HCTs were taken over the next 24 hours. Her fluid infusion was slowed further to 3 mL/kg, and six hours later her haematocrit was 41%. She continued to improve and after 48 hours her intravenous fluids were stopped and she was discharged home the following day.

SUMMARY BOX

Dengue

Dengue is a member of the flavivirus family, and is transmitted by *Aedes* mosquitoes. There are four distinct but closely related serotypes. The global burden of dengue has increased fourfold in the last decade. It is now endemic in over 100 countries and there are an estimated 390 million cases a year, of which 96 million are clinically apparent.[1] The vast majority of dengue infections are either asymptomatic or present with a self-limiting febrile illness; however, a minority can develop severe disease. Severe dengue may manifest with organ impairment, bleeding and capillary leakage which can lead to intravascular volume depletion and shock. There are three clinical phases: the febrile phase, which usually lasts 2–5 days, presenting with high fever, headache, severe myalgias, thrombocytopenia and leukopenia. This is followed by the critical phase, which is the 48 hours around defervescence when the patient is at risk of capillary leakage leading to fluid accumulation, shock and occasionally bleeding. Finally there is the recovery phase, where the patient starts to improve clinically; platelets and white cell count begin to rise and any extravascular fluid will gradually be resorbed. If intravenous fluids are continued into the recovery phase there is a high risk of iatrogenic fluid overload.[2] Although a mild rise in hepatic transaminases is usually present, rarely ALT levels above 1000 U/L are seen with associated liver dysfunction. Specific organ impairment can occur without any other features of severe disease, including hepatitis, encephalitis and myocarditis.

The severe manifestations occur relatively late in the course of the illness, around fever resolution, which coincides with the virus being cleared from the peripheral blood. This observation plus the association that severe dengue is more common in patients with a secondary infection with a different serotype has lead to theories of an immune-mediated pathogenesis.[3]

There are no licensed antivirals and no available vaccine. The mainstay of treatment is careful fluid replacement and haemodynamic monitoring.

Prevention of dengue relies on vector control, mainly by controlling the small water container breeding sites of *Aedes* mosquitoes and during outbreaks larvicides and occasionally adulticides can be used.

Further Reading

1. Yacoub S, Farrar J. Dengue. In: Farrar J, editor. Manson's Tropical Diseases. 23rd ed. London: Elsevier; 2013 [chapter 15].
2. Simmons CP, Farrar JJ, Nguyen V, et al. Dengue. N Engl J Med 2012;366(15):1423–32.
3. Yacoub S, Mongkolsapaya J, Screaton G. The pathogenesis of dengue. Curr Opin Infect Dis 2013;26(3):284–9.

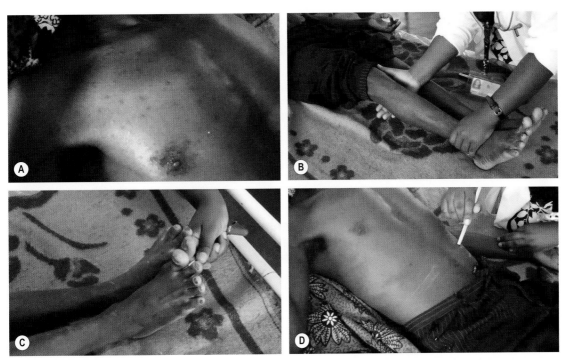

FIGURE 11-1 Physical examination of a Malawian patient with back pain and difficulties walking. (A) Tattoos from a traditional healer on the chest of the patient. (B) Severe spasticity and contractures of both lower limbs. (C) Upgoing plantar reflexes (so-called Babinski's sign). (D) Sensory level for pain and temperature at T9.

Discussion

A 45-year-old Malawian man presents with chronic back pain and slowly progressive spastic paraparesis. On examination there is tenderness over the lower thoracic spine and a thoracic sensory level. The patient denies any constitutional symptoms. His past medical history is unremarkable. His HIV status is unknown.

ANSWER TO QUESTION 1

What is the Neuroanatomical Syndrome and What is Your Differential Diagnosis?

The clinical signs – spastic paraparesis with hyperreflexia, upgoing plantar reflexes and thoracic sensory level – localize the lesion unequivocally to the spinal cord.[1] The bladder is usually involved in spinal cord disease, but the absence of bladder symptoms does not rule out spinal cord involvement, particularly in slowly progressive lesions, as in our case.

The differential diagnosis of spinal cord disease is broad. It can be traumatic or non-traumatic. Nothing in the patient's history suggests trauma. Non-traumatic spinal cord disease can be compressive or non-compressive. Compressive disease is sometimes amenable to spinal surgery.

Common causes of adult non-traumatic compressive spinal cord disease in sub-Saharan Africa are spinal tuberculosis ('Pott's disease'), spinal metastases and degenerative spinal disease including slipped disc.[2] Common causes of non-compressive spinal cord disease are schistosomiasis, autoimmune transverse myelitis and HIV-associated vacuolar myelopathy.

ANSWER TO QUESTION 2

What is the Further Management?

The diagnosis of spinal cord disease in resource-limited settings is often clinical, based on history and physical examination (Table 11-1). Management should focus on diagnosis and treatment of the underlying etiology and, equally important, on prevention and treatment of the complications of spinal cord disease. Diagnostic clues and possible treatment regimens are summarized in Table 11-2.

TABLE 11-1   Important Causes of Spinal Cord Disease in the Tropics and Their Typical Clinical Features

	Typical Onset and Course	Clinical Features
Spinal tuberculosis	Insidious onset, chronically progressive over weeks, with months of back pain	Spasticity common, bladder may be spared, spinal deformity on examination
Spinal metastases	Subacute onset, chronically progressive over weeks	Spasticity or flaccidity, bladder may be spared
Transverse myelitis (incl. autoimmune)	Acute onset, often non-progressive	Bladder involvement common
Schistosomiasis	Acute (days) or subacute (a couple of weeks)	Often flaccid paresis, bladder involvement common

TABLE 11-2   Diagnostic Clues and Possible Treatment Regimens for Important Causes of Spinal Cord Disease in Resource-Limited Settings

	Diagnostic Clues	Treatment
Spinal tuberculosis	Typical spinal radiograph (see Box) Epidemiological evidence	Anti-tuberculous treatment Spinal surgery if available and applicable (see Box)
Spinal metastases	Clinical evidence of the primary tumour (e.g. prostate, breast)	Very limited options: radiotherapy rarely available; corticosteroids to decrease oedema
Transverse myelitis (incl. autoimmune)	Young adults Inflammatory CSF	Corticosteroids
Schistosomiasis	Blood in urine or stool Young adults Evidence of ova in urine, stool or rectal biopsy Exposure to freshwater in endemic regions CSF eosinophilia	Praziquantel, corticosteroids

TABLE 11-3   Common Complications of Spinal Cord Disease and Their Prevention and Management

Complication	Prevention/Management
Pressure sores	Nursing, training and counselling of guardians (two hourly turning)
Urinary retention	Catheterization
Contractures	Physiotherapy, training of guardians for home-based physiotherapy
Pain	Pain relief by NSAID/opiates, involvement of local palliative care team
Immobilization	If available, prescription of walking aids/wheelchairs
Depression	Spiritual and mental support, occupational therapy/community projects, pharmacotherapy, involvement of local palliative care team

All patients should be tested for HIV, ova of *Schistosoma* spp. in urine and stool, and evidence of tuberculosis or neoplasia on chest and spinal radiography. If available, ultrasound examination of the abdomen is very valuable in tumour-screening and tuberculosis work-up. CSF should be examined, which is of particular importance in immunosuppressed patients.

Realistically, most patients admitted to hospital with paraplegia due to spinal cord disease will leave the hospital paraplegic. The prognosis is overall poor, and often the secondary complications rather than the primary pathology dictate the further course of the disease. The prevention of complications of spinal cord disease is therefore of paramount importance. Health workers should work hand in hand with guardians, physiotherapists and the local palliative care team (Table 11-3).

THE CASE CONTINUED ...

The patient was tested and found to be reactive for HIV. His urine dipstick was normal and there were no ova of *Schistosoma* spp. detected in his urine and stool. The spinal radiograph showed a

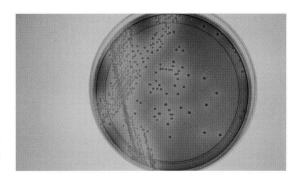

Figure 14-1 Stool culture growing *Vibrio cholerae* producing typical golden-yellow colonies on thiosulphate citrate bile salt sucrose (TCBS) agar.

Stool culture grows *V. cholerae* (Figure 14-1) and the organism was typed as *V. cholerae* O1, Serotype Ogawa, biotype El Tor. The organism was susceptible to tetracycline, furazolidone and quinolone groups of antibiotics.

QUESTIONS

1. How was the infection most likely acquired? Is there an outbreak?
2. How is dehydration assessed and managed?

Discussion

A 22-year-old Bengali woman who has recently visited a religious festival in her home village is brought into hospital in a stuporous condition with a history of rapid onset of severe, acute watery diarrhoea. There is no associated fever, vomiting or abdominal pain. On clinical examination she is severely dehydrated and biochemical parameters show hypokalaemia, elevated creatinine and lactic acidosis. The microscopic examination of her stool indicates cholera which is confirmed on culture. A number of other people who attended the same festival have also fallen ill with diarrhoea.

ANSWER TO QUESTION 1

How Was the Infection Most Likely Acquired? Is There an Outbreak?

Cholera transmission is closely linked to inadequate environmental management.[1] Typical at-risk areas include peri-urban slums, where basic infrastructure is not available, rural and urban areas in endemic countries where sanitation is limited, as well as camps for internally displaced people or refugees or during natural disasters, where minimum requirements of clean water and sanitation are not met.

An outbreak is defined as the occurrence of disease episodes in greater numbers than would be expected at a particular time and place.

In this case, there seems to be a typical cholera outbreak. The source is most probably contaminated water consumed from the metal containers during the village festival, with the likelihood that unless control measures for disease prevention and appropriate case management are instituted rapidly, there will be spread, significant morbidity and, possibly, mortality.

ANSWER TO QUESTION 2

How is Dehydration Assessed and Managed?

The WHO has recommended an assessment based on the general clinical condition of the patient (Table 14-2). Depending on their degree of fluid depletion, patients are assigned to rehydration at home, supervised oral rehydration or intravenous rehydration (Table 14-3).[2]

Adequate fluid and electrolyte replacement is the cornerstone of cholera management and differs substantially from the approach to patients with gastroenteritis of other aetiologies. Patients with severe cholera present with a higher degree of initial dehydration, have more rapid continuing losses and proportionately greater electrolyte depletion than patients with other forms of gastroenteritis. The

TABLE 14-2 Clinical Assessment of Dehydration in Patients with Suspected Cholera			
	No Dehydration (<5%)	**Some Dehydration (5–10%)**	**Severe Dehydration (>10%)**
General Appearance	Well, alert	Restless, irritable	Lethargic or unconscious
Eyes	Normal	Sunken	Sunken
Thirst	Drinks normally	Thirsty, drinks eagerly	Drinks poorly or is unable to drink
Skin Turgor	Instantaneous recoil	Non-instantaneous recoil	Very slow recoil (>2 s)
Pulse	Normal	Rapid, low volume	Weak or absent

Source: *After Harris et al.*[2]

TABLE 14-3 Approach to Rehydration in Patients with Cholera Depending on the Degree of Clinical Dehydration			
	No Dehydration (<5%)	**Some Dehydration (5–10%)**	**Severe Dehydration (>10%)**
Requirement for Fluid Replacement	Ongoing losses only	75 ml/kg in the first 24 hours in addition to ongoing losses	>100 ml/kg in the first 24 hours in addition to ongoing losses
Preferred Route of Administration	Oral	Oral or intravenous	Intravenous
Timing	Usually guided by thirst	Replace fluids over 3–4 hours	As rapidly as possible until circulation is restored, then complete the remainder of fluids within 3 hours
Monitoring	Observe until ongoing losses can definitely adequately replaced by ORS	Observe every 1–2 hours until all signs of dehydration resolve and patient urinates	Once circulation is established monitor every 1–2 hours

ORS = oral rehydration solution.
Source: *After Harris et al.*[2]

most common error is for clinicians to underestimate the speed and volume of fluids required for rehydration.[2]

Up to 80% of sufferers can be treated successfully through prompt administration of oral rehydration salts (WHO/UNICEF ORS standard sachets). In adults, 2–4 litres of ORS may be required in the first four hours.[1]

Patients with severe cholera typically require an average of 200 ml/kg of isotonic oral or IV fluids in the first 24 hours (Table 14-2). The initial fluid deficit should be replaced within 3–4 hours of initial presentation and patients should ideally be given more than one large-bore IV cannula. Cholera cots can help estimate continuing losses, but in their absence, 10–20 mL/kg bodyweight should be calculated for each diarrhoeal stool or episode of vomiting.[2]

Antibiotic therapy in cholera is secondary, but in patients with severe disease appropriate antibiotics diminish the duration of diarrhoea, reduce the volume of rehydration fluids needed and shorten the duration of *V. cholerae* excretion.

THE CASE CONTINUED ...

The patient was admitted immediately and started on intravenous rehydration with Ringer's lactate solution. After receiving 2 L in the first 30 minutes her pulse rate dropped to 90 bpm and her blood pressure rose to 90/60 mmHg. She was given another 1 L in 45 minutes and her pulse rate and blood pressure further picked up to 84 bpm and 100/70 mmHg, respectively. Over the next three hours she was given an additional 2 L and became alert and responsive. She was then started on oral rehydration and given a single dose of 300 mg doxycycline. She was discharged on the third day, by which time stool consistency had returned to normal.

The local health authorities investigated the village the woman had visited and identified an additional 44 cases of cholera. All were treated, health education carried out and the overhead tanks were chlorinated. An additional two cases were identified three days later, but there were no subsequent cases.

SUMMARY BOX

Cholera

Cholera, caused by *Vibrio cholerae*, is a major cause of acute dehydrating diarrhoea, particularly in South and South-east Asia, where it is endemic; it also occurs as large-scale outbreaks in Africa and Latin America.[1,2]

Seven cholera pandemics have been recorded since the early nineteenth century. The current 'seventh' cholera pandemic started in 1961 and is still continuing. This pandemic, due to the emergence of *V. cholerae* biotype El Tor, first appeared in Indonesia and has since spread worldwide, leading to the re-emergence of cholera in Africa in the early 1970s and in Central and South America in the early 1990s. A new group, *V. cholerae* O139, emerged in the early 1990s and spread to several parts of the world.

Vibrio cholerae is an aerobic Gram-negative bacillus with typical darting motility. It produces golden yellow colonies on a selective medium. Man is the only natural host of *V. cholerae* and asymptomatic carriage is possible. The main source of transmission is from a contaminated water source. In some parts of the world, copepods are responsible for maintaining *Vibrio* spp. in a viable but non-cultivable state.

The incubation period ranges between 12 hours and five days. Patients are usually afebrile and do not have any abdominal pain. The major clinical challenge is dehydration, ranging from mild to severe, and electrolyte imbalance leading on to renal failure in severe cases.

In epidemics, the diagnosis of cholera may be presumptive on clinical and epidemiological grounds following the WHO clinical case definition. Laboratory confirmation may be required when sporadic cases occur or when an extensive outbreak requires confirmation and typing of the etiological agent.

Treatment typically involves isolation of the patient, correction of dehydration and antimicrobial treatment. Fluid therapy must be carefully balanced to correct the electrolyte and acid base imbalance and to keep the urine output adequate. In most cases oral replacement solutions may be used. Antimicrobial therapy is secondary; it is shown to decrease shedding of the bacteria and also hastens clinical resolution of illness. Tetracycline and doxycycline are the preferred drugs in adults, but ciprofloxacin or macrolides can also be used depending on availability and local resistance pattern.

Public health measures to improve water and sanitation are essential for long-term control. WHO has endorsed the inclusion of oral vaccines[3] in cholera control programmes in endemic areas in conjunction with other preventive and control strategies.

Further Reading

1. Kang G, Hart CA, Shears P. Bacterial enteropathogens. In: Farrar J, editor. Manson's Tropical Diseases. 23rd ed. London: Elsevier; 2013 [chapter 24].
2. Harris JB, LaRocque RC, Qadri F, et al. Cholera. Lancet 2012;379(9835):2466–76.
3. Holmgren J, Svennerholm AM. Vaccines against mucosal infections. Curr Opin Immunol 2012;24(3):343–53.

15

A 3-YEAR-OLD BOY FROM LAOS WITH RIGHT SUPPURATIVE PAROTITIS

Sayaphet Rattanavong / Viravong Douangnoulak / Buachan Norindr / Paul N. Newton / Caoimhe Nic Fhogartaigh

Clinical Presentation

HISTORY

A 3-year-old rural Lao boy, whose parents are rice farmers, presents to the ENT clinic with a ten-day history of gradual, painful swelling of the right cheek with associated fever and poor appetite. Three days previously his mother noticed a purulent discharge from the ear. He has no cough, vomiting or diarrhoea. There is no history of previous ear infection or dental problems, and no known history of trauma. The child is developing normally and is up to date with vaccinations.

CLINICAL FINDINGS

The child looks unwell, with a fever of 39.5°C. There is a localized, fluctuant, hot, tender swelling below and anterior to the right ear, 6–8 cm in diameter, extending from the lower cheek to the submandibular region, consistent with a parotid mass (Figure 15-1). Ear examination reveals purulent discharge in the auditory canal and a suspicion of a small fistula from which the pus is arising, with a right lower motor neuron facial nerve palsy. The oral cavity and throat are unremarkable. There is no lymphadenopathy and no hepatosplenomegaly. Heart sounds are normal and the chest is clear.

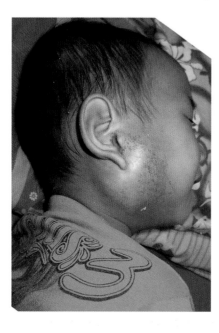

FIGURE 15-1 A Lao boy with a unilateral parotid mass showing signs of local inflammation.

QUESTIONS

1. What are your differential diagnoses?
2. What investigations would you perform?

Discussion

A 3-year-old boy from rural Laos presents to a local hospital because of unilateral parotid swelling, high fever and purulent discharge from his ear. The little boy has previously been well.

ANSWER TO QUESTION 1

What Are Your Differential Diagnoses?

Acute, suppurative, unilateral parotitis in children is usually bacterial, the most common pathogens being *Staphylococcus aureus*, *Streptococcus pyogenes* and *Haemophilus influenzae*, although the latter has declined since widespread vaccination. Neonates are at risk of parotitis caused by Gram-negative bacteria, and *Streptococcus pneumoniae* parotitis may occur in HIV-infected children.

In an endemic area like Laos, *Burkholderia pseudomallei*, the causative agent of melioidosis, must also be considered. Studies in neighbouring countries have shown melioidosis to be the commonest cause of suppurative parotitis in children.[1] Actinomycosis and cat-scratch disease (*Bartonella henselae*) are more unusual bacterial causes.

Mumps was the commonest cause of parotid swelling in children until the introduction of vaccination, which is still not commonly available in some countries, including Laos. Swelling is painful, but is non-suppurative, and becomes bilateral in the majority of cases. Other less common viral agents that cause parotitis include parainfluenza viruses, influenza A, cytomegalovirus, Epstein–Barr virus and enteroviruses, but these do not cause the degree of inflammation and suppuration seen here.

Granulomatous parotitis, caused by *Mycobacterium tuberculosis*, *M. avium-intracellulare* and other mycobacteria, is rare, and presents with a more chronic, painless, enlarging mass without surrounding inflammation. Salivary stones and malignancies are very rare in children.

ANSWER TO QUESTION 2

What Investigations Would You Perform?

Samples for bacterial culture before commencing antimicrobial therapy are crucial. Gram stain and bacterial culture of pus from the ear is quick and non-invasive. Blood cultures should be taken as the results have therapeutic and prognostic implications in cases of melioidosis.

A throat swab may detect causative bacterial pathogens, and has been used to diagnose melioidosis in children.[2] Deep pus from incision and drainage of the parotid abscess is the most useful diagnostic material, and drainage may be necessary for management of the abscess. This may be performed under ultrasound guidance.

Full blood count may help differentiate between bacterial and viral causes. When melioidosis is suspected, chest radiograph and abdominal ultrasound should be requested to look for other foci of infection. In this patient a radiograph of the skull would be useful to detect any osteomyelitis.

The laboratory must be informed if melioidosis is suspected, as selective media are used to isolate *B. pseudomallei* from non-sterile sites, and suspected growth must be handled under containment level 3 conditions when available.

If melioidosis is confirmed, investigations should look for underlying predisposing conditions such as diabetes mellitus, although these are found less commonly in children with *B. pseudomallei* parotitis than in adults with melioidosis.

THE CASE CONTINUED ...

The patient had a raised white cell count at 16.5 x10^9/L (4–10 x10^9/L), of which 90% were neutrophils. He was anaemic with a haemoglobin of 9.4 g/dL (13–15 g/dL), but otherwise all blood tests were normal.

Pus culture from the right ear and parotid abscess isolated *B. pseudomallei*. Blood culture was negative. Chest radiography and abdominal ultrasound were normal.

The patient had incision and drainage of the parotid with removal of copious pus. Intravenous ceftazidime was administered for ten days followed by oral co-amoxiclav for 16 weeks with good clinical response. No complications occurred, and no underlying disease was identified. Being from a rice farming family, the boy was likely to have been frequently exposed to soil and water containing *B. pseudomallei* in the paddy fields.

SUMMARY BOX

Melioidosis

Melioidosis is an infectious disease caused by *Burkholderia pseudomallei*, a saphrophytic Gram-negative environmental bacterium endemic in South-east Asia and northern Australia. It is the third most common cause of death in north-east Thailand after HIV and tuberculosis.[1]

In endemic areas it is readily isolated from soil and surface water. The disease is highly seasonal and most cases present during the rainy season.[1]

The clinical presentation ranges from mild localized infection to severe septicaemia. In endemic areas, 60–80% of children have evidence of seroconversion to *B. pseudomallei* by the age of four years and most paediatric infections are mild or asymptomatic.[1]

Septicaemic melioidosis occurs in more than one-third of paediatric cases, with a similar clinical presentation to adults. The lung is the most common organ involved, and septic shock is associated with a high mortality.[2] Multiple organ involvement and disseminated infections are well described. Localized disease, however, accounts for the majority of paediatric melioidosis, with the parotid gland being the most common site involved in 40% of Thai children.[2] Skin and soft tissue abscesses are also common. Parotitis is uncommon in adults, and has not been seen in children in Australia.

It is believed that ingestion of water contaminated with *B. pseudomallei* may cause colonization of the oropharynx and ascending infection to the parotid gland, particularly where drinking water is obtained from bore holes.[3] Suppurative inflammation and parotid abscess formation ensues. Less than 10% of children have a predisposing condition. The prognosis is usually favourable, although complications include spontaneous rupture into the auditory canal, facial nerve palsy, septicaemia and osteomyelitis.[2]

The aims of treatment are to reduce mortality and morbidity, prevent recurrence and drain abscesses. Referral to a surgeon for consideration for drainage should be arranged; however, such surgery risks damage to the facial nerve. There is little evidence to inform the choice and duration of antimicrobial treatment for localized melioidosis in children. The authors recommend precautionary intravenous ceftazidime, meropenem or impimem for the acute phase (10–14 days); however, parenteral therapy is very expensive.[4] This is followed by co-trimoxazole monotherapy for the eradication phase (12–20 weeks), which has recently been shown to be non-inferior to dual therapy with co-trimoxazole and doxycycline, and avoids adverse effects of doxycycline in children.[5]

Further Reading

1. Dance DAB. Melioidosis. In: Farrar J, editor. Manson's Tropical Diseases. 23rd ed. London: Elsevier; 2013 [chapter 34].
2. Lumbiganon P, Viengnondha S. Clinical manifestations of melioidosis in children. Pediatr Infect Dis J 1995;14(2): 136–40.
3. Stoesser N, Pocock J, Moore CE, et al. Paediatric suppurative parotitis in Cambodia between 2007 and 2011. Paediatr Infect Dis J 2012;31(8):865–8.
4. Phetsouvanh R, Phongmany S, Newton P, et al. Melioidosis and Pandora's box in the Lao People's Democratic Republic. Clin Infect Dis 2001;32(4):653–4.
5. Chetchotisakd P, Chierakul W, Chaowagul W, et al. Trimethoprim-suplhamethoxazole versus trimethoprim-sulphamethoxazole plus doxycycline as oral eradicative treatment for melioidosis (MERTH): A multicentre, double-blind, non-inferiority, randomised controlled trial. Lancet 2013;doi:10.1016/S0140-6736(13)61951-0.

A 25-YEAR-OLD FEMALE SCHOOL TEACHER FROM MALAWI WITH ABRUPT ONSET OF A FEBRILE CONFUSIONAL STATE

Emma C. Wall

Clinical Presentation

HISTORY

A 25-year-old Malawian primary school teacher presents to a local central hospital. She was reported to be well at 8 a.m., confused by 10 a.m. and drowsy with a high fever and convulsions on admission at 11 a.m.

She is HIV-reactive and has been on antiretroviral therapy (ART) with tenofovir, lamivudine and efavirenz for six months with good adherence. Her CD4 count on starting ART was 320 cells/μL. She completed treatment for pulmonary tuberculosis two months ago.

CLINICAL FINDINGS

The patient is restless and agitated; Glasgow Coma Scale 10/15. Pupils are equal and reactive with photophobia, the neck is stiff and there is no rash. Plantar responses are down-going, Kernig's sign is positive. Chest and abdominal examinations are unremarkable.

Observations: temperature 40°C, pulse 125 bpm, blood pressure 125/68 mmHg, oxygen saturation 93% on room air. During the physical examination she suffers renewed seizure.

LABORATORY RESULTS

Her blood results are shown in Table 16-1. A spinal tap is done. The CSF appears hazy; CSF results are shown in Table 16-2. Rapid antigen test for *Plasmodium falciparum* is negative.

TABLE 16-1 Blood Results on Admission		
Parameter	Patient	Reference
WBC (x10⁹/L)	10.5	4–10
Neutrophil count (x10⁹/L)	8.9	2.5–6
Haemoglobin (g/dL)	8.9	12–14
MCV (fL)	85	78–90
Platelets (x10⁹/L)	255	150–400
Creatinine (μmol/L)	106	35–106
Random blood glucose (mmol/L)	5.6	3.9–7.8

TABLE 16-2 CSF Results on Admission		
Parameter	Patient	Reference
Leukocytes (cells/μL)	35 (60% neutrophils)	0–5/μL
Protein (g/L)	2.6	0.15–0.42
Glucose (mmol/L)	1.2	2.5–5

1. What are your treatment priorities for this woman?
2. What adjunctive interventions should be used in this setting?

Discussion

A 25-year-old Malawian woman, known to be HIV-positive and on ART, presents with acute severe symptoms including a high fever, a rapid decline in consciousness and new onset convulsions, suggesting a severe neurological infection. Her CSF is hazy and shows a neutrophilic pleocytosis, as well as a high CSF-protein and low glucose.

Bacterial meningitis is the most likely diagnosis; cryptococcal meningitis and tuberculous meningitis are possibilities, though much less likely.

ANSWER TO QUESTION 1

What Are Your Treatment Priorities for This Woman?

The suspected diagnosis is acute bacterial meningitis. In Africa outside of the meningitis belt, *Streptococcus pneumoniae* is the most common cause of meningitis in adults and children.[1] The immediate treatment priority is emergency resuscitation, including rapid administration of antibiotics. A third generation cephalosporin such as ceftriaxone at a high dose to penetrate the CSF is appropriate; where this is not available, high dose benzylpenicillin plus chloramphenicol is a suitable alternative. Resistance rates of *S. pneumoniae* to both penicillins and chloramphenicol are rising, hence local advice about resistance patterns should be sought. Data to guide resuscitation in adults are lacking, but careful fluid resuscitation, airway support, oxygenation and seizure control are all indicated. Public health services are required for case management to ensure that appropriate vaccination programmes and case notification for outbreak monitoring are done.

ANSWER TO QUESTION 2

What Adjunctive Interventions Should be Used in This Setting and What Are Your Differential Diagnoses?

Several meta-analyses suggest that while in well-resourced countries dexamethasone should be given to adults and children presenting to hospital with meningitis, steroids should not be used in resource-limited hospitals in Africa given their lack of efficacy.[2] Glycerol has been tested in paediatric meningitis with mixed results, but was shown to be harmful in adults with meningitis in Malawi.[3] No other adjuncts have been tested in clinical trials to date; adjunctive treatment is not indicated.

In cases of suspected meningitis a lumbar puncture (LP) must be undertaken to obtain a diagnosis. Despite clinical contraindications to lumbar puncture in this patient (seizures and altered conscious level), the risk of causing harm by doing an LP is low. LP should not be delayed by attempts to obtain cerebral imaging unless obvious signs of a space-occupying lesion are present. CT scan of the brain is of limited value in bacterial meningitis. Administration of antibiotics should not be delayed while the LP is undertaken, particularly in resource-limited settings.

The main differential diagnoses for this patient are cryptococcal meningitis (CCM) and TB meningitis (TBM). However, her CD4 count is too high for CCM and her recent completion of TB treatment makes TBM less likely. In addition, both of these infections classically have a more chronic course.

She is not pregnant, therefore meningitis caused by *Listeria monocytogenes* is very unlikely. Bacterial pathogens that cause meningitis in HIV-infected adults include *S. pneumoniae*, group A streptococci, *Staphylococcus aureus*, non-typhoidal salmonellae, *Salmonella typhi*, *Escherichia coli* and *Haemophilus influenzae*; all will be treated with a third-generation cephalosporin. European guidelines recommend 14 days of antibiotics in HIV-infected adults with bacterial meningitis. However, in sub-Saharan Africa often shorter courses are given, determined by the patient's recovery rate, local guidelines and availability of antibiotics for long courses. In children with bacterial meningitis in Malawi, five days of ceftriaxone was shown to be non-inferior to ten days, with substantial savings shown, and shorter courses are now commonly used.

THE CASE CONTINUED ...

In the emergency department the patient received ceftriaxone 2 g IV, 1 litre of Ringer's lactate IV, 10 mg of diazepam IV and 600 mg of phenobarbitone IV. Her oxygen saturations improved with resuscitation. She received ten days of IV ceftriaxone and recovered consciousness by day 3. CSF culture grew *S. pneumoniae*. Audiometry revealed a minor hearing loss in her right ear. No further neurological impairment or seizures were noted; anticonvulsants were weaned by day 3.

SUMMARY BOX

Acute Bacterial Meningitis

In resource-rich settings, acute bacterial meningitis in adults and children is declining in incidence due to successful vaccination campaigns, but sporadic cases continue to occur. In contrast, many countries with high HIV-prevalence have reported an increase in patients presenting with acute bacterial meningitis (ABM) since the start of the HIV epidemic.

Mortality rates in resource-rich settings have improved from 45–50% to 11–25% over the past 50 years, associated with early administration of broad-spectrum antibiotics and better supportive care. In contrast, adult ABM mortality rates in sub-Saharan Africa are reported to vary between 50 and 70% without any change over time, and survivors experience higher rates of neurological disabilities.

Adjunctive treatments have failed to impact on mortality in large randomized controlled trials in Africa despite efficacy elsewhere. In well-resourced settings, important risk factors for poor outcome include advanced age, hyperglycaemia and immunosuppression. In Africa, coma, seizures, anaemia and delayed presentation to hospital are poor prognostic features. Antibiotic treatment depends on local sensitivities. A third-generation cephalosporin at high dose given as early as possible is the treatment of choice.

Further Reading

1. Heckmann JE, Bhigjee AI. Tropical neurology. In: Farrar J, editor. Manson's Tropical Diseases. 23rd ed. London: Elsevier; 2013 [chapter 71].
2. van de Beek D, Farrar JJ, de Gans J, et al. Adjunctive dexamethasone in bacterial meningitis: a meta-analysis of individual patient data. Lancet Neurol 2010;9(3):254–63.
3. Wall EC, Ajdukiewicz KM, Heyderman RS, et al. Osmotic therapies added to antibiotics for acute bacterial meningitis. Cochrane Database Syst Rev 2013;(3):CD008806.

A 34-YEAR-OLD MAN FROM THAILAND WITH FEVER AND A PAPULAR RASH

Juri Katchanov / Hartmut Stocker

Clinical Presentation

HISTORY

A 34-year-old man from Phuket, Thailand, presents to a European hospital with a two-week history of fever. He has also noticed a papular rash affecting his whole body, particularly his face and trunk. When asked, he reports having lost 7 kg in the last three months.

He lives in Thailand and arrived in Europe only three days previously to visit friends.

CLINICAL FINDINGS

On examination, the patient is febrile with a temperature of 38.2°C. His conjunctivae are pale. He is very wasted, with a body mass index of 14 kg/m².

The patient has a generalized non-pruritic rash, predominantly on his face and trunk, which consists of small umbilicated papules (Figure 17-1). There is generalized lymphadenopathy with visibly swollen lymph nodes in the left supraclavicular region (Figure 17-2); his inguinal and axillary lymph nodes are also enlarged. On abdominal examination, the spleen is palpable two fingers below the left costal margin. The liver span was 15 cm in the midclavicular line.

LABORATORY RESULTS

Full blood count: WBC 2.1 x10⁹/L (reference range 4–10), haemoglobin 9.8 g/dL (13–16), platelets 110 x10⁹/L (150–350). C-reactive protein 150 mg/L (<5).

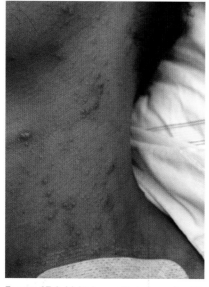

FIGURE 17-1 Multiple umbilicated papular skin lesions on the neck.

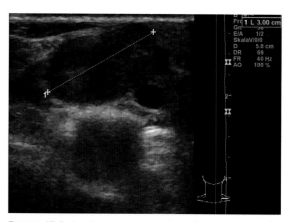

FIGURE 17-2 An ultrasound examination of the supraclavicular region showing an enlarged lymph node of 3 cm in diameter. (*Courtesy of G. Branding.*)

1. What is the single most important test to be done in this patient?
2. What is your differential diagnosis?

Discussion

A 34-year-old man from Thailand presents with a two-week history of fever and a three-month history of wasting. On examination, he has mild hepatosplenomegaly, generalized lymphadenopathy and a papular rash. The laboratory results reveal pancytopenia and an elevated C-reactive protein.

ANSWER TO QUESTION 1

What is the Single Most Important Test to be Done in This Patient?

The most important test to be done is an HIV serology. The patient presents with fever, unexplained weight loss, lymphadenopathy and a umbilicated papular rash; his blood results show pancytopenia. Each of these conditions alone should warrant HIV testing.

ANSWER TO QUESTION 2

What is Your Differential Diagnosis?

Common causes of fever, generalized lymphadenopathy and hepatosplenomegaly are infectious diseases and neoplasms.

Apart from HIV, CMV and EBV infection should be considered. All three of these viral infections may present with a maculopapular rash, but umbilicated papular lesions are not part of the clinical picture. However, in HIV-infected individuals, mollusca contagiosa are common, which resemble the lesions seen in this patient.

Disseminated tuberculosis and infections with atypical mycobacteriae are important differential diagnoses. Both can also present with cutaneous manifestations. An infection that resembles mycobacterioses in many ways is melioidosis. Melioidosis is one of the leading causes of community-acquired septicaemia in Thailand. It may present with lymphadenitis and disseminated papular skin lesions.

Bartonella spp. (*B. henselae*, *B. quintana*) cause bacillary angiomatosis in immunosuppressed individuals. Bacillary angiomatosis presents with nonspecific systemic symptoms and umbilicated papular skin lesions. However, these papules are usually erythematous.

Fungal infections to consider in this patient are cryptococcosis, histoplasmosis and penicilliosis, which are all commonly associated with immunosuppression but may also rarely occur in non-immunosuppressed individuals. All three may also present with umbilicated, papular skin lesions.

Neoplasms to consider include lymphomas and non-malignant neoplastic conditions such as HHV-8-associated Castleman's disease.

THE CASE CONTINUED ...

The HIV test came back reactive. The patient was found to be highly immunosuppressed, with a CD4 cell count of 2/µL (normal range: 500–1000/µL).

Blood cultures were taken. A fine needle aspirate of the lymph node and a skin biopsy were performed and the material was sent for microbiological and pathological work-up. Histopathology of the lymph node biopsy showed multiple yeast-like structures (Figure 17-3). There were no acid-fast bacilli seen. The blood culture, and cultures from the skin biopsy and lymph node, all grew *Penicillium marneffei*.

The diagnosis of penicilliosis was made and the patient was started on a two-week course of intravenous liposomal amphotericin B followed by oral itraconazole. On three-week follow-up he was afebrile and gaining weight. Antiretroviral therapy (ART) was initiated.

Six months later the patient presented with a recurrence of his cervical lymphadenopathy. A penicilliosis relapse was suspected. However, this time an infection with atypical mycobacteriae was found.

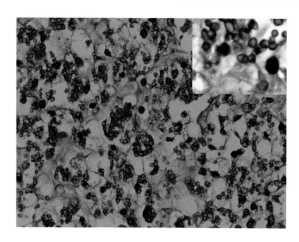

FIGURE 17-3 Histology of the supraclavicular lymph node showing multiple round-shaped yeast-like structures (PAS stain, ×400). *Inset:* Prominent septal wall ('septation') as a result of reproduction by fission. *(Courtesy U. Zimmermann, M. Grünbaum and H. Herbst.)*

His CD4 count had come up to 102/μL and the viral load was suppressed. This second infection within six months after starting ART was interpreted as an immune reconstitution inflammatory syndrome (IRIS) of the unmasking type.

SUMMARY BOX

Penicilliosis

Penicilliosis is caused by *Penicillium marneffei*, a dimorphic fungus endemic to East and South-east Asia. Incidence of penicilliosis has increased in parallel with the AIDS pandemic.[1] It is the third commonest AIDS-related opportunistic infection in Thailand and Vietnam after tuberculosis and cryptococcosis.[2,3] Penicilliosis has also been reported in immunosuppressed travellers to endemic areas. Its environmental reservoir and the mode of transmission are still unknown.

Penicilliosis usually affects severely immunocompromised individuals who frequently have other concurrent opportunistic infections. Patients present with nonspecific symptoms such as prolonged fever, fatigue, weight loss and diarrhoea. Clinical signs are lymphadenopathy, hepatosplenomegaly and anaemia. Generalized umbilicated papular skin lesions can help the clinician narrow down the differential diagnosis. The papules are often located in the face, on the chest and extremities. Lung involvement is common and chest radiography may reveal diffuse reticulonodular or alveolar infiltrates.

Diagnosis is made by identification of the fungus by microscopy and culture. Blood, bronchoalveolar lavage fluid, or biopsies of skin, lymph nodes or bone marrow are appropriate clinical specimens. Microscopical examination reveals extracellular and intracellular yeasts. The extracellular forms often have a transverse septum as a result of binary fission.

Treatment is usually with intravenous amphotericin B for two weeks (0.6 mg/kg bodyweight) followed by oral itraconazole 200 mg bid for ten weeks. Secondary prophylaxis in HIV-infected patients with itraconazole (200 mg od) has been suggested until a CD4+ count of ≥100 cells/μL has been maintained for at least six months.

Further Reading

1. Wood R. Clinical features and management of HIV/AIDS. In: Farrar J, editor. Manson's Tropical Diseases. 23rd ed. London: Elsevier; 2013 [chapter 10].
2. Hay RJ. Fungal infections. In: Farrar J, editor. Manson's Tropical Diseases. 23rd ed. London: Elsevier; 2013 [chapter 38].
3. Chakrabarti A, Slavin MA. Endemic fungal infections in the Asia–Pacific region. Med Mycol 2011;49(4):337–44.

A 43-YEAR-OLD MALE TRAVELLER WITH FEVER AND EOSINOPHILIA

18

Gerd-Dieter Burchard

Clinical Presentation

HISTORY

A 43-year-old German man presents to a local travel clinic on 21 May because of fever. He had been in Mozambique from 16 April to 30 April, afterwards in Chile from 30 April to 17 May. He did not take any malaria chemoprophylaxis in Mozambique and reports self-treatment for malaria with atovaquone/proguanil because of fever (27 April to 29 April). He is now complaining of renewed fever for the past three days. The day prior to presentation his temperature was as high as 39.8°C. He also has some headache and diarrhoea.

He reports freshwater contact in a small lake near Maputo. His past medical history is unremarkable.

CLINICAL FINDINGS

The patient is a 43-year-old man, febrile, with a temperature of 39.2°C. The rest of the physical examination is normal and there is no rash, no hepatomegaly, no splenomegaly and no lymphadenopathy.

LABORATORY RESULTS

The relevant laboratory results on admission are shown in Table 18-1.

FURTHER INVESTIGATIONS

Electrocardiogram is normal. Chest radiography reveals some nodular lesions ranging in size from 2 mm to 5 mm in the periphery of the lower lung zones bilaterally (Figure 18-1); this finding is confirmed by a CT scan of his chest.

TABLE 18-1 Laboratory Results on Admission		
Parameter	**Patient**	**Reference**
WBC (×10⁹/L)	9.0	4–11.3
Eosinophils (×10⁹/L)	2.1	<0.5
LDH (U/L)	422	135–225
Creatinine (μmol/L)	88.4	53–106
AST(U/L)	106	10–50
ALT(U/L)	179	10–50
GGT (U/L)	186	<65
C-reactive protein (mg/L)	57.9	<5

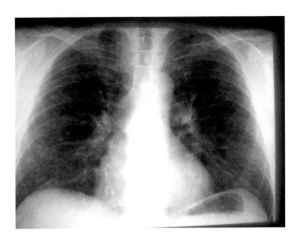

FIGURE 18-1 Chest radiograph showing nodular changes in the periphery of both lungs.

QUESTIONS

1. What are your differential diagnoses and which investigations would you like to do?
2. What is the significance of eosinophilia in returning travellers?

Discusssion

A 43-year-old man presents with of a three-day history of high fever. He has recently returned from a five-week trip to Mozambique and Chile. He did not take any malarial chemoprophylaxis, but he took antimalarial stand-by therapy when feeling febrile about three weeks ago. He reports freshwater contact in Mozambique. On examination he is febrile. His FBC shows eosinophilia with a normal total white cell count. His liver enzymes, lactate dehydrogenase (LDH) and C-reactive protein (CRP) are slightly raised. Chest radiography and CT-chest show small nodular changes in the periphery of both lungs.

ANSWER TO QUESTION 1

What Are Your Differential Diagnoses and which Investigations Would You Like to Do?

The patient has travelled in Mozambique without taking any malaria chemoprophylaxis. Thus, first of all malaria has to be excluded – irrespective of any other symptoms or lab results.

The differential diagnosis of pyrexia is long, but typhoid fever and amoebic liver abscess should always be excluded since they are common and potentially life-threatening diseases, therefore blood cultures should be taken and an abdominal ultrasound should be done. In contrast to what was seen in this patient though, typhoid fever usually causes eosinopenia.

The further differential diagnosis of fever after a stay in tropical areas relies on the presence of focal symptoms and signs, and laboratory results.

The patient has slighty elevated liver enzymes. The differential diagnosis of acute infections involving the liver includes viral hepatitis, including hepatitis E.

EBV and CMV infections seem less likely in the absence of a mononucleosis-like syndrome with hepatosplenomegaly and lymphadenopathy.

Leptospirosis, rickettsioses and Q-fever are bacterial infections to consider, as well as brucellosis, secondary syphilis and relapsing fever. Yet, none of these infections as such would explain the patient's pronounced eosinophilia.

ANSWER TO QUESTION 2

What is the Significance of Eosinophilia in Returning Travellers?

In any patient returning from the tropics with eosinophilia a helminth infection should be ruled out. The most relevant differential diagnosis in this patient who presents with eosinophilia and fever

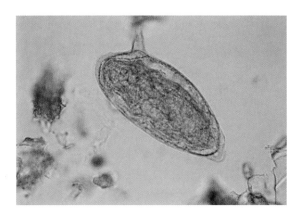

FIGURE 18-2 *Schistosoma mansoni* egg.

reporting freshwater contact is acute schistosomiasis, also known as Katayama syndrome.[1] Another rare cause of fever, eosinophilia and elevated liver transaminases is acute fascioliasis.[2]

THE CASE CONTINUED ...

Thick films for *Plasmodium* spp. were negative. Microscopy of stool and urine samples for *Schistosoma* eggs (3×) were negative.

The patient was tested for antischistosomal antibodies using an enzyme-immunoassay and an immunofluorescence assay (IFA); both came back negative.

Four weeks later antischistosomal antibodies could be detected (IFA 1:1280, cercarial- and egg-ELISA positive). *S. mansoni* ova were detected in the stool and a diagnosis of schistosomiasis was established. The patient was treated with praziquantel.

SUMMARY BOX

Acute Schistosomiasis (Katayama Syndrome)

Acute schistosomiasis (Katayama syndrome) is an acute hypersensitivity reaction thought to be the result of initial egg deposition by adult female schistosoma trematodes.[1] It is named after the Katayama region in Japan, where it was first described.

Katayama syndrome usually occurs 2–12 weeks after *Schistosoma* infection. It is characterized by fever, urticaria and a dry cough sometimes accompanied by a wheeze. Patchy pulmonary infiltrates or micronodular changes in the lower lung zones may be present on chest radiograph. Full blood count in the majority of cases shows eosinophilia, but of note, eosinophilia can occur with a delay of several weeks after the onset of symptoms.[3] Most patients recover spontaneously after 2–10 weeks. Rarely, neurological complications can occur, e.g. transverse myelitis, or a conus medullaris or cauda equina syndrome.

Diagnosis of acute schistosomiasis can be challenging. *Schistosoma* ova (Figure 18-2) may still be absent from urine or stool at this early stage and serological tests can take up to three months to become positive.[4] As a consequence, these investigations have to be repeated several times after the diagnosis has been clinically suspected. Novel PCR-based methods seem to be promising for the diagnosis of acute *Schistosoma* infection in recently exposed populations such as travellers.

Praziquantel has a lack of activity against immature flukes and severe reactions have been reported following praziquantel treatment during the acute phase. Therefore, antiparasitic treatment should be delayed until the flukes are adult, i.e. until eggs can be detected in stool or urine.

Under certain circumstances, such as neurological complications, supportive steroid therapy may be useful in Katayama syndrome.

Of note, different stages of the parasite life cycle may overlap in a patient who is infected with many schistosomulae. There-fore, control examinations after several months are necessary and treatment with praziquantel may have to be repeated.[5]

Further Reading

1. Bustinduy AL, King CH. Schistosomiasis. In: Farrar J, editor. Manson's Tropical Diseases. 23rd ed. London: Elsevier; 2013 [chapter 52].
2. Checkley AM, Chiodini PL, Dockrell DH, et al. Eosinophilia in returning travellers and migrants from the tropics: UK recommendations for investigation and initial management. J Infect 2010;60(1):1–20.
3. Jaureguiberry S, Paris L, Caumes E. Acute schistosomiasis, a diagnostic and therapeutic challenge. Clin Microbiol Infect 2010;16(3):225–31.
4. Logan S, Armstrong M, Moore E, et al. Acute schistosomiasis in travelers: 14 years' experience at the Hospital for Tropical Diseases, London. Am J Trop Med Hyg 2013;88(6):1032–4.
5. Ross AG, Vickers D, Olds GR, et al. Katayama syndrome. The Lancet Infect Dis 2007;7(3):218–24.

A 40-YEAR-OLD MAN FROM TOGO WITH SUBCUTANEOUS NODULES AND CORNEAL CHANGES

19

Guido Kluxen

Clinical Presentation

HISTORY

A 40-year-old man from Togo presents to a local clinic. He has noticed changes in both of his eyes over the past four years. There are no visual disturbances, but he is worried. In his village there are adults in each family who have turned completely blind after their eyes had shown features very similar to the changes he has noticed in his own eyes.

He has also observed some painless bumps under his skin which have developed over the past two decades. The patient also complains of suffering from intense itching of his skin that keeps him awake at night.

The patient has always lived in a village in the savannah near a fast-flowing river. He reports that small biting flies are common near the river.

CLINICAL FINDINGS

Opacities are noticeable in the cornea of both eyes. The patient's left eye is shown in Figure 19-1.

The skin shows evidence of atrophy in some areas (thinning with loss of elasticity), and there are multiple scratch marks. Subcutaneous nodules are palpable in various regions of his body, especially over bony prominences like the ribs (Figure 19-2), iliac crest, femoral trochanters and on the head. The nodules are firm, non-tender and measure 1–3 cm in diameter.

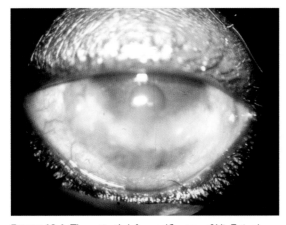

FIGURE 19-1 The patient's left eye. *(Courtesy of Hj. Trojan.)*

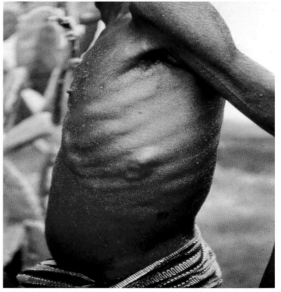

FIGURE 19-2 Subcutaneous nodule over the costal arch. *(Courtesy of Hj. Trojan.)*

1. What is your most important differential diagnosis?
2. What investigations would you like to carry out?

Discussion

The patient presents with a triad of ocular changes, skin changes and subcutaneous nodules, mainly located over bony prominences. He comes from a village in Togo, West Africa, located close to a rapidly flowing river. Many adults in the village are blind.

ANSWER TO QUESTION 1

What is Your Most Important Differential Diagnosis?

The clinical triad of ocular changes, itchy dermatitis with atrophy of the skin and subcutaneous nodules in a patient from rural Togo makes onchocerciasis (river blindness) the most likely differential diagnosis. A fast-flowing river is the preferred breeding site for *Simulium* blackflies, which transmit the disease.

The picture of his left eye shows keratitis semilunaris, a form of band-shaped sclerosing keratopathy commonly seen in onchocerciasis. The central and upper part of the cornea is initially clear, but may become affected as the disease progresses.

Subcutaneous nodules can resemble lipomas and cysticerci of *Taenia solium* may present in a similar way.

Pruritic dermatitis may also be caused by scabies or be seen in papular pruritic eruptions associated with HIV infection. In patients from West Africa, infection with *Mansonella streptocerca* can also cause pruritus. Chronic dermatitis can also be seen in yaws, leprosy, mycotic infections and eczema[1].

ANSWER TO QUESTION 2

What Investigations Would You Like to Carry Out?

The patient's presentation appears very typical for onchocerciasis. In an endemic resource-limited setting his diagnosis would most probably be made on clinical grounds alone.

INVESTIGATIONS

Skin-snips taken from the vicinity of a subcutaneous nodule may show microfilariae of *O. volvulus*.
Slit-lamp examination of the eyes may reveal microfilariae in the anterior chamber of the eye and in the cornea.
Nodulectomy of subcutaneous nodules may show adults of *O. volvulus*, but this is not routinely done.
Serological tests are not useful in patients from endemic areas, because antibody test results are not clearly linked to clinical disease.

THE CASE CONTINUED ...

The patient was treated with ivermectin (150 μg/kg) which was repeated after three months and after one year. He also received doxycycline 100 mg/d for six weeks (see Summary Box).

SUMMARY BOX

Onchocerciasis

Onchocerciasis ('river blindness') is an infection caused by *Onchocerca volvulus*, a filarial nematode. It is transmitted by biting *Simulium* spp. blackflies, which breed in rapidly flowing freshwater. It is estimated that 17.7 million people have onchocerciasis, 99% of them living in sub-Saharan Africa. There is focal disease in Latin America and in Yemen.

Continued on following page

Adult females of *O. volvulus* live in human subcutaneous tissue and shed living microfilariae. Microfilariae migrate through the skin and often into the eyes. Most pathology is caused by reactions to dead and dying microfilariae and perhaps to their endo-symbiontic *Wolbachia*.

Typical clinical features of onchocerciasis are:

1. Non-tender subcutaneous nodules located mainly over bony prominences
2. Dermatitis, depigmentation of the skin ('leopard skin'), lichenification and thickening of the skin ('lizard skin'), and skin atrophy at times leading to 'hanging groins'. The skin changes may be stigmatizing and the unrelenting itch may cause sleep distur-bances, depression and even lead to suicide
3. Ocular changes may present as pear-shaped pupil, punctate subepithelial stromal keratopathy, sclerosing keratitis, iritis, uveitis, 'flecked retina' or scarred choroidoretinal fundus (Hissette–Ridley fundus) or as optic nerve atrophy.

Ivermectin is now the drug of choice for individual and mass treatment of onchocerciasis. Ivermectin kills microfilariae but has little impact on adult worms apart from reducing embryogenesis. It has to be given repeatedly throughout the lifespan of the adult worm (10–14 years).

For individual treatment, ivermectin is provided as a single dose of 150 µg/kg PO. Treatment should be repeated at three to six-month intervals. In mass treatment programmes it is usually provided annually. Ivermectin should not be given to patients with heavy *Loa loa* infections (with microfilaria counts greater than 30,000), as this sometimes causes fatal encephalitis; it can also cause significant adverse events in patients with lower microfilaria counts, and consultation with an expert in tropical medicine may be helpful for managing patients with loiasis. Ivermectin is also contraindicated in pregnancy and in children below the age of five or below a height of 90 cm.

Doxycyclin at a dosage of 100–200 mg/d for four to six weeks kills the Wolbachia endosymbionts, permanently sterilizes adult worms, and blocks embryogenesis and slowly kills approximately 60% of adult worms.

Onchocerciasis control has progressed rapidly in recent years thanks to successful public–private partnerships, sustained funding and technical advances. The key strategy for disease control in affected communities is annual community-directed mass treatment with ivermectin.[1–3]

Further Reading

1. Simonsen P, Fischer PU, Hoerauf A, et al. The filariases. In: Farrar J, editor. Manson's Tropical Diseases. 23rd ed. London: Elsevier; 2013 [chapter 54].
2. Taylor MJ, Hoerauf A, Bockarie M. Lymphatic filariasis and onchocerciasis. Lancet 2010;376(9747):1175–85.
3. Kluxen G, Hoerauf A. Keratitis caused by onchocerciasis: *Wolbachia* play a key role. In: Srinivasan M, editor. Keratitis. Rijeka, Croatia: Intech Open Access; 2012. p. 31–44.

A 56-YEAR-OLD MAN RETURNING FROM A TRIP TO THAILAND WITH EOSINOPHILIA

20

Sebastian Dieckmann / Ralf Ignatius

Clinical Presentation

HISTORY

A 56-year-old European man is referred to a local specialist clinic for further work-up of peripheral eosinophilia. Clinically, he suffers from fatigue and back pain. The patient returned from a three-week round trip to Thailand four months ago.

He is known to have mild hypertension and suffered a transient ischaemic attack (TIA) five years ago. He has never experienced any allergic reactions. The patient has taken aspirin since suffering the TIA and an angiotensin receptor blocker (sartan) for one year.

CLINICAL FINDINGS

The vital signs are normal, he is afebrile. His physical examination does not reveal any pathological findings.

LABORATORY RESULTS

The patient's full blood count is shown in Table 20-1.

TABLE 20-1 Full Blood Count Results on Admission		
Parameter	**Patient**	**Reference**
WBC ($\times 10^9$/L)	8.6	4–10
Haemoglobin (g/dL)	14	12–15
Platelets ($\times 10^9$/L)	400	150–450
Basophils (%)	2	0–2
Eosinophils (%)	32	0–6
Total eosinophil count ($\times 10^9$/L)	2.75	<0.45
Neutrophils (%)	38	20–50
Band neutrophils (%)	0	0–5
Lymphocytes (%)	21	20–40
Monocytes (%)	7	0–10

QUESTIONS

1. How is eosinophilia defined and what is the differential diagnosis?
2. How do you narrow down your differential diagnosis in a traveller with eosinophilia?

Discussion

A 56-year-old European man presents with nonspecific symptoms and pronounced peripheral blood eosinophilia. He has recently travelled to Thailand. He is on a medication with low-dose aspirin and an angiotensin receptor blocker. His physical examination is unremarkable and he is afebrile.

ANSWER TO QUESTION 1

How is Eosinophilia Defined and What is the Differential Diagnosis?

Eosinophilia is usually defined as a total peripheral blood eosinophil count $>0.45 \times 10^9/L$.[1] It can be caused by a whole variety of aetiologies (Table 20-2) and the differential diagnosis is wide.[2]

In travellers or migrants from tropical and subtropical areas, the most common identifiable cause of eosinophilia is helminth infection.[1] Ectoparasitic diseases such as scabies and myiasis may also cause eosinophilia, which usually is mild. Protozoal infections usually do not cause eosinophilia, with the exception of *Isospora belli* and *Sarcocystis* spp. infections, which may be accompanied by a mostly mild eosinophilia.

Bacterial, viral and fungal infections may cause eosinopenia. One important exception is HIV infection, where immune dysregulation can lead to eosinophilia. Endemic fungal infections associated with eosinophilia are coccidioidomycosis and paracoccidioidomycosis.

TABLE 20-2   **Causes of Eosinophilia**
Infections, in particular infections with tissue-invasive helminths
Convalescence from any infection
Allergies
Drug-induced
Connective tissue diseases
Idiopathic hypereosinophilic syndromes
Leukaemias and lymphomas
Paraneoplastic

ANSWER TO QUESTION 2

How Do You Narrow Down Your Differential Diagnosis in a Traveller With Eosinophilia?

It is crucial to get a detailed history of possible exposures and concomitant symptoms. The travel history should include recent and past travel, since some causes of eosinophilia such as *Strongyloides stercoralis* infection or schistosomiasis may present after years, even decades.

Exposure to food items (salads, watercress, crabs, raw fish, snails, frogs) should be explicitly enquired after. Patients should be asked about freshwater exposure (schistosomiasis) and contact with sand or soil (soil-transmitted helminths, *Fasciola hepatica* and other flukes). However, negative exposure history does not rule out risk, as many patients simply do not recall their exposure.[3]

Concomitant symptoms may also help to narrow down the differential diagnosis. However, eosinophilia is asymptomatic in up to one-third of returning travellers and migrants. Common causes of asymptomatic eosinophilia include intestinal helminths (following migration through tissues), schistosomiasis and filarial infections.

THE CASE CONTINUED …

Serology revealed antibodies against *Ascaris lumbricoides* while the serological tests for other helminth infections, including *S. stercoralis*, remained negative. However, larvae of *S. stercoralis* were detected in sediments of stool samples (Figure 20-1). Upon single-dose treatment with ivermectin, the absolute eosinophil count (AEC) declined and the *A. lumbricoides* serology (most likely cross-reactive antibodies against *S. stercoralis*) turned negative.

The patient's symptoms, however, did not settle, and it was later discovered that his backpain was caused by a slipped disc.

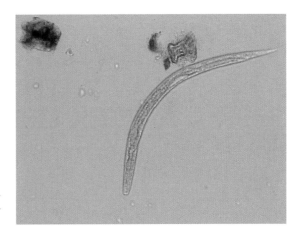

FIGURE 20-1 Rhabditiform larva of *Strongyloides stercoralis* in a stool preparation (ether-based concentration, magnification 100×).

SUMMARY BOX

Strongyloidiasis

Strongyloides stercoralis is a human nematode without an animal reservoir. It is usually acquired by invasion of the intact skin or by auto-infection via the intestinal mucosa or perianal skin.[4] Faecal–oral transmission is also possible.

Upon invasion, larvae of *S. stercoralis* migrate within the bloodstream, exit the blood vessels in the pulmonary alveoli and enter the airways where they are coughed up and swallowed to eventually reach the small intestine where they complete their life cycle.

Only female adults live in the small intestine and reproduce asexually by parthenogenesis (i.e. production of fertile eggs without fertilizing males). They release eggs from which hatch non-infectious rhabditiform larvae that are excreted in the stool. Eggs are rarely seen in stool specimens; the normal finding is live larvae.

Outside of the human host, larvae either mature into free-living male and female adult worms, which reproduce sexually, or transform into infectious filariform larvae ready to invade another host.

Alternatively, autoinfection is possible: in the gastrointestinal tract some larvae moult into infective filariform larvae and penetrate the gut wall or the perianal skin to enter the circulation. Autoinfection may result in decades of ongoing disease.

Strongyloidiasis may cause nonspecific gastrointestinal symptoms, and sometimes swiftly moving cutaneous eruptions are noticed, especially on the trunk, which correspond to subcutaneously migrating larvae, a phenomenon called 'larva currens'. In the majority of patients, however, strongyloidiasis is asymptomatic.[5]

In severely immunocompromised hosts, e.g. in association with steroid therapy, malignancies, chemotherapy or infection with HTLV-I, strongyloidiasis may disseminate and cause overwhelming life-threatening disease ('hyperinfection syndrome'). In HIV infection, strongyloides hyperinfection syndrome has been described but seems to be uncommon.

Definitive diagnosis is made by detection of larvae in stool specimens using various techniques; however, false-negative results often occur due to intermittent larval excretion and low infectious burden. Indirect evidence may be provided by serology, but false-negative results are possible, as seen in our case. Furthermore, most serological tests become positive only 4–12 weeks post infection and may be negative when eosinophilia is first detected.[1] False-positive serological results may occur due to cross-reacting antibodies against other helminths, particularly other nematodes.

The diagnosis is supported by clinical signs, such as 'larva currens', and eosinophilia, although the latter is not always present during chronic infection.

Treatment of choice is ivermectin (200 µg/kg stat). Patients with *Strongyloides* infection returning from West or Central Africa and who might be co-infected with *Loa loa* should be screened for microfilaraemia before receiving ivermectin. In patients unable to receive ivermectin, albendazole 400 mg bd for three days is an alternative.

Since the diagnosis of strongyloidiasis is difficult, presumptive treatment with ivermectin or albendazole may be justified in individuals with eosinophilia, larva currens or a positive serology and a possible exposure to *S. stercoralis*.

Further Reading

1. Checkley AM, Chiodini PL, Dockrell DH, et al. Eosinophilia in returning travellers and migrants from the tropics: UK recommendations for investigation and initial management. J Infect 2010;60:1–20.
2. Afshar K, Vucinic V, Sharma OP. Eosinophil cell: pray tell us what you do! Curr Opin Pulmon Med 2007;13:414–21.
3. Whitty CJ, Carroll B, Armstrong M, et al. Utility of history, examination and laboratory tests in screening those returning to Europe from the tropics for parasitic infection. Trop Med Int Health 2000;5:818–23.
4. Brooker S, Bundy DAP. Soil-transmitted helminths (Geohelminths). In: Farrar J, editor. Manson's Tropical Diseases. 23rd ed. London: Elsevier; 2013 [chapter 55].
5. Greaves D, Coggle S, Pollard C, et al. *Strongyloides stercoralis* infection. BMJ 2013;347:f4610.

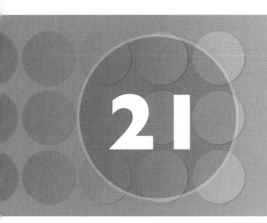

21

A 35-YEAR-OLD AMERICAN MAN WITH FATIGUE AND A NECK LESION

Mary E. Wright | Arthur M. Friedlander

Clinical Presentation

HISTORY

A 35-year-old Caucasian male presents to a clinic in the United States with fatigue and a rash on his neck that started as a papule two days earlier. The lesion is non-pruritic, but it is associated with significant nonpainful swelling and a pressure sensation in the neck. There is no history of fever, but the patient reports at least one episode of diaphoresis with mild confusion and headache.

The patient recalls a break in the skin at the site of the lesion three days before while shaving, and is sure that he has not been bitten by an insect. He has had no contact with animals or foreign travel within the previous year.

He had come to the clinic 24 hours earlier with similar symptoms. After blood cultures were obtained he was given one dose of a first-generation cephalosporin and discharged on a ten-day oral course. He returns because of worsening malaise and neck swelling associated with mild difficulty breathing.

The past medical history is unremarkable. The patient is a postal worker by profession.

CLINICAL FINDINGS

Examination reveals a 2 cm irregularly shaped, indurated non-tender patch on the left anterior neck with mild overlying erythema and several 2–3 mm vesicles. The main lesion has a 6 mm shallow ulceration. There is massive neck oedema making lymph nodes difficult to assess (see Figure 21-1). His neck circumference had increased from 57 cm at baseline to a peak of 81 cm. Temperature is 36.9°C, pulse 118 bpm, blood pressure 138/90 mmHg and respiratory rate 20 breath cycles per minute. The remainder of the initial physical examination is normal.

INVESTIGATIONS

Full blood count, Na$^+$, K$^+$, Cl$^-$ HCO$_3$, BUN, creatinine and random glucose are normal except for a mildly elevated haemoglobin at 18.7 g/dL (reference range: 13.0–18.0 g/dL).

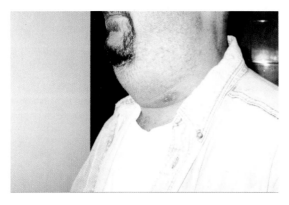

FIGURE 21-1 Papulovesicular lesion with extensive neck oedema two days after the onset of a small papule.

QUESTIONS

1. What are the distinguishing features of this lesion that help narrow down your differential diagnosis?
2. What investigations need to be performed to establish early diagnosis and appropriate treatment?

Discussion

A 35-year-old male postal worker presents to a clinic in the United States with a papulovesicular lesion on his neck associated with massive neck swelling. There is no fever but diaphoresis. The patient's condition is worsening despite antibiotic therapy with an oral cephalosporin.

ANSWER TO QUESTION 1

What Are the Distinguishing Features of This Lesion that Help Narrow Down Your Differential Diagnosis?

The differential diagnosis of an ulcerative skin lesion with concomitant massive soft tissue swelling and systemic symptoms depends upon the epidemiological setting and the individual exposure; it includes bacterial ecthyma (*Streptococcus pyogenes*, *Staphylococcus aureus*), rickettsial diseases, necrotic arachnidism (bite by brown recluse spider), rat-bite fevers (*Spirillum minus*), ulceroglandular tularaemia and bubonic plague.[1]

At the time of the patient's presentation, the United States is in the process of investigating a possible event of bioterrorism. Therefore, the most important, though overall rare, diagnosis to consider is cutaneous anthrax. There may be few distinguishing features at the time of presentation, depending on the age of the lesion. While it is commonly known that cutaneous anthrax is manifested by a central black eschar, this is not seen until approximately a week after inoculation. The anthrax lesion begins as a painless papule that lasts 1–2 days before becoming a vesicle that later ruptures. It then develops the classic necrotic central ulcer and may be surrounded by smaller peripheral vesicles. Therefore, a patient may present with a nonspecific localized papulovesicular eruption. Key associated findings include a preceding history of a break in the skin at the affected site, the presence of systemic symptoms such as malaise and headache, and extensive, non-tender oedema. Fever and leukocytosis may not be present. In parts of the world where anthrax is endemic, zoonotic exposure to infected animals or contaminated animal products is important to establish, whereas exposure from a bioterrorism act may not be immediately apparent.

ANSWER TO QUESTION 2

What Investigations Need to be Performed to Establish Early Diagnosis and Appropriate Treatment?

Aspirate of fluid from the skin lesion should be sent for Gram stain, culture and susceptibilities along with blood cultures in patients with systemic symptoms regardless of fever status. In the absence of preceding antimicrobial therapy, numerous Gram-positive rods in high concentration will grow within 24 hours. Empiric antibacterial treatment with a quinolone or doxycycline should be instituted while awaiting microbiological results. Because negative cultures do not exclude anthrax, full-thickness punch biopsy from the vesicle and the eschar should be obtained, fixed in 10% buffered formalin and sent to a specialized laboratory for nucleic acid amplification and immunohistochemical (IHC) staining to detect *Bacillus anthracis* antigens. Serum should also be tested for antibodies to the protective antigen at baseline and four weeks later.

THE CASE CONTINUED ...

Blood cultures taken at the first clinic visit grew Gram-positive rods. Gram stain and culture of the skin lesion obtained at the second visit were negative for *B. anthracis*. The patient was admitted and received intravenous levofloxacin and ampicillin-sulbactam and recovered. Stains for bacteria and IHC of the skin biopsy performed at a reference laboratory showed abundant bacilli in the dermis and the presence of *B. anthracis* antigens respectively. Serology revealed that antibody to protective antigen was present in convalescent serum.

The patient was exposed during his occupation as a postal worker, handling contaminated mail. Overall, 22 cases were identified, of which 11 presented with cutaneous anthrax, and a further 11 fell ill with the inhalational form. Five people died; all deaths occurred secondary to inhalational anthrax.

SUMMARY BOX

Anthrax

Anthrax is caused by *Bacillus anthracis*, a Gram-positive rod that forms spores under certain environmental conditions.[1] It is primarily a disease of domestic and wild herbivores. Anthrax remains endemic in animals worldwide, most importantly in Asia, Africa and south-eastern Australia, as well as parts of the southern United States.

Humans usually acquire the infection when they are exposed to infected animals or animal products, but anthrax has also been used as an agent of bioterrorism.[1,2] In the developed world, cases usually tend to be sporadic. In resource-limited countries anthrax remains a relevant public health problem. Habitats of humans and animals commonly overlap, handling of animal carcasses dying of unknown causes lacks supervision by health authorities and there is insufficient health surveillance, particularly in rural areas. Large outbreaks can occasionally occur.[1,3]

Depending on the route of entry, *B. anthracis* can cause cutaneous, gastrointestinal or inhalational disease. Cutaneous anthrax is the most common form worldwide, accounting for 95% of all human cases. While only a small percentage develop systemic disease, it can be lethal if not treated quickly.

The clinical marker lesion is a painless central ulcer with vesicles and extensive surrounding edema but the initial lesion will appear as a nonspecific papulovesicular eruption.

History includes recent exposure to infected animals or contaminated animal products, unless the setting is a bioterrorism event, a previous break in the skin at the affected site and the presence of systemic symptoms in disseminated disease. A high index of suspicion is critical to the diagnosis. Differential diagnosis of cutaneous anthrax depends upon the setting and the individual exposures; it includes bacterial ecthyma, rickettsial diseases, rat-bite fevers, necrotic arachnidism, ulceroglandular tularaemia and bubonic plague.[1]

Gram stain and culture of affected fluids (blood, skin lesion aspirate, pleural fluid) and paired serological testing for antibodies to protective antigen remain the cornerstone of diagnosis. However, negative cultures do not exclude anthrax. In cutaneous anthrax, full-thickness punch biopsy from the vesicle and eschar should be fixed and sent to a specialized laboratory for PCR and immunohistochemical staining.

Empiric antibacterial treatment with a quinolone or doxycycline should be instituted while awaiting results for limited cutaneous infection.[4] When disseminated infection or other forms of anthrax are suspected, multi-drug therapy that includes those with CNS penetration should be used.

Whilst 7–10 days of antibiotic treatment are usually sufficient in cutaneous anthrax, up to 60 days of antibiotics are needed in inhalational disease due to the possibility of retained ungerminated spores in the lungs. Prevention of anthrax involves either prevention of exposure in occupational settings or immunization. In the setting of a suspected bioterrorism event, those at risk of exposure should receive a 60-day course of oral antibiotics.

Further Reading

1. Eitzen E. Anthrax. In: Farrar J, editor. Manson's Tropical Diseases. 23rd ed. London: Elsevier; 2013 [chapter 31].
2. Shieh WJ, Guarner J, Paddock C, et al. The critical role of pathology in the investigation of bioterrorism-related cutaneous anthrax. Am J Pathol 2003;163(5):1901–10.
3. Hang'ombe MB, Mwansa JC, Muwowo S, et al. Human–animal anthrax outbreak in the Luangwa valley of Zambia in 2011. Trop Doctor 2012;42(3):136–9.
4. Carucci JA, McGovern TW, Norton SA, et al. Cutaneous anthrax management algorithm. J Am Acad Dermatol 2002;47(5):766–9.

A 32-YEAR-OLD WOMAN FROM NIGERIA WITH JAUNDICE AND CONFUSION

22

Christopher J.M. Whitty

Clinical Presentation

HISTORY

A 32-year-old, previously fit woman of African ethnicity but born in Europe travelled to rural Jos in Nigeria to visit relatives. According to her husband, 18 days after her return to Europe she developed a fever, and three days later became very unwell with abnormal behaviour.

CLINICAL FINDINGS

On examination she has a temperature of 37.5°C, is mildly jaundiced and confused, Glasgow Coma Scale 14/15. She has no rash or palpable lymph nodes, and throat and sclerae are not injected. She has some fine crepitations at the lung bases.

LABORATORY RESULTS

The laboratory refuses to undertake tests because of recent rural exposure in an area known to have viral haemorrhagic fever (Lassa).

QUESTIONS

1. What is the differential diagnosis?
2. Is viral hemorrhagic fever (VHF) a real risk, and which single test is the most important?

Discussion

A young woman presents with a fever, jaundice and confusion almost three weeks after returning from a visit to rural Nigeria. The patient is of African ethnicity but was born in Europe.

ANSWER TO QUESTION 1

What is the Differential Diagnosis?

The differential diagnosis is wide, but by some distance the most common cause of fever and jaundice, or fever and confusion, from West Africa is severe falciparum malaria. The fact that the patient had a low grade fever at presentation is not a reason to exclude malaria, as the temperature swings in malaria and a significant proportion of cases are apyrexial at presentation. A common misdiagnosis is acute viral hepatitis; there, fever precedes the jaundice, and this rapid fulminant course would not be typical. Other causes of acute fever and jaundice include typhoid fever, leptospirosis and ascending cholangitis. Patients with advanced HIV disease and Gram-negative sepsis can also present like this.

People returning from visiting friends and relatives constitute a large proportion of imported malaria and are at high risk of not taking antimalarial prophylaxis. A woman born in Europe would be unlikely to have any immunity to malaria.

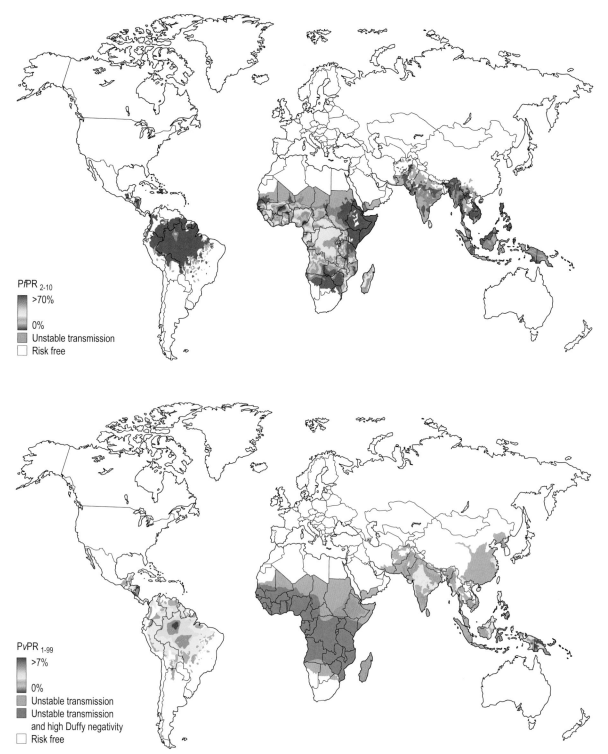

FIGURE 22-1 Global distribution of *Plasmodium falciparum* and *Plasmodium vivax* malaria. Upper panel shows the model-based geostatistical point (MBG) estimates of the *Plasmodium falciparum* annual mean parasite rate PfPR2–10 (defined as the predicted proportion of 2–10-year-olds with patent parasitaemia) for 2010 within the spatial limits of stable *P. falciparum* malaria transmission. Lower panel shows equivalent estimates of the *Plasmodium vivax* annual mean parasite rate (PvPR1–99). Note this prediction is for all age groups (1–99). Areas in which the Duffy negativity gene frequency is predicted to exceed 90% are shown in hatching. *(Reproduced from Farrar J, editor. Manson's Tropical Diseases. 23rd ed. London: Elsevier; 2013. Fig. 43.1. © Elsevier.)*

ANSWER TO QUESTION 2

Is Viral Hemorrhagic Fever (VHF) a Real Risk, and which Single Test is Most Important?

The laboratory is right to raise VHF as a possible diagnosis, but VHF is very rare and 18 days (or more) since leaving the high-risk area is at the outer limit of the incubation period of Lassa fever and other VHF (generally up to 21 days). The absence of injected sclerae or rash is also against the diagnosis. A malaria blood film would be mandatory in this case. If it is positive, the woman could be treated as malarial and other tests taken with standard universal precautions.

THE CASE CONTINUED ...

The patient was found to have a *Plasmodium falciparum* parasite count of 18% and a plasma creatinine of 430 μmol/L (reference range 45–90 μmol/L), demonstrating acute kidney injury. Urine output failed to respond to fluid challenges, therefore pre-renal failure could be ruled out. She was treated with intravenous artesunate and the parasite count dropped to 5% but she lapsed into deep coma. Renal function deteriorated and she needed haemofiltration. After the parasites had cleared on day 5 her consciousness level began to improve, but she developed laboured breathing. The chest radiography findings were suggestive of ARDS and she required prolonged respiratory support. She eventually made a full recovery.

SUMMARY BOX

Malaria

Malaria is the most common life-threatening infection in patients who have recently arrived from Africa. It is also common, but much less so, from South and South-east Asia (Figure 22-1). A history of fever is usual in non-immune patients, but other features of the presentation are nonspecific and overlap with many other infections, with headache and malaise. Malaria should always be high on the list of differential diagnoses for any unwell patient from the tropics, as there are many misleading presentations.

The only way to exclude malaria is a malaria blood test. Diagnosed early before complications begin, falciparum malaria is relatively easily treated with antimalarial drug combinations. In patients with severe malaria, artesunate is the drug of choice; if this is not available locally, artemether or quinine are the alternatives.

In adults, cerebral malaria (for practical purposes altered consciousness, seizures), acute renal failure and pulmonary oedema or ARDS are the most common manifestations of severity, and may occur together or in any combination. Renal failure, and in particular ARDS, often present later in treatment, and may first become apparent after all parasites have cleared. Disseminated intravascular coagulation and shock (often with co-existing bacteraemia) are rare complications. Elderly patients have a high mortality. Various adjunctive treatments for malaria complications have been tried but to date none shows survival advantage. The key to malaria management is to diagnose it early and get effective antimalarial drugs into the patient as soon as possible.[1-3]

Further Reading

1. White NJ. Malaria. In: Farrar J, editor. Manson's Tropical Diaseses. 23rd ed. London: Elsevier; 2013 [chapter 43].
2. Checkley AM, Smith A, Smith V, et al. Risk factors for mortality from imported falciparum malaria in the United Kingdom over 20 years: an observational study. BMJ 2012;344:e2116.
3. WHO Global Malaria Programme. Management of Severe Malaria – A Practical Handbook. 3rd ed. Geneva: WHO; 2013.

23

A 31-YEAR-OLD HIV-POSITIVE MAN WITH EXTENSIVE TRAVEL HISTORY, WITH COUGH AND NIGHT SWEATS

Katherine Woods / Robert F. Miller

Clinical Presentation

HISTORY

You are on-call in a London hospital and are referred a 31-year-old HIV-positive man from Accident and Emergency. He has a six-week history of drenching night sweats, dry cough and increasing shortness of breath on exertion. He also reports general fatigue and a loss of about 10 kg in weight over the past five months.

He works in the retail industry and travels extensively for business. In the past six months he has had work trips to Europe, China, Korea, Japan, Singapore and the United States. He lives with his male partner, denies any recreational drug use and has never smoked tobacco. He was diagnosed with HIV six years ago. He says that one month ago his CD4 was 280/μL. He is not yet on antiretroviral therapy (ART), or any other regular medications. There is no other significant past medical history.

CLINICAL FINDINGS

On examination, he is alert, short of breath at rest but able to complete full sentences. He has a temperature of 39.2°C. Respiratory rate is 26 breath cycles per minute, oxygen saturation is 87% on air, 97% on 15 L O_2 via reservoir bag. Pulse 100 bpm, blood pressure 120/70 mmHg. Chest is clear on auscultation. The rest of the physical examination is unremarkable.

LABORATORY RESULTS

His arterial blood gases on air are shown in Table 23-1, the full blood count and blood chemistry results are given in Table 23-2.

CHEST RADIOGRAPHY

His chest radiograph is shown in Figure 23-1.

TABLE 23-1 Arterial Blood Gases on Ambient Air		
Parameter	**Patient**	**Reference Range**
pH	7.44	7.35–7.45
PO_2 (kPA)	7.6	10.67–13.33
PCO_2 (kPA)	3	4.67–6.00
HCO_3 (mmol/L)	19	22–26
Base excess (mmol/L)	−3.8	±2
Lactate (mmol/L)	1.6	0.5–1.6

TABLE 23-2 Full Blood Count and Blood Chemistry Results on Admission

Parameter	Patient	Reference Range (Units)
Haemoglobin (g/dL)	13.0	12–16
MCV (fL)	81.1	80–99
Platelets (x10⁹/L)	233	150–400
WBC (x10⁹/L)	5.31	4–10
Neutrophils (x10⁹/L)	2.42	2–7.5
Lymphocytes (x10⁹/L)	2.72	1.20–3.65
C-reactive protein (mg/L)	6.7	<5
Urea (mmol/L)	2.8	1.7–8.3
Creatinine (μmol/L)	59	66–112
Bilirubin (μmol/L)	4	0–20
ALT (U/L)	28	10–50
ALP (U/L)	97	40–129
Albumin (g/L)	35	34–50

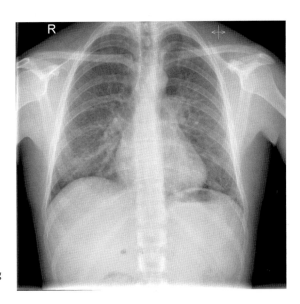

FIGURE 23-1 Chest radiograph on admission, showing bilateral perihilar infiltrates.

QUESTIONS

1. What further investigations would you perform in order to confirm the diagnosis?
2. What is your immediate management of the patient?

Discussion

An HIV-positive man who was well up until five months ago and is not yet on ART presents with progressive shortness of breath, dry cough and drenching night sweats, with associated significant weight loss. He has a history of extensive work-related travel. He is febrile with type 1 respiratory failure and bilateral perihilar infiltrates seen on chest radiography. Routine laboratory tests are normal, except for a very slightly elevated CRP.

ANSWER TO QUESTION 1

What Further Investigations Would You Perform in Order to Confirm the Diagnosis?

Pneumocystis pneumonia (PCP) should be high up in the differential of any ART-naive HIV-positive patient with a low CD4 count who presents with progressive shortness of breath on exertion and dry cough, with patchy perihilar infiltrates on the chest radiograph. In this case the normal bloods and single organ failure despite a number of weeks of illness make this the most likely diagnosis, although tuberculosis, atypical bacterial pneumonia, cryptococcosis or histoplasmosis should also be considered. Bronchoscopy and immunofluorescence or Grocott methenamine silver staining of bronchoalveolar lavage (BAL) specimens is the diagnostic test of choice. Ziehl–Neelsen staining of the BAL fluid for acid-fast bacilli (AFB) should also be requested. Similar staining of induced sputum is a less sensitive alternative. CD4 count and HIV viral load should be requested as well.

ANSWER TO QUESTION 2

What is Your Immediate Management of the Patient?

Correction of hypoxia with high flow oxygen aiming for saturations above 95% is the first priority. Early intensive care review should be requested, as some patients will require CPAP or ventilatory support in addition to oxygen therapy. High-dose co-trimoxazole is first-line treatment for PCP (see Summary Box) – this may be given IV in severe respiratory failure or if the patient is unable to tolerate oral therapy. In moderate to severe PCP (Table 23-2) steroids should be added. Standard starting dose is prednisolone 40 mg bid or methylprednisolone 30 mg bid, IV if unable to tolerate PO.

THE CASE CONTINUED ...

The patient was treated with high flow oxygen and started on high-dose co-trimoxazole plus prednisolone combined with a proton-pump inhibitor for gastrointestinal protection. His tachycardia settled with reversal of his hypoxia and he remained otherwise stable. He did not require any more intensive ventilatory or other organ support. In view of his multiple recent long-haul flights a CT-pulmonary angiogram was performed to rule out pulmonary embolism (Figure 23-2). This showed extensive ground-glass opacity in both lungs, especially in the lower lobes, but no evidence of pulmonary emboli or cavitations.

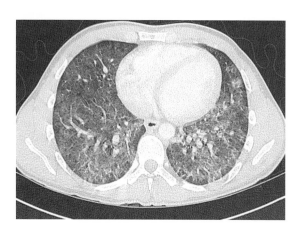

FIGURE 23-2 CT angiogram of the chest showing bilateral ground-glass opacities but no pulmonary emboli.

TABLE 23-3	**Grading of Severity of *Pneumocystis* Pneumonia**		
	Mild	**Moderate**	**Severe**
Clinical features	Increasing exertional dyspnoea ± cough and sweats	Dyspnoea on minimal exertion, occasional dyspnoea at rest, fever ± sweats	Dyspnoea at rest, tachypnoea at rest, persistent fever, cough
Arterial blood gas (room air)	PaO_2 normal, SaO_2 falling on exercise	PaO_2 = 8.1–11 kPa	PaO_2 < 8.0 kPa
Chest radiography	Normal or minor perihilar infiltrates	Diffuse interstitial shadowing	Extensive interstitial shadowing ± diffuse alveolar shadowing ('white out'), sparing costophrenic angles and apices

Source: After Miller RF, Doffman S. Pneumocystis jirovecii infection. In Farrar J, editor. Manson's Tropical Diseases, 23rd ed. London: Elsevier; 2013. ch. 39.

The day after admission bronchoscopy was performed, which was macroscopically normal but cytology and Grocott staining revealed *Pneumocystis jirovecii* cystic forms. CD4 on admission was 150/μL with an HIV viral load of 1.500 000 copies/mL. HIV resistance testing revealed fully sensitive virus.

Oxygen was gradually weaned over ten days and the patient was discharged on oral co-trimoxazole to complete a 21-day total course. Ten days into PCP treatment the patient commenced antiretroviral therapy with tenofovir, emtricitabine and efavirenz. A few days post-discharge, two weeks into PCP treatment, he developed a widespread pruritic maculopapular rash most likely attributable to either co-trimoxazole or efavirenz. As a result co-trimoxazole was changed to clindamycin and primaquine for the final week of treatment and efavirenz was replaced by a protease inhibitor. After completing PCP treatment he was started on dapsone and pyrimethamine for secondary prophylaxis.

SUMMARY BOX

Pneumocystis Pneumonia

Pneumocystis jirovecii, a fungus found worldwide, causes *Pneumocystis* pneumonia (PCP) in immunocompromised individuals. Classic symptoms are subacute onset of malaise, non-productive cough and progressive exertional dyspnoea; fever may also be present. On examination desaturation on exertion is the classic sign; the chest is often clear on auscultation. Complications include respiratory failure and pneumothorax. Without treatment PCP is progressive and usually fatal.

Grading of severity at presentation is important to guide management decisions (Table 23-3).

Diagnosis is by visualizing *P. jirovecii* on bronchoalveolar lavage fluid (>90% sensitivity, and sensitivity maintained up to ten days into treatment). Induced sputum has lower sensitivity (50–90%). PCR of respiratory secretions has variable specificity. Chest imaging can support the diagnosis, but changes are nonspecific and the chest radiograph may be normal in up to 40% of PCP cases at presentation. The classic finding is of diffuse perihilar interstitial infiltrates, which may progress rapidly over 2–3 days.

First-line treatment is with co-trimoxazole (120 mg/kg/day in three to four divided doses for the first three days, then 90 mg/kg/day), which in severe cases should initially be intravenous. The addition of high-dose corticosteroids in moderate to severe PCP improves outcomes if started within 72 hours of starting specific PCP treatment. In HIV-positive patients co-trimoxazole should be continued for a total of 21 days, in other types of immunosuppression 14 days may be sufficient. Steroids are weaned over 20 days. ART should be started within the first 14 days of PCP treatment in ART-naive HIV-positive patients.

In resource-limited settings, the diagnosis of PCP is most commonly made on clinical grounds. Differentiating PCP from pulmonary TB is often challenging. TB in immunosuppressed patients may present with similar clinical features, a normal chest radiograph and negative sputum smears for AFB. Dual infections with both TB and PCP also need to be considered. In the absence of intensive care options severely ill patients may have to be empirically treated for both infections. Co-trimoxazole is often available as an oral formulation only.

Adverse effects with co-trimoxazole are common and usually occur at 6–14 days of treatment, e.g. cytopenias (40%), rash (25%), fever (20%) and abnormal liver profile (10%). Second-line treatment is with primaquine and clindamycin. IV pentamidine is another option but not without side-effects. For mild to moderate cases dapsone-trimethoprim or atovaquone may be given. Patients with G6PD deficiency should not receive co-trimoxazole, dapsone or primaquine due to increased risk of haemolysis. In resource-limited settings alternative treatments are mostly unavailable. In case of a mild rash, the only option may be desensitization with cautious re-exposure to co-trimoxazole.

Secondary prophylaxis with co-trimoxazole (480 mg or 960 mg od) should be given until patients regain their cell-mediated immunity, or in HIV once a CD4 count above 200/μL has been maintained for at least three months. Atovaquone, nebulized pentamidine or dapsone-pyrimethamine are alternatives in resource-rich settings.

Further Reading

1. Huang L, Cattamanchi A, Davis J, et al. HIV-associated *Pneumocystis* pneumonia. Proc Am Thorac Soc 2011;8:294–300.
2. Miller RF, Doffman S. *Pneumocystis jirovecii* infection. In: Farrar J, editor. Manson's Tropical Disease. 23rd ed. London: Elsevier; 2013 [chapter 39].
3. Miller RF, Huang L, Walzer PD. *Pneumocystis* pneumonia associated with human immunodeficiency virus. Clin Chest Med 2013;34(2):229–41.

24

A 14-YEAR-OLD BOY FROM RURAL TANZANIA WITH DIFFICULTIES IN WALKING

William P. Howlett

Clinical Presentation

HISTORY

A 14-year-old boy presents to his local hospital in rural Tanzania with a history of difficulty in walking. He had been well up until just over two years earlier when his illness suddenly started. He describes that he was walking home from school when he first noticed that his legs began to feel heavy and started to tremble, which caused him difficulty in walking, with a tendency to fall over. He slowly completed the journey home and since that day has been unable to stand or walk unaided. He now stands on his toes and drags his legs around with the aid of a stick (Figure 24-1). He denies any history of fever, pain, sensory, bladder or bowel symptoms or disease progression.

His past history is otherwise unremarkable. He lives in a village in northern Tanzania in a rural area with limited agricultural suitability where the main staple food crop is cassava. His diet for the two months before the illness was almost exclusively cassava. He has three other siblings, one of whom is similarly affected, whereas their parents remained fine. He mentions that identical cases had occurred in his own and neighbouring villages at around the same time.

CLINICAL EXAMINATION

Clinically he is well nourished with normal vital signs. General examination is unremarkable. On neurological examination he is fully orientated and higher mental function appears normal. Cranial nerves are normal but bilateral optic pallor was noted on fundoscopy. Limbs reveal signs of spastic

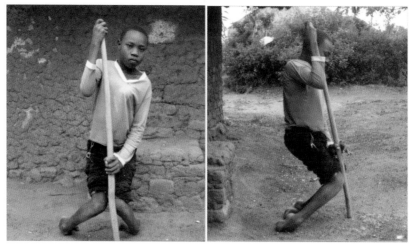

FIGURE 24-1 A 14-year-old boy from rural Tanzania with spastic paraparesis. His illness started about two years earlier and had an acute onset.

paraparesis with flexion contractures at both ankles and knees. Power in the legs is graded 3–4/5 (= just overcoming gravity) with the knee extensors and foot dorsiflexors involved to the greatest extent (Figure 24-1). There is bilateral hypertonia, hyperreflexia and sustained ankle clonus with extensor plantar responses. The arms are normal apart from generalized hyperreflexia. There is no impairment or loss of sensation. A lumbar lordosis with thoracic kyphoscoliosis is noticeable only on standing.

INVESTIGATIONS

Full blood count, erythrocyte sedimentation rate, blood glucose and creatinine are normal. Urine analysis is normal. Microscopy of urine and stool specimens does not show any ova of *Schistosoma* spp. HIV serology and VDRL are negative. Lumbar puncture is normal. Radiographs of the chest and thoracolumbar spine are normal.

QUESTIONS

1. What is the clinical diagnosis and the likely cause in this patient?
2. How do you plan to manage this patient?

Discussion

A 14-year-old boy from rural northern Tanzania presents with acute onset non-progressive spastic paraplegia. There is no history of back pain. On examination there is no sensory impairment and no bladder dysfunction. The main staple food crop in his village is cassava.

ANSWER TO QUESTION 1

What is the Clinical Diagnosis?

The clinical syndrome is spastic paraparesis. The main differential diagnosis in Africa includes spinal tuberculosis (Pott's disease), transverse myelitis, spinal cord infections such as schistosomiasis and tuberculous myelitis, spinal malignancy (mainly metastases) and tropical nutritional myeloneuropathies.

There are three important features in our case: (1) the isolated involvement of motor neurons without any sensory and bladder involvement; (2) the absence of back pain; (3) the acute onset with no progression over two years. These three clinical points make spinal tuberculosis, spinal cord infection or spinal malignancy very unlikely. Of note, his diet (and probably that of his siblings and other children in the village) for the two months before the illness was almost exclusively cassava, and the same disease has affected one of his siblings and more children in the neighbourhood. Hence, a nutritional cause must be suspected.

The tropical myeloneuropathies that are nutritional in origin are konzo and lathyrism. Lathyrism in Africa occurs exclusively in Ethiopia. The clinical diagnosis in our patient is konzo. Konzo is a distinct form of tropical spastic paraparesis which occurs exclusively in cassava-growing areas in Africa (see Summary Box).[1–3]

ANSWER TO QUESTION 2

How Do You Plan To Manage this Patient?

There is no cure for patients with konzo as it results in a permanent spastic paraparesis. Management is therefore directed at support, symptomatic improvement and disease prevention. The majority of patients can walk with the aid of a stick or crutches and some will benefit from a wheelchair. Muscle relaxants have a limited role because of relative ineffectiveness due to the severity of the spasticity and these agents' high long-term cost. Surgical treatment involving Achilles' tendon lengthening operations have proved useful in improving mobilization in selected patients with konzo. Because of the severity of contractures in this patient, he should be assessed for surgery.

THE CASE CONTINUED ...

At follow-up examination at 6 and 12 months the findings were unchanged, with a permanent spastic paraparesis. The patient had not been referred for surgery because of the lack of resources and the extent of the epidemic, with many other similar cases in the community. He uses one stick with very restricted mobility and works as a shoe repairer in his village.

SUMMARY BOX

Konzo

Konzo is a distinct form of tropical spastic paraparesis which occurs exclusively in cassava growing areas in Africa.[1–3] It is characterized by an abrupt onset of a permanent but non-progressive form of spastic paraparesis related to cassava consumption. It occurs mainly as epidemics, typically during droughts, famines or armed conflict when there is an overreliance on cassava as a staple food for weeks or months. It also occurs in an endemic form but at much lower rates. It affects mainly children and breastfeeding mothers.

The following are the clinical criteria for diagnosing konzo:

- symmetrical spastic paraparesis without sensory or genitourinary involvement
- abrupt onset in less than one week with a non-progressive course
- occurring in a cassava-growing area, usually with other cases emerging at the same time
- no other cause found.

Its cause is attributed to chronic high dietary exposure of cyanogenic glycosides from insufficiently processed cassava tubers, but the exact pathogenic mechanisms of konzo remain unknown.

Cassava is a staple food for more than 600 million people. It grows well in poor soils and is resistant to drought, plant diseases, insects and animal predators,[4] but it contains cyanogenic glycosides, mainly linamarin. Processing disrupts the tubers releasing cyanide, which makes the food safe for human consumption. Konzo is associated with high intake of insufficiently processed cassava tubers in combination with low or absent levels of the essential amino acids methionine or cysteine. Oxidative stress and glutamate-mediated neuro-excitatory cell death appears likely to be the final pathogenic mechanism. This results in a clinically exclusive pattern of upper motor neurone disease.

Further Reading

1. Aronson JK. Plant poisons and traditional medicines. In: Farrar J, editor. Manson's Tropical Diseases. 23rd ed. London: Elsevier; 2013 [chpter 76].
2. Howlett WP, Brubaker GR, Mlingi N, et al. Konzo, an epidemic upper motor neuron disease studied in Tanzania. Brain 1990;113(Pt 1):223–35.
3. Howlett WP. Paraplegia. Neurology in Africa. Kilimanjaro Christian Medical Centre and University of Bergen; 2012.
4. Tshala-Katumbay D, Mumba N, Okitundu L, et al. Cassava food toxins, konzo disease, and neurodegeneration in sub-Sahara Africans. Neurology 2013;80(10):949–51.

A 72-YEAR-OLD MALE FARMER FROM LAOS WITH EXTENSIVE SKIN LESIONS ON THE LOWER LEG

Günther Slesak / Saythong Inthalad / Paul N. Newton

Clinical Presentation

HISTORY

A 72-year-old male farmer is admitted to a provincial hospital in northern Laos with extensive, painful verrucous skin lesions on his left foot and lower leg.

Ten years prior he had a leech bite on the dorsum of his left foot. One week later a small painless red nodule developed at the site of the bite. Over the following years the lesion slowly increased in size; further lesions developed and spread up to his knee. Three days before admission his ankle became painful and swollen.

CLINICAL FINDINGS

Vital signs are normal and the patient is afebrile. His left lower leg and foot are grossly swollen (Figure 25-1); the skin is hyperaemic and feels hot. There are several cauliflower-like masses and oval plaque-like lesions on his left lower leg and foot. The lesions are partly erythematous, partly fungating and purulent, oozing a bad odour.

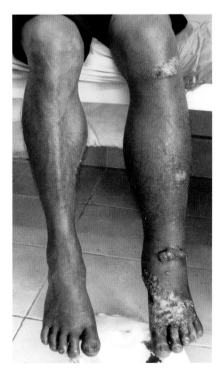

FIGURE 25-1 Lower legs of the patient at presentation with fungating lesions on his left foot that spread centripetally up to his knee. The left lower leg is also swollen and hyperaemic.

INVESTIGATIONS

Radiography of the left leg and foot showed no bone involvement.

QUESTIONS

1. What are the important differential diagnoses?
2. Which diagnostic tests should be done?

Discussion

A male Lao farmer presents with several verrucous, partially fungating skin lesions on his left leg and foot which have been growing over the past ten years following a minor trauma. The affected leg has additionally swollen up and become painful over the previous three days.

ANSWER TO QUESTION 1

What Are the Important Differential Diagnoses?

Chronic verrucous skin lesions can typically be seen in fungal infections such as sporotrichosis (*Sporothrix schenckii*) and chromoblastomycosis, which is caused by various pigmented fungi.

Mycobacterial infections (cutaneous tuberculosis, lepromatous leprosy and infections with atypical mycobacteria) also need to be considered. Cutaneous leishmaniasis can present with verrucous lesions, however it has not been reported in Laos.

Non-infectious causes such as squamous cell carcinoma, sarcoidosis, chronic eczema and psoriasis should be borne in mind.

Acute localized inflammatory signs are indicative of bacterial superinfection or deep vein thrombosis.

ANSWER TO QUESTION 2

Which Diagnostic Tests Should be Done?

Direct microscopy of skin scrapings taken from the lesions can help detect pigmented fungi in chromoblastomycosis and may be useful to visualize amastigotes in cutaneous leishmaniasis.

Sporotrichosis differs from the other subcutaneous mycoses in that culture is the most reliable mode of diagnosis because there are few organisms present in lesions and these may be difficult to find.

In leprosy, slit skin smears are fairly easy to obtain; however, for other mycobacterial infections biopsy and/or culture may be necessary.

THE CASE CONTINUED ...

Secondary bacterial superinfection was suspected and so iodine-based antiseptics were applied locally and oral antibiotics were started, initially cloxacillin and metronidazole. After bacterial culture of the pus grew *Escherichia coli*, antibiotics were changed to co-trimoxazole, guided by susceptibility testing.

Simple direct microscopic investigations of wet film lesion scrapings revealed characteristic brownish, round, thick-walled, multiseptate sclerotic cells typical of chromoblastomycosis (Figure 25-2). Use of 10% potassium hydroxide solution made the fungal cells more readily visible. Antifungal treatment was initiated with itraconazole (400 mg/d for seven days monthly pulse therapy) and surgical debridement of all lesions performed. PCR from skin tissue was positive and sequencing revealed 100% similarity with *Fonsecaea pedrosoi*, *F. monophora* and *F. nubica*. When oral terbinafine could be obtained this was added (initially 500 mg/d, later 750 mg/d) for nine months and local terbinafine ointment was applied for six months. Liver function tests and serum glucose were monitored during treatment and remained normal. The lesions healed uneventfully with some residual swelling and hypopigmentation.

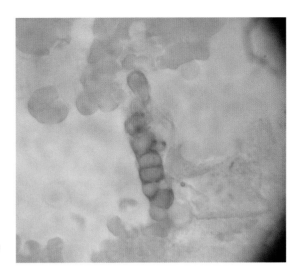

FIGURE 25-2 Characteristic brownish sclerotic cells in skin scrapings (100×, oil immersion, wet film).

SUMMARY BOX

Chromoblastomycosis

Chromoblastomycosis is a chronic fungal infection of the skin and subcutaneous tissue, most commonly of hands, feet and lower legs.[1-4] It is typically caused by traumatic percutaneous inoculation of the genera *Fonsecaea*, *Phialophora* and *Cladophialophora* which are found in plant debris or forest detritus. Infection occurs worldwide but is most common in rural tropical and subtropical areas. Male agricultural workers are most commonly affected.

Painless lesions develop slowly over years from the site of inoculation as veruccous nodules or plaques, gradually spreading centripetally by lymphatic or cutaneous dissemination. Typical complications are ulcerations, chronic lymphoedema, even elephantiasis and bacterial superinfection.

Diagnosis is made by direct microscopic detection of pathognomonic sclerotic cells in skin scrapings ('Medlar bodies', fumagoid or muriform cells). These are brownish, round, thick-walled structures of 4–12 µm length, which are already visible on a simple wet film. Hyphae can be more readily seen on a potassium hydroxide preparation. More sophisticated techniques such as culture as well as serology and PCR are rarely available in endemic areas and are often reserved for research purposes, but species identification can also guide treatment schemes.[5]

Treatment is challenging and effectiveness depends on the causative agent, the clinical form and the severity of the lesions. Antifungal therapy commonly comprises oral itraconazole (200–400 mg/d) alone or in combination with terbinafine or flucytosine (which may be hard to obtain). Antifungals have to be given for at least 6–12 months and in advanced stages for years in order to avoid relapse. Cure rates range from 15 to 80%. Multidrug therapy seems more effective but is expensive. Itraconazole pulse therapy (7 d/month) is cost-saving.

In addition, topical heat therapy, phototherapy, cryosurgery, surgical debridement and/or combination therapy may be helpful.

Further Reading

1. Hay RJ. Fungal infections. In: Farrar J, editor. Manson's Tropical Diseases. 23rd ed. London: Elsevier; 2013 [chapter 38].
2. Lu S, Lu C, Zhang J, et al. Chromoblastomycosis in mainland China: a systematic review on clinical characteristics. Mycopathologia 2013;175(5–6):489–95.
3. Slesak G, Inthalad S, Strobel M, et al. Chromoblastomycosis after a leech bite complicated by myiasis: a case report. BMC Infect Dis 2011;11:14.
4. Correia RT, Valente NY, Criado PR, et al. Chromoblastomycosis: study of 27 cases and review of medical literature. An Bras Dermatol 2010;85(4):448–54.
5. Queiroz-Telles F, Santos DW. Challenges in the therapy of chromoblastomycosis. Mycopathologia 2013;175(5–6):477–88.

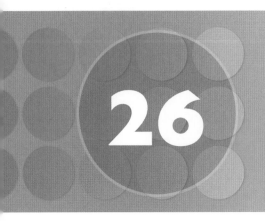

26

A 14-YEAR-OLD BOY FROM MALAWI WHO HAS BEEN BITTEN BY A SNAKE

Gregor Pollach

Clinical Presentation

HISTORY

A 14-year-old Malawian boy presents to a local hospital because of an extensive necrotic wound on his right foot.

Three weeks earlier he was playing with his friends on a path leading through rocky grassland to the maize field of his family when he stepped on a snake. The snake was brown with V-shaped black bands on its back, and it was approximately one metre long. His friends told his mother later that the snake had hissed loudly but did not move away before biting him – which the boy did not even realize, being busy chasing a football. Shortly after the bite, haemorrhagic bullae formed on the right leg. His gums started to bleed and he vomited extensively. He was taken to a local traditional healer for treatment. His bleeding and vomiting settled, however, he developed intense pain and swelling at the site of the bite.

CLINICAL FINDINGS

The patient is a 14-year old boy, who appears weak and is in respiratory distress. His vital signs are: temperature 39.4°C, pulse 126 bpm, blood pressure 85/60 mmHg, respiratory rate 30 breath cycles per minute. There is an extensive foul-smelling necrosis affecting his right foot and ankle where the tendons are exposed (Figure 26-1). The right lower leg is swollen and he is unable to bend the ankle of his right foot. The inguinal lymph nodes are enlarged on the right side.

The urine is clear, rectal exam does not show any signs of bleeding and upon provoked coughing there is no haemoptysis. Fundoscopy is normal.

INVESTIGATIONS

The 20 minute whole blood clotting test is normal. The results of the other blood tests are shown in Table 26-1.

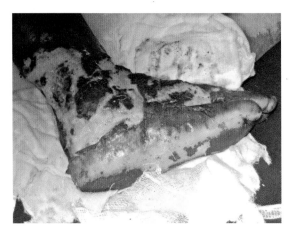

FIGURE 26-1 The right foot and ankle with extensive tissue necrosis three weeks after a snake bite.

TABLE 26-1	**Laboratory Results on Admission**	
Parameter	Patient	Reference Range
WBC (x10^9/L)	19	4–10
Haemoglobin (mg/dL)	9.5	12–14
Platelets (x10^9/L)	60	150–400
K$^+$ (mmol/L)	4.2	3.5–5.2

QUESTIONS

1. Which snake was most probably responsible for the bite?
2. What first-aid measures should have been taken?

Discussion

A 14-year-old boy from rural Malawi who was bitten by a snake three weeks earlier presents to a local hospital. He is septic with an extensive foul-smelling necrotic wound on the right ankle, exposed tendons and oedema of the right leg.

ANSWER TO QUESTION 1

Which Snake Was Most Probably Responsible for the Bite?

The African puff-adder (*Bitis arietans*) is the most likely snake to have caused his bite. Puff-adders are about one metre long and stout. They show a distinctive 'V' or 'U' pattern on their back. When disturbed they behave aggressively, hissing loudly and inflating their body. The puff-adder is a highly dangerous snake, with large quantities of a potent venom and long fangs. It commonly lives in densely populated areas.[1,2] Throughout the whole African savannah this species is responsible for the high number of serious bites. The main problem is massive local swelling, which may spread to involve the whole limb and cause hypovolaemic shock. Bullae filled with haemorrhagic fluid may develop at the site of the bite. Extensive necrosis may occur. Cardiotoxic effects of the venom may lead to arrhythmias. The venom may cause systemic haemorrhage.

The puff-adder, along with the saw-scaled or carpet viper (*Echis* spp.), which produce similar symptoms, are responsible for the most fatalities following snake bites in Africa. In contrast, bites by mambas, the most feared snakes in Africa, are relatively uncommon.

ANSWER TO QUESTION 2

What First-Aid Measures Should Have Been Taken?

First-aid should include reassurance of the victim. Paracetamol should be used for pain relief since aspirin might aggravate haemorrhage and morphine can enhance respiratory depression caused by the venom. Any tight jewellery should be removed. The affected limb should be immobilized along with the whole patient, since any muscular contractions will increase the absorption of the venom.

In cases where a neurotoxic venom cannot be excluded, a pressure immobilization technique should be used. For example, a long elastic bandage can be wrapped around the affected limb incorporating a splint.[3] However, in cytotoxic venoms the local effects may be worsened through such pressure techniques.

The wound itself should be left alone to avoid infection and absorption of the venom.
The patient should gently but quickly be taken to the nearest appropriate health facility. Patients should be placed in a recovery position when vomiting or when their level of consciousness is reduced. All patients bitten by snakes should ideally be observed in hospital for at least 24 hours.

Finally, helpers should not try to kill the snake, risking further bites. However, if the snake has already been killed it should be taken to the healthcare facility for identification. Even a dead snake needs to be handled with great caution as it still may bite by reflex.

Some widely popular first-aid measures have never been proven to be of any help in the management of snake bites; these include local cuts with a knife or razor blade, attempts to suck the venom out of the wound, the often disastrous application of an arterial tourniquet, cauterization, chemicals, ice, electric shocks and the use of 'magic stones'.[3]

THE CASE CONTINUED ...

The snake bite had occurred three weeks earlier, therefore application of antivenom was not deemed useful. Since the boy was septic on admission he was managed according to the international sepsis treatment guidelines, crucially including early start of broad-spectrum antibiotics, 'ventilator support' and fluid resuscitation.[4] He also received tetanus prophylaxis.

The wound was treated surgically. After several debridements (Figure 26-2) it stayed clean and mesh-grafting was successfully performed. Further reconstructive surgery was not necessary and severe local complications (e.g. compartment syndrome, deep tissue infections, ischaemia) did not develop. The boy was discharged several weeks later. Some functional impairment of his right foot remained and he was booked for outpatient physiotherapy.

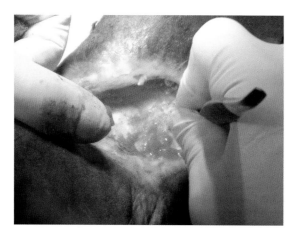

FIGURE 26-2 After several debridements the wound looks clean.

TABLE 26-2	**Principal Effects of African Snake Venoms in Humans**	
Venom Activity	**Clinical Manifestations**	**African Snake Responsible**
Cytotoxic	Massive local swelling, blistering, necrosis; plasma extravasation with consecutive fluid loss, hypotension Eye: keratoconjunctivitis, corneal ulcer, blindness (spitting cobra)	Puff-adder and other large *Bitis* spp., saw-scaled vipers (*Echis*), burrowing asps (*Atractaspis* spp.); spitting cobra
Autopharmacological	Release of vasoactive compounds (e.g. NO, histamine, serotonin, bradykinin); anaphylaxis, acute profound hypotension, urticaria, vomiting, diarrhoea	Burrowing asps (*Atractaspis* spp.), *Bitis* spp., boomslang
Haematotoxic	Spontaneous systemic bleeding (gums, brain, gastrointestinal, uterine), bleeding from trauma and recent wounds	Puff-adder and other large *Bitis* spp., saw-scaled vipers, boomslang, vine snake
Cardiotoxic	Hypotension, shock, arrhythmias, conduction abnormalities	Puff-adder and other large *Bitis* spp., burrowing asps
Neurotoxic	Cranial nerve palsies, bulbar and respiratory paralysis	Elapids (mamba, cobra, rinkhals) berg adder, Peringuey's adder
Myotoxic	Trismus; rhabdomyolysis with myalgias, myoglobinuria, renal failure, hyperkalaemia, respiratory failure	Sea snake
Nephrotoxic	Acute kidney injury, renal necrosis	Boomslang, vine snake, saw-scaled vipers

Source: after Warrell, 2013[3]

SUMMARY BOX

Snake Bite

Snake bite is a common problem in rural areas of many tropical countries. The true numbers are unknown since many patients may never reach the official health system and rather seek the help of a traditional practitioner. Snake bites are most common amongst farm workers, herdsmen, plantation workers and their children. Most bites occur at the beginning of the rainy season. Even though there is a large variety of venomous snakes, the toxic effects of snake bites can be classified into one or more of seven groups (see Table 26-2).[3]

The therapeutic approach in hospital has to consider local and systemic effects of the bite and the complications that might arise. Tetanus prophylaxis, antibiotic coverage, wound cleansing and sterile dressing are mandatory.

Antivenom should be given in systemic envenoming, indicated by clinical signs and symptoms or deranged laboratory parameters.

Of note, loosening of tourniquets or improvement of circulation may lead to an increased systemic load of venom. In severe local envenoming, antivenom should be given if the swelling involves more than half of the bitten limb and in patients bitten by snakes known to cause local necrosis.[1]

Antivenom is most effective when administered by slow IV injection or infusion. Children need the same dose as adults since the same amount of venom has been injected. Antivenom mostly consists of non-human hyperimmunoglobulin; it therefore can lead to severe side-effects including fever, anaphylaxis or late serum sickness-like reactions.

Necrotic wounds require careful debridement. Wound infection, compartment syndrome or osteomyelitis must be suspected and treated early. Skin grafts, reconstructive surgery, fasciotomy or amputation may be necessary. Massive local oedema carries the risk of hypovolaemic shock.

In severe haemorrhagic complications with hypotension, patients should be transfused; if blood is unavailable sufficient IV fluids should be administered.

For neurotoxic complications mechanical ventilation is often required and anticholinesterase drugs should be attempted.

Further Reading

1. Warrell DA. Venomous and poisonous animals. In: Farrar J, editor. Manson's Tropical Diseases. 23rd ed. London: Elsevier; 2013 [chapter 75].
2. Warrell DA. Treatment of bites by adders and exotic venomous snakes. BMJ 2005;331(7527):1244–7.
3. Warrell DA. Venomous and other dangerous animals. In: Mabey D, Gill G, Parry E, et al., editors. Principles of Medicine in Africa. 4th ed. Cambridge: Cambridge University Press; 2013. p. 849–74.
4. Dellinger RP, Levy MM, Rhodes A, et al. Surviving sepsis campaign: international guidelines for management of severe sepsis and septic shock: 2012. Crit Care Med 2013;41(2):580–637.

A 16-YEAR-OLD BOY FROM SRI LANKA WITH FEVER, JAUNDICE AND RENAL FAILURE

Ranjan Premaratna

Clinical Presentation

HISTORY

A 16-year-old Sri Lankan boy presents to a local hospital with fever, frontal headache and severe body aches for two days. He has vomited two to three times during the illness and has not passed any urine for the previous 12 hours. He does not have a cough, coryza or shortness of breath. He has been attending school until his illness. He had been fishing in an urban water stream five days prior to falling ill.

CLINICAL EXAMINATION

The boy looks ill and drowsy. He is jaundiced and has subconjunctival haemorrhages (Figure 27-1). There is no neck stiffness, however there is severe muscle tenderness, mainly involving the abdominal wall and in the calves so that the patient finds it difficult to walk. There is no lymphadenopathy. The liver is palpable at 4 cm below the right costal margin and is tender. The spleen is not palpable. There is mild bilateral renal angle tenderness. Body temperature is 38.3°C. The pulse rate is 100 bpm and is low in volume. The blood pressure is 90/60 mmHg. The cardiac apex is not shifted. Examination of the lungs and the CNS are normal.

FURTHER INVESTIGATIONS

The laboratory findings are summarized in Table 27-1. The urine microscopy shows 20 red blood cells per high-power field, proteins '+' and granular casts '+'. A chest radiograph is normal. An ECG shows sinus tachycardia.

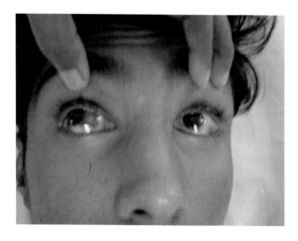

FIGURE 27-1 Jaundice and subconjunctival haemorrhages.

TABLE 27-1   Laboratory Results on Admission

Parameter	Patient	Reference
WBC (×10⁹/L) (neutrophils : lymphocytes)	5.7 (68%: 31%)	4–10
Haemoglobin (g/dL)	14.8	12–16
Platelets (×10⁹/L)	96	150–350
AST (IU/L)	64	13–33
ALT (IU/L)	58	3–25
ALP (IU/L)	246	40–130
Serum bilirubin total (µmol/L)	77	13.7–30.8
Serum bilirubin direct (µmol/L)	54.7	<5
Blood urea nitrogen (µmol/L)	20.7	2.5–6.4
Serum creatinine (µmol/L)	212.2	71–106
C-reactive protein (mg/L)	48	<5

QUESTIONS

1. What is the most likely diagnosis and what are your differentials?
2. What tests are indicated to confirm the diagnosis?

Discussion

A Sri Lankan teenage boy presents with fever, severe body aches and a reduced urine output. He is jaundiced with subconjunctival haemorrhages and has a tender hepatomegaly. He has had contact with a water stream prior to ill health.

His laboratory results show signs of cholestasis with only mildly elevated transaminases. The creatinine is increased twofold and there is thrombocytopenia. The leukocyte count is normal.

ANSWER TO QUESTION 1

What is the Most Likely Diagnosis and What Are Your Differentials?

An acute febrile illness accompanied by jaundice, renal failure and conjunctival haemorrhages should raise the suspicion of leptospirosis, particularly in case of a history involving exposure to potentially contaminated water.

Scrub typhus is another very common infection in South Asia. It may present with an acute onset of fever, hepatomegaly and renal failure. There usually is lymphadenopathy and on careful examination one may spot an eschar. Subconjunctival haemorrhages have been described but are less common than in leptospirosis and complications such as renal failure tend to occur late in the infection (after about seven days).

Hantavirus infection may cause a haemorrhagic fever with renal syndrome. It has a similar epidemiology to leptospirosis and is also associated with contact to rodent excreta.

Dengue haemorrhagic fever (DHF) is another differential diagnosis to consider. It also presents with fever, severe myalgias, thrombocytopenia and haemorrhages. Jaundice is uncommon for DHF.

ANSWER TO QUESTION 2

What Tests Are Indicated to Confirm the Diagnosis?

A definitive diagnosis of leptospirosis is based upon the isolation of *Leptospira* spp. or a positive microscopic agglutination test (MAT).

Isolation of the bacteria from blood or CSF is only possible during the first week of the disease. Culture results may take 2–3 weeks and need to be examined weekly by dark field or phase-contrast microscopy since the bacteria stain poorly. This technique is not routine practice in a standard microbiological laboratory.[1]

The MAT cannot differentiate between current or past infections. Therefore two consecutive serum samples should be examined to look for seroconversion or an at least fourfold rise in titre. The significance of titres in single serum specimens is a matter of debate.

THE CASE CONTINUED ...

Severe leptospirosis was suspected and the patient was commenced on empirical benzylpenicillin. Despite rehydration he developed acute renal failure warranting haemodialysis (HD). He developed myocarditis and atrial fibrillation, but luckily tolerated further HD. He gradually recovered over ten days with intensive care management.

SUMMARY BOX

Leptospirosis

Leptospirosis is a zoonotic disease that occurs worldwide. It is caused by pathogenic *Leptospira* spp.,[1–3] which belong to the spirochaetes. The most common species causing disease in humans and animals are *L. interrogans* and *L. borgpetersenii*.

Humans become infected through direct contact with urine of infected mammalian hosts, animal abortion products, or contact with contaminated water. The major reservoirs are rodents, canines, livestock and wild mammals. The people most at risk are slum dwellers and those with an occupational or recreational exposure involving animal contact or immersion in water. Also, natural disasters such as hurricanes and floods may put people at risk.

The bacteria enter the human body through cuts or abrasions of the skin or through intact mucous membranes. The incubation period is 2–30 days. The spectrum of disease ranges from asymptomatic to severe infection.

The classical presentation of leptospirosis is that of a biphasic illness. The initial leptospiraemic phase usually starts abruptly. Symptoms are nonspecific with fever, headache, sore throat, abdominal pain and a rash. Severe myalgias, most notably of the calf and the lumbar area and conjunctival suffusions, have been mentioned as distinguishing physical findings.[3] This first phase lasts for a week and is followed by a second phase dominated by immune-mediated pathology.

Five to ten per cent of those with clinical infection will develop severe leptospirosis with cholestatic jaundice, acute kidney injury and haemorrhagic diathesis (Weil's syndrome). Further complications include pulmonary involvement, aseptic meningitis and myocarditis.

A definitive diagnosis of leptospirosis is based upon the isolation of *Leptospira* spp. from blood or CSF, or the positive microscopic agglutination test (MAT). Both are laborious and not widely available.

Leptospirosis is usually treated with antibiotics, although the usefulness of antibiotic treatment in particular during the second, immune-mediated phase of illness has been disputed.

For uncomplicated cases, oral doxycycline is the drug of choice. Alternatives include amoxicillin and azithromycin. In severe infection benzylpenicillin, IV doxycycline, ceftriaxone or cefotaxime seem to have similar efficacy. Doxycycline 200 mg weekly has been suggested as exposure prophylaxis.

Further Reading

1. Chierakul KW. Leptospirosis. In: Farrar J, editor. Manson's Tropical Diseases. 23rd ed. London: Elsevier; 2013 [chapter 37].
2. WHO. Human leptospirosis: guidance for diagnosis, surveillance and control. In: World Health Organization and International Leptospirosis Society, editors. Geneva: WHO; 2003.
3. Bharti AR, Nally JE, Ricaldi JN, et al. Leptospirosis: a zoonotic disease of global importance. Lancet Infect Dis 2003;3(12):757–71.

A 67-YEAR-OLD FEMALE EXPATRIATE LIVING IN CAMEROON WITH EOSINOPHILIA AND PERICARDITIS

28

Sebastian Dieckmann / Ralf Ignatius

Clinical Presentation

HISTORY

A 67-year-old German woman who has lived as an expatriate in Cameroon for the past four years presents with palpitations at a tropical medicine clinic in Germany. She also reports transient subcutaneous swellings for the past year. There is no history of fever or constitutional symptoms and the past medical history is otherwise unremarkable.

A 24-hour ECG was done elsewhere, which showed paroxysmal supraventricular extrasystoles. Echocardiography revealed a minimal pericardial effusion.

CLINICAL FINDINGS

Vital signs are normal and the patient is afebrile. There are no visible subcutaneous swellings. Heart sounds are clear and regular and there are no murmurs. No pathological findings are noted on physical examination.

LABORATORY RESULTS

Full blood count results are shown in Table 28-1.

FURTHER INVESTIGATIONS

The chest radiograph does not show any abnormalities.

TABLE 28-1 Full Blood Count Results at Presentation		
Parameter	Patient	Reference
WBC ($\times10^9$/L)	6.20	4–10
Haemoglobin (g/dL)	13.8	12–15
Platelets ($\times10^9$/L)	155	150–450
Neutrophils (%)	45	20–50
Eosinophils (%)	14	0–6
Absolute eosinophil count ($\times10^9$/L)	0.868	<0.45
Band neutrophils (%)	1	0–5
Lymphocytes (%)	36	20–40
Monocytes (%)	4	0–10
Basophils (%)	0	0–2

QUESTIONS

1. What are the key findings?
2. What are your differential diagnoses?

Discussion

A 67-year-old expatriate living in Cameroon for four years presents with eosinophilia and reports transient subcutaneous swellings. Additionally, the patient suffers from cardiac arrhythmia.

ANSWER TO QUESTION 1

What Are the Key Findings?

The pattern of transient subcutaneous swellings, eosinophilia and the history of living in Cameroon for several years are the key pieces of clinical information suggestive of a filarial infection.

Some filarial infections may affect the heart, and chronic eosinophilia is known to be cardiotoxic and may cause endomyocardial fibrosis. The cardiac findings in this patient, however, may warrant further work-up.

ANSWER TO QUESTION 2

What Are the Differential Diagnoses?

The differentials of skin swellings and eosinophilia include nonspecific urticaria, calabar swellings in loiasis, cysticercosis, larva currens in *Strongyloides stercoralis* infection and infection with *Mansonella perstans*.

Acute schistosomiasis (Katayama syndrome) may present with fever and an urticarial rash; however, this patient is afebrile and the migratory swellings she describes do not fit the clinical picture of schistosomiasis.

Gnathostomiasis and sparganosis may also cause eosinophilia and migratory swellings; however, these infections are more common in East Asia than in Africa. Sparganosis has been reported from Kenya and Tanzania and gnathostomiasis occurs in the Okavango Delta.

THE CASE CONTINUED ...

Serology for filarial infections was positive. Day-blood samples were collected, filtered and stained with Giemsa, which revealed sheathed microfilariae with a tapered tail characteristic for *Loa loa* (Figure 28-1). (In contrast, microfilariae of *M. perstans*, another filarial nematode endemic in West and Central Africa, which may cause similar symptoms, would have been smaller and unsheathed with a blunt tail.) The microfilarial count was 1400/mL.

The patient was first treated with albendazole followed by ivermectin (see Summary Box). Therapy was tolerated well. The absolute eosinophil count (AEC) returned to normal and the microfilarial count declined (Figure 28-2). No sequelae were observed and the palpitations settled.

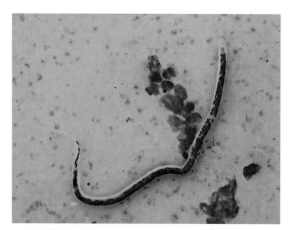

FIGURE 28-1 Sheathed microfilaria of *Loa loa*. The tail is tapered and nuclei are extending into the tip of the tail. (Giemsa staining; magnification 200×.)

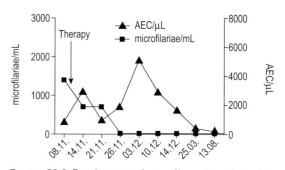

FIGURE 28-2 Development of microfilaraemia and absolute eosinophil count (AEC) in the patient following treatment.

TABLE 28-2 Treatment of Loiasis Matched to Levels of Microfilaraemia[2]

Level of Microfilaraemia	Drug Regimen
High (>8000 mf[a]/mL)	Albendazole 200 mg bd for 21 days, followed by ivermectin 150–200 µg/kg stat, then DEC at slowly increasing doses[b]
Moderate (1000–8000 mf/mL)	Ivermectin 150–200 µg/kg stat, followed by DEC[b]
Low (<1000 mf/mL)	DEC[b]

[a]mf = microfilariae.
[b]DEC: start with low doses of 6.25–12.5 mg/d, slowly increase to up to 300–400 mg/d. Several 3–4 week courses of DEC administered at intervals of 2–3 weeks may be required to achieve a complete cure.

Follow-up echocardiography three months later was normal, the pericardial effusion had disappeared, 24-hour ECG was also normal.

Loiasis has been implicated in the development of endomyocardial fibrosis; however, it remains unclear in this case whether there was any association between the infection and the patient's transient cardiac problems.

SUMMARY BOX

Loiasis

Loiasis is the symptomatic infection with the filarial nematode *Loa loa*. It is common in West and Central Africa. The infective larvae of *L. loa* are transmitted by female *Chrysops* spp. flies.[1,2]

Inside the human host larvae develop into adult worms, which takes several months. Adult *L. loa* migrate through the subcutaneous and connective tissues of the human body. Migration may cause urticaria and transient painless subcutaneous swellings ('Calabar swellings'), angioedemas, which last from several hours to a few days.

Adult worms may be spotted when migrating through the bulbar conjunctiva, which is noticed by the patient as intense itching of the eye, pain and photophobia. Passage of the palpebral conjunctiva is associated with swelling of the eyelid and the periorbital region.

Loiasis may cause renal complications (glomerulonephritis, nephrotic syndrome etc.) and a wide range of neurological symptoms.[2]

The female worms release sheathed microfilariae that are detectable in the peripheral blood during daytime with a peak around noon, but are usually absent at night. This diurnal periodicity corresponds to the day-biting habits of the *Chrysops* vectors.

Microfilaraemia in *L. loa* infection tends to be higher than in other filarial infections; however, there is also a high percentage of amicrofilaraemic individuals ('occult loiasis') in endemic areas, which poses a diagnostic challenge.

Clinical diagnosis in loiasis relies on the typical passage of the adults through the bulbar conjunctiva ('eye worm').

Microfilariae of *L. loa* may be detected in a thick blood film or filtered blood using day-blood samples. PCR (polymerase chain reaction) is currently the best diagnostic method for amicrofilaraemic patients with occult loiasis. Serology has to be interpreted with caution. Serological tests for *L. loa* are usually based on antigens derived from another filarial species, e.g. *Dirofilaria immitis*. Therefore serology is unable to distinguish between the different filarial diseases. Furthermore, cross-reactions with antibodies against other nematodes are common.

For treatment of loiasis, DEC, ivermectin and albendazole are used. DEC is effective against microfilariae of *L. loa* and also kills a proportion of the adult worms. It has long been considered the drug of choice for the treatment of loiasis; however, it may have severe side-effects in patients with high levels of microfilariae and in individuals co-infected with onchocerciasis (see below). Furthermore, DEC is difficult to access in non-endemic countries and repeated courses of treatment may be required for final cure. Ivermectin is only microfilaricidal, and albendazole may have embryostatic activity;[3] however, the precise mechanism of action and the nature and degree of its impact on adult *L. loa* remain to be elucidated.

When patients with high microfilaraemia are treated with DEC or ivermectin, the rapid death of microfilariae can lead to severe side-effects, including glomerulonephritis, encephalopathy, coma or death. Sequential treatment has since been suggested, depending upon the degree of microfilaraemia (Table 28-2).[2]

Further Reading

1. Simonsen P, Fischer PU, Hoerauf A, et al. The filariases. Manson's Tropical Diseases. 23rd ed. London: Elsevier; 2013 [chapter 54].
2. Boussinesq M. Loiasis. Ann Trop Med Parasitol 2006;100:715–31.
3. Klion AD, Massougbodji A, Horton J, et al. Albendazole in human loiasis: results of a double-blind, placebo-controlled trial. J Infect Dis 1993;168:202–6.

29

A 35-YEAR-OLD WOMAN FROM MALAWI WITH FEVER AND PROGRESSIVE WEAKNESS

Camilla Rothe

Clinical Presentation

HISTORY

A 35-year-old Malawian woman presents to a local hospital because of fever and weakness.

The fever started three days earlier, but the weakness has progressed over the past several months. There is no cough and no night sweats but she reports some weight loss. There is no diarrhoea, no dysuria and no history of abnormal bleeds.

Two months earlier she presented to a local health centre because of her weakness. She was found to be clinically pale and was prescribed iron tablets, which she took. Nevertheless, the weakness progressed. Otherwise, the patient does not report any abnormalities.

She is divorced, with three children (17, 15 and 12 years old), who are all well. She works as a small-scale farmer and sells vegetables on the local market. The family can afford three meals a day and occasionally meat or fish.

CLINICAL FINDINGS

A 35-year-old woman, wasted, body mass index 17 kg/m². Blood pressure 90/60 mmHg (difficult to measure on the wasted arm), pulse 110 bpm, temperature 37.8°C, respiratory rate 25 breath cycles per minute, oxygen saturation 97% on ambient air, Glasgow Coma Scale 15/15.

Her conjunctivae are very pale, but there is no jaundice. The examination of her mouth is normal, there is no oral thrush, no Kaposi's sarcoma lesions and no oral hairy leukoplakia. The chest is clear. The abdomen is soft, with slight diffuse tenderness, but no guarding. The spleen is palpable 3 cm below the left costal margin. The rectal examination is normal.

INVESTIGATIONS

The malaria rapid diagnostic test is negative. The HIV serology comes back reactive.

The results of her full blood count are shown in Table 29-1.

TABLE 29-1 Laboratory Results on Admission		
Parameter	Patient	Reference
WBC (×10⁹/L)	3.0	4–10
Haemoglobin (mg/dL)	4.8	12–14
MCV (fL)	90	80–99
Platelets (×10⁹/L)	112	150–400

QUESTIONS

1. What is the suspected diagnosis?
2. How would you manage this patient?

Discussion

A 35-year-old Malawian woman presents in a state of sepsis without any clear focal symptoms. She is wasted and severely anaemic and she newly tests HIV-positive.

This is a very common scenario and any physician working in a busy hospital in a high-prevalence setting for HIV in sub-Saharan Africa will encounter similar patients several times a day.

ANSWER TO QUESTION 1

What is the Suspected Diagnosis?

The patient presents with a septic picture; she is newly diagnosed HIV-positive and her wasting and anaemia suggest advanced immunosuppression and/or possible concomitant tuberculosis.

The most common cause of sepsis in HIV-reactive adults in many parts of sub-Saharan Africa is infection with invasive non-typhoidal salmonellae (iNTS).[1,2] The slight abdominal tenderness and her splenomegaly would also fit with this diagnosis.

Enteric fevers (typhoid or paratyphoid) are clinically indistinguishable from infection with iNTS, but typhoid is far less common than iNTS in HIV-positive patients in sub-Saharan Africa. Interestingly, HIV infection seems to protect against typhoid, even though the protection is not absolute. The reason for this phenomenon is unknown.

The severe anaemia that led to the feeling of progressive 'weakness' in this patient is most likely a consequence of infection of her bone marrow with HIV, salmonellae and possibly also with *Mycobacterium tuberculosis*.[3]

Other causes of severe anaemia, such as iron deficiency, worm infections and malaria, are less common in an HIV-positive urban adult population but may have to be considered in other patients, in particular children, pregnant women or in the rural poor.[3] Thalassaemia usually leads to a microcytic anaemia.

Severe anaemia is very common in sub-Saharan Africa. Often patients only present to health care facilities when they are developing heart failure secondary to their anaemia.

ANSWER TO QUESTION 2

How Would You Manage This Patient?

Sepsis is a life-threatening condition and immediate action needs to be taken to prevent organ damage.

Treatment principles for sepsis are the same all over the world; they are based upon early administration of sufficient amounts of fluids and broad-spectrum antibiotics. Both need to be started immediately in the emergency room. Before starting antibiotic treatment blood cultures should be taken.

Since severe anaemia commonly is a sign of tuberculosis, the patient should be assessed for underlying TB. A chest radiograph and an abdominal ultrasound scan should be done.

Of note, anaemia may be the only finding in a patient with TB hiding in the bone marrow and even if all routine investigations are unremarkable, TB should still be high on the list of possible diagnoses if the patient does not make a satisfactory recovery, i.e. remains febrile and/or anaemic or continues to lose weight.

The CD4 count should be checked and the patient should be started on co-trimoxazole preventive treatment as prophylaxis against *Pneumocystis pneumonia*, toxoplasmosis and other opportunistic infections. Antiretroviral therapy (ART) should be started once the acute infection is under control. Her children and her current and past sexual partners should be encouraged to go for an HIV test.

THE CASE CONTINUED ...

Blood cultures were taken and the patient was started on IV ceftriaxone 2 g od, as well as on fluid resuscitation with 2000 mL of normal saline in the first hour. Her blood pressure picked up and she was continued on maintenance fluids.

Blood cultures grew *Salmonella enterica* var Typhimurium. Her antibiotic treatment was changed to oral ciprofloxacin 500 mg bid which was continued for 14 days. TB screening revealed prominent hilar lymph nodes and the patient was also commenced on antituberculous treatment and on antiretroviral therapy. She also received co-trimoxazole prophylaxis, vitamin B6 to prevent peripheral neuropathy and therapeutic feeding.

She was discharged after four weeks in hospital. On review in ART clinic three months later she was feeling much better. She had gained weight and her haemoglobin levels were picking up. Her three children tested negative for HIV. Her ex-husband refused to go for testing.

SUMMARY BOX

Invasive Non-Typhoidal-Salmonellae (iNTS) Infection

Non-typhoidal salmonellae (NTS) usually cause a self-limiting enterocolitis in immunocompetent individuals in industrialized countries. In contrast, in sub-Saharan Africa (SSA) NTS commonly cause invasive disease resulting in sepsis and death.[1,2,4]

There is a pronounced bimodal age distribution in iNTS infection in SSA. It commonly affects children under the age of three with malaria, malnutrition, HIV or sickle cell disease and adults with advanced HIV infection. In Asia, typhoid fever still prevails as a cause of invasive salmonellosis, which may be associated with the lower prevalence of *Plasmodium falciparum* malaria and HIV.

Non-typhoidal salmonellae have a broad host-range, including humans and many vertebrate animals. This is in contrast to the typhoidal serotypes *S. typhi* and *S. paratyphi* which are restricted to humans. In resource-rich countries, transmission is commonly driven by industrialized production of food such as meat, eggs and processed food items. In the developing world commercialized food production and large-scale rearing of animals is still uncommon and both the reservoir and source of infection for iNTS remain unclear. *S. typhimurium* and *S. enteritidis* are the most common serovars, but it is unknown if the same strains cause invasive and diarrhoeal disease and if the modes of transmission are the same.

Infection with iNTS commonly presents as a non-specific septic state. Some patients report abdominal pain or a history of diarrhoea, but often the focus remains clinically unclear. Mild splenomegaly occurs in more than one-third of patients, hepatomegaly is less common. About 30% of patients with iNTS have a concomitant lower respiratory tract co-infection, with pathogens such as *M. tuberculosis* or *Streptococcus pneumoniae*. Severe anaemia is common and should prompt the clinician to look carefully for signs of TB co-infection.

Diagnosis is by proof of the pathogen in blood cultures and all febrile patients in SSA should have blood cultures irrespective of the result of their malaria test.

Management of patients with iNTS infection who commonly are septic on admission includes early initiation of antibiotic treatment and appropriate fluid resuscitation, as in any other septic condition.

Antibiotic choice depends upon the local resistance pattern but usually empirical management includes either a fluoroquinolone or, if oral intake is not possible, a third generation cephalosporin. Azithromycin is an alternative. Effective antibiotic treatment should be given for 10–14 days. Antiretroviral therapy should be started urgently to prevent relapses. The case fatality rate of patients with iNTS is high (22–47%).[2]

Further Reading

1. Feasey NA, Gordon MA. Salmonella infections. In: Farrar J, editor. Manson's Tropical Diseases. 23rd ed. London: Elsevier; 2013 [chapter 25].
2. Feasey NA, Dougan G, Kingsley RA, et al. Invasive non-typhoidal salmonella disease: an emerging and neglected tropical disease in Africa. Lancet 2012;379(9835):2489–99.
3. Lewis DK, Whitty CJ, Walsh AL, et al. Treatable factors associated with severe anaemia in adults admitted to medical wards in Blantyre, Malawi, an area of high HIV seroprevalence. Trans R Soc Trop Med Hyg 2005;99(8):561–7.
4. Reddy EA, Shaw AV, Crump JA. Community-acquired bloodstream infections in Africa: a systematic review and meta-analysis. Lancet Infect Dis 2010;10(6):417–32.

A 12-YEAR-OLD BOY FROM RURAL KENYA WITH PAINFUL EYES

30

Hillary K. Rono / Andrew Bastawrous / Nicholas A.V. Beare

Clinical Presentation

HISTORY

A 12-year-old boy is brought to a health centre in rural north-west Kenya. He reports a two-month history of pain, watering and redness of both eyes. The watering of his eyes is worse in the sun and he is struggling to keep his eyes open.

Six months previously he was treated at a dispensary for similar, but less severe symptoms. He was given a course of tetracycline ointment but his symptoms did not improve. Following this, he went to a traditional healer who applied some herbal medication made from juice extracts from the ecucuka plant (*Aloe vera* species). After instillation he experienced severe eye pain and discharge, both eyes became red and his vision was reduced.

The boy lives with his parents in the hot, dusty and dry area of Loima in Turkana County. They keep large herds of cows and sheep and the boy helps with herding and watering the animals. They fetch water for domestic use from a dried river bed about 6 kilometres from their home.

CLINICAL FINDINGS

A 12-year-old boy who appears systemically fit and well. Visual acuity is markedly reduced in both eyes. He can only perceive hand movements in the right eye and the vision is 6/60 in the left eye. The findings on inspection of his eyes are shown in Table 30-1 and Figures 30-1, 30-2.

QUESTIONS

1. What are your differential diagnoses?
2. What features fit the criteria for trachoma?

TABLE 30-1	Findings on Inspection of Both Eyes	
	Right Eye	**Left Eye**
Lid	Upper lids swollen, eyelashes turned inwards. Crusts	
Conjunctiva	Severely inflamed	
	>5 follicles identified on eversion	
	Scarring of the upper tarsal conjunctivae	
	Right eye: Limbal (peri-corneal) follicle	
Cornea	Multiple corneal scars with whitening/opacification	Corneal scars
	Central cornea thin	Central cornea thin
	Fibrovascular pannus on the upper cornea	Perforated corneal ulcer with adherent leucoma (white, opaque scar)
Anterior chamber	Deep, other details not clearly seen	Shallow
		Pupil constricted and deformed

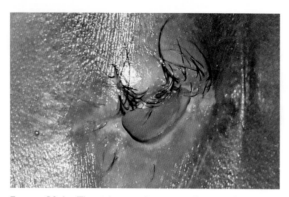

FIGURE 30-1   The right eye showing trichiasis and extensive corneal opacification.

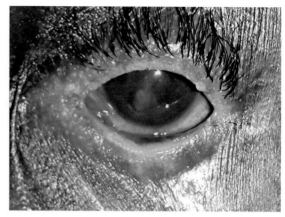

FIGURE 30-2   The left eye with a perforated corneal ulcer and adherent leucoma.

Discussion

A 12-year-old Kenyan boy from a pastoralist community, who lives in a hot and arid area, presents with pain and redness of his eyes, eye discharge and poor vision. He has a history of using traditional eye medicine. On examination he has trichiasis, conjunctival follicles and scarring, limbal follicles and corneal opacities. One eye has got a perforating ulcer with adherent leucoma.

ANSWER TO QUESTION 1

What Are Your Differential Diagnoses?

The most important diagnoses to consider given the clinical presentation and the setting are:

1. Corneal ulcer from use of traditional medicine.
2. Trachomatous trichiasis.
3. Vitamin A deficiency.

Important further information needed would include the daily dietary intake, previous history of measles predisposing to vitamin A deficiency, a full blood count and, ideally, blood retinol levels.

ANSWER TO QUESTION 2

What Features Fit the Criteria for Trachoma?

For the diagnosis of trachoma, two out of five clinical criteria need to be fulfilled. This boy is showing all five criteria:

1. Follicles on the flat tarsal conjunctiva.
2. Conjunctival scarring at the upper tarsal conjunctiva.
3. Limbal follicles or Herbert's pits.
4. Fibrovascular Pannus, mostly at the upper limbus.
5. Trichiasis on the upper lid.

THE CASE CONTINUED ...

The child was diagnosed with bilateral trachomatous trichiasis (TT), corneal opacity (CO) of the right eye and a perforating corneal ulcer of the left eye.

He was admitted and given oral azithromycin. He was referred to the ophthalmologist for trichiasis surgery and for a conjunctival flap to seal the corneal defect.

SUMMARY BOX

Trachoma

Trachoma, caused by *Chlamydia trachomatis*, is the leading infectious cause of blindness in the world.[1] It accounts for about 3% of the world's blindness, with currently 8 million people being irreversibly visually impaired.

Trachoma is common in poor rural communities, where there is scarcity of water, poor sanitation and low socioeconomic status. The spread occurs due to overcrowding within households. Women are affected more than men and younger children are at greater risk of infection, especially children under five years.[2]

After repeated infections in childhood, signs of trachoma progress from inflammation to conjunctival scarring. Scarring of the tarsal conjunctiva leads to inversion of the lid resulting in trichiasis, corneal scarring and consecutive visual impairment.

A simplified scheme for assessing and classifying trachoma based on clinical signs has been developed. The stages are:
Trachomatous inflammation with follicles (TF)
Intense trachomatous inflammation (TI)
Trachomatous conjunctival scarring (TS)
Trachomatous trichiasis (TT) and
Corneal opacity due to trachoma (CO).[3]

TF and TI are prevalent in young children and are manifestations of moderate and severe active disease, respectively, while TT is common in adults.[2]

The WHO initiated a global programme to eliminate trachoma as a disease of public health importance by 2020 (GET 2020). This programme includes mass antibiotic administrations to reduce the prevalence of *Chlamydia* infections, facial cleanliness, surgery and environmental improvement – the SAFE strategy:[4]

S Surgery for advanced cases.

A Antibiotic treatment.

F Facial cleanliness to reduce transmission.

E Environmental improvements.

Both tetracyclines and macrolides are effective against trachoma in its acute stage (TF and TI). Tetracycline eye ointment can be given twice daily for six weeks. However, in practice compliance with this treatment is poor. A single dose of azithromycin is equally effective and more convenient (20 mg/kg for children, 1 g for adults). The WHO recommends three years of azithromycin-distribution as part of a trachoma control programme in communities where active trachoma is present in >10% of children. However, without additional environmental improvements antibiotic treatment will not have a permanent effect. Communities need to secure suitable water supply, build and use well-designed latrines, safely dispose of their rubbish, and house animals some distance apart from the family home.[1]

Further Reading

1. Beare NV, Bastawrous A. Ophthalmology in the tropics and sub-tropics. In: Farrar J, editor. Manson's Tropical Diseases. 23rd ed. Lomndon: Elsevier; 2013 [chapter 67].
2. Mabey DC, Solomon AW, Foster A. Trachoma. Lancet 2003;362(9379):223–9.
3. Negrel AD, Mariotti SP. Trachoma rapid assessment: rationale and basic principles. Community Eye Health/Int Cent Eye Health 1999;12(32):51–3.
4. Emerson PM, Burton M, Solomon AW, et al. The SAFE strategy for trachoma control: using operational research for policy, planning and implementation. Bull WHO 2006;84(8):613–19.

A 6-YEAR-OLD BOY FROM MALAWI WITH FEVER, COUGH AND IMPAIRED CONSCIOUSNESS

Charlotte Adamczick

Clinical Presentation

HISTORY

You review a 6-year-old boy in the paediatric high dependency unit of a Malawian Central Hospital. The boy was admitted the night before because of a high fever, dyspnoea and a dry cough which started three days before. On admission he was started on antibiotics and presumptive antimalaria treatment; the results of the malaria smear are pending.

The boy is known to be HIV-reactive. Antiretroviral therapy (ART) was deferred on his last visit to the clinic six months ago when his CD4 count was high and he was clinically not deemed eligible for ART (WHO clinical stage 2).

CLINICAL FINDINGS

Examination reveals a sick child with a temperature of 39.8°C and laboured breathing. The Blantyre coma score is 3/5. The boy has coryza and a bilateral conjunctivitis. Behind both ears and on the forehead you notice a fine maculopapular rash that has not been described before. There is bilateral axillary lymphadenopathy.

QUESTIONS

1. What is your most important differential diagnosis?
2. What complications should you expect and how do you manage the patient?

Discussion

An HIV-positive boy presents with high fever, dry cough, coryza, conjunctivitis and impaired level of consciousness together with a fine maculopapular rash on the neck and face.

ANSWER TO QUESTION 1

What is Your Most Important Differential Diagnosis?

At initial presentation his symptoms and signs are rather nonspecific and the list of differential diagnoses is long, ranging from malaria and typhoid fever to atypical pneumonia and various viral infections.

However, in hospital the boy develops a rash which, in combination with the three 'Cs' of cough, coryza and conjunctivitis, should raise the suspicion of measles. He has passed the prodromal stage and is showing signs of the following exanthematous stage.

Bright red spots with a whitish centre ('Koplik's spots') on the buccal mucosa would be pathognomic, however, they may be absent or may appear only for a short period of time. In this case they were not seen.

Other infections that present with an exanthema and are often mistaken for measles are scarlet fever, meningococcaemia, rickettsial spotted fever, rubella, entervoirus infection and infectious mononucleosis.

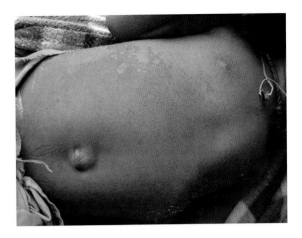

FIGURE 31-1 Scaling of the erythematous rash.

ANSWER TO QUESTION 2

What Complications Should You Expect and How Do You Manage the Patient?

This boy is immunocompromised by his HIV infection, even though he was deemed clinically stable and not eligible for ART six months ago. Complications in measles are much more common in individuals with cellular immune defects than in the immunocompetent. Severe diarrhoea, septicaemia, giant cell pneumonia, superimposed bacterial pneumonia, encephalitis, otitis media and corneal ulcerations can complicate the course of disease. In this case, with a reduced Blantyre Coma Scale and laboured breathing, encephalitis and pulmonary involvement have to be considered.

Since the rash has only just appeared, the boy is still contagious. He needs to be separated from other patients, but still monitored closely with supplementation of fluids and oxygen.

Exposed patients on the ward without vaccination coverage should receive vaccination within three days if not they are too sick. Human gamma-globulin would protect contacts as well, but is not readily available in most settings.

THE CASE CONTINUED ...

The patient was put on IV fluids because his oral intake was insufficient. Vitamin A was added to the treatment for corneal protection. The malaria smear came back negative and antimalarial treatment was stopped. After three days the rash had spread over the trunk, and skin scaling appeared over the abdominal wall (Figure 31-1). The boy developed severe pneumonia, which was treated with antibiotics to cover for bacterial superinfection. The CD4 count came back below 300/μL. Antiretroviral therapy was started in clinic after full recovery.

SUMMARY BOX

Measles

Measles is a highly contagious viral infection, caused by a paramyxovirus and transmitted through droplets.[1,2] There is no animal reservoir. The course of disease is strongly influenced by both nutritional and immune status of the affected individual.[3]

Around 232 000 measles cases were reported in 2012, but WHO estimate that the true number of people affected may be as high as 20 million.

The Case Fatality Rate (CFR) in Europe is 0.3 per 1000 whereas worldwide CFRs range between 3 and 5%. In settings such as refugee camps the CFR can be as high as 30%. More than 95% of deaths occur in developing countries, mostly in children below the age of five years.[3] Recent outbreaks have even been reported from industrialized countries where the vaccination coverage is waning, often due to parental hesitancy.

The incubation period is approximately 8–12 days. The initial prodromal stage presents with fever, conjunctivitis, rhinitis and cough. On day 3–4, a maculopapular rash starts on the forehead and neck, spreading over the trunk and limbs. The rash lasts for 5–6 days, followed by severe desquamation. The patient is highly contagious from about four days before up to four days after the appearance of the exanthema.

Continued on following page

Immunocompromised individuals may not show the rash ('white measles') but are very vulnerable to developing complications,[4] such as giant cell pneumonitis, superimposed bacterial or viral pneumonia, otitis media, severe keratoconjunctivitis and encephalomyelitis. Furthermore, a sub-acute 'inclusion-body' measles encephalitis has been described in the immunocompromised, which occurs a few months after the acute measles infection.

A late complication is sub-acute sclerosing panencephalitis (SSPE), which appears several years after measles infection and is invariably fatal. Estimates as to the incidence of SSPE vary between one per 10000 and one per million cases of measles.

There is no specific antiviral treatment. In developing countries, all children with measles should receive vitamin A supplementation which prevents blindness and death. Vaccination, or application of human immunoglobulin within six days of exposure,[1] can protect non-vaccinated contacts.

Routine measles vaccination of children is recommended by WHO. Almost 100% of children vaccinated with two doses of this live vaccine will have protective immunity if the first dose is given after 12 months of age. Maternal transplacental antibodies may inhibit vaccine efficacy up to the age of 6–12 months. However, in areas of high endemicity, the first dose is usually given at nine months of age and even vaccination at six months may be used in high risk-situations, such as outbreaks, despite lower seroconversion rates. Ideally, children who receive their first dose in the first year of life should receive two additional doses, separated by a minimum of four weeks after their first birthday.

The measles vaccine is safe in most children. Asymptomatic and not severely immunocompromised HIV-positive children may receive measles vaccine because the risk of acquiring wild virus disease outweighs the risks of the vaccine. Severely immunocompromised HIV infected persons should not receive measles vaccine.

Further Reading

1. Munoz FM. Viral exanthemas. In: Farrar J, editor. Manson's Tropical Diseases. 23rd ed. London: Elsevier; 2013 [chapter 20].
2. Solomon T. Virus infections of the nervous system. In: Farrar J, editor. Manson's Tropical Diseases. 23rd ed. London: Elsevier; 2013 [chapter 21].
3. Minetti A, Kagoli M, Katsulukuta A, et al. Lessons and challenges for measles control from unexpected large outbreak, Malawi. Emerg Infect Dis 2013;19(2):202–9.
4. Taha TE, Graham SM, Kumwenda NI, et al. Morbidity among human immunodeficiency virus-1-infected and -uninfected African children. Pediatrics 2000;106(6):E77.

A 44-YEAR-OLD MALE FARMER FROM LAOS WITH DIABETES AND A BACK ABSCESS

32

Sayaphet Rattanavong / Valy Keoluangkhot /
Siho Sisouphonh / Vatthanaphone Latthaphasavang /
David Dance / Caoimhe Nic Fhogartaigh

Clinical Presentation

HISTORY

A 44-year-old male rice farmer presents to a provincial hospital in Southern Laos in the rainy season with a one-month history of fever, headache, generalized myalgia and arthralgia, and a painful swelling over the left scapula. The swelling has gradually increased in size, without any history of preceding trauma. He has not noticed any lesions elsewhere. He was diagnosed with type 2 diabetes four years previously, but was not compliant with oral antidiabetic drugs or follow-up. The lesion on his back was incised and drained at a local health centre the previous week, since when he has been taking cloxacillin 1 g four times daily. However, there has been no improvement and during the two days prior to admission he has deteriorated, with high fever, chills and severe malaise.

CLINICAL FINDINGS

The patient appears septic, with a fever of 40°C, a heart rate of 136 bpm, blood pressure of 140/80 mmHg and a respiratory rate of 30 breath cycles per minute. He is pale and jaundiced. In the left scapular region there is an erythematous swelling of 2.5×4 cm with pus discharging from a central wound (Figure 32-1). There is no regional lymphadenopathy. On chest auscultation there are bilateral crepitations and reduced breath sounds at both lung bases. Heart sounds are normal. The abdomen is soft, without any palpable organomegaly.

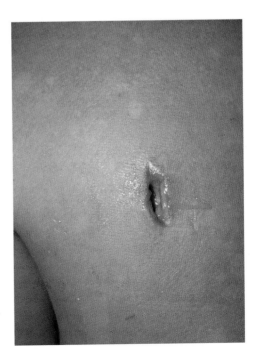

FIGURE 32-1 Wound on the patient's left shoulder, after incision and drainage of the abscess. (Side finding: hypopigmented macular skin lesions of Pityriasis versicolor (Malassezia spp.), commonly seen in humid tropical climates.)

TABLE 32-1   Laboratory Results

Parameter	Patient	Reference Range
WBC (×10⁹/L)	16.2	6.0–8.0
Polymorphs (%)	92.1	45–70
Haemoglobin (g/dL)	12.5	12.0–16.0
Platelets (×10⁹/L)	112	150–300
Glucose (mmol/L)	20.6	4.1–6.1
Serum creatinine (µmol/L)	56	62–120
Urea (mmol/L)	6.8	5.4–16.1
AST (U/L)	131	0–37
ALT (U/L)	83	0–40
Serum total bilirubin (µmol/L)	111.2	1.71–20.5
Serum direct bilirubin (µmol/L)	56.4	0–7

LABORATORY RESULTS

The laboratory results are shown in Table 32-1.

QUESTIONS

1. What are your differential diagnoses?
2. What additional investigations would you like to do?

Discussion

A male Lao rice famer presents during the rainy season with prolonged fever, jaundice, a back abscess and chest signs. He is a known type 2 diabetic but has been non-compliant with his antidiabetic medication.

ANSWER TO QUESTION 1

What Are Your Differential Diagnoses?

Bacterial abscess with sepsis may be caused by *Staphylococcus aureus*, *Streptococcus pyogenes* or other *Streptococcus* spp., *Klebsiella pneumoniae*, *Vibrio vulnificus* or anaerobes. This patient, however, has epidemiological and clinical risk factors for melioidosis, caused by *Burkholderia pseudomallei*. This may cause a spectrum of disease in immunocompromised patients, especially diabetics, ranging from localized abscesses to pneumonia and septicaemia with disseminated abscess formation and high mortality. There is often no history of an inoculation injury or trauma.

Tuberculosis should also be considered with the sub-acute history of abscess with respiratory findings, however tuberculous abscesses are usually 'cold', without much pain, erythema or warmth.

Disseminated fungal infection seems unlikely, but would be possible if there was additional immunocompromise such as HIV.

ANSWER TO QUESTION 2

What Additional Investigations Would You Like to Do?

Essential investigations include blood culture and abscess swab (or deep pus) for microscopy and culture. A throat swab, or sputum sample if there is pulmonary involvement, may also be cultured on selective media, such as Ashdown's agar. A chest radiograph (CXR) should be done looking for evidence of pneumonia or pleural effusion. An ultrasound of the abdomen, or other imaging such as CT or MRI scan, should also be considered, as the findings of liver and splenic abscesses would strongly support a diagnosis of melioidosis while culture results are awaited. Biochemistry assays to check glucose and creatinine are important to optimize glycaemic control and adjust drug dosage, respectively. Depending on the CXR findings, sputum, pleural fluid and pus may be sent for staining for acid-fast bacilli (e.g. Ziehl–Neelsen stain).

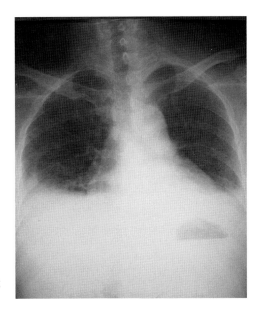

FIGURE 32-2 Admission chest radiograph of the patient, showing bilateral pleural effusions.

THE CASE CONTINUED ...

Pus culture yielded *B. pseudomallei* after 48 hours, and later his blood culture also grew the same bacterium. Three throat swabs were cultured on selective media but failed to grow the organism. The CXR revealed bilateral pleural effusions (Figure 32-2). A shoulder radiograph showed no evidence of bony involvement. Abdominal ultrasound showed hepatosplenomegaly without evidence of liver or splenic abscesses.

The patient was empirically treated with ceftriaxone and gentamicin while awaiting the culture results. Treatment was switched to ceftazidime after 48 hours when the laboratory alerted the clinicians to the suspicion of melioidosis. The patient improved after seven days of treatment and was afebrile by day 14, when he was switched to oral co-trimoxazole plus doxycycline to complete 20 weeks. Glycaemic control was established. No other foci of infection were detected by locally available investigations. The patient was discharged after 21 days of hospitalization and continued on oral 'eradication' treatment for five months. He remains well.

SUMMARY BOX

Melioidosis

Melioidosis is an infectious disease caused by *Burkholderia pseudomallei*, an environmental saprophyte endemic to South-east Asia and northern Australia. The disease is being described with increasing frequency, probably due to a combination of greater awareness, improving laboratory facilities in endemic areas and possibly a genuine increase in incidence.[1,2] North-eastern Thailand and northern Australia are highly endemic areas, where *B. pseudomallei* is an important cause of community-acquired sepsis and pneumonia.[3,4] It is probably widely distributed elsewhere in the tropics and may be greatly under-diagnosed.[1]

Humans are thought usually to become infected by inoculation through cuts and abrasions (e.g. whilst working in rice fields), inhalation during heavy monsoon rain and winds, and possibly ingestion, although it is often difficult to determine precisely the mode of acquisition.[2] Host factors are very important; the majority of cases occur in those who are immunocompromised, especially with diabetes mellitus, but also renal disease, thalassaemia, steroid use, but surprisingly not HIV infection.[2,4] The disease is highly seasonal, with 80% of cases presenting during the wet season.[4]

Clinical presentation varies from benign localized infection to rapidly progressive septicaemia. The bacteraemic form accounts for 40–60% of cases and carries a mortality of 19–65%,[2] but even with appropriate treatment this may be as high as 80% in advanced infections with septic shock.[4] The organism may localize in the lungs, liver, spleen, prostate, parotid, skin and soft tissue, bones and joints, or the central nervous system, causing abscesses and granulomas, but approximately 15% of bacteraemic cases have no evident clinical focus.[4] It is important to use available imaging to identify the extent of infection and monitor the course of treatment. The confirmation of the diagnosis of melioidosis is based on the isolation and identification of *B. pseudomallei* in clinical samples, and in endemic areas it may be possible to reduce the time to diagnosis using immunofluorescence on pus or sputum, and *B. pseudomallei* antigen latex agglutination on isolates. Serology and PCR have relatively low sensitivity and specificity.

Continued on following page

Parenteral antibiotics (e.g. ceftazidime, meropenem) are usually given for two weeks in the acute phase, followed by oral co-trimoxazole to complete 12–20 weeks eradication therapy to minimize risk of relapse. This recommendation is based upon a recently published randomised controlled trial which demonstrated that co-trimoxazole monotherapy was non-inferior to, and better tolerated than, co-trimoxazole and doxycycline dual therapy.[5] For patients unable to take co-trimoxazole, co-amoxiclav is an alternative but has higher relapse rates. Supportive treatment of sepsis and surgical drainage of abscesses are important in optimizing outcome.

Further Reading

1. Dance DAB. Melioidosis. In: Farrar J, editor. Manson's Tropical Diseases. 23rd ed. London: Elsevier; 2013 [chapter 34].
2. Cheng AC, Currie BJ. Melioidosis: epidemiology, pathophysiology and management. Clin Microb Rev 2005;18(2): 383–416.
3. Limmathurotsakul D, Wongrattanacheewin S, Teerawatanasook N, et al. Increasing incidence of human melioidosis in Northeast Thailand. Am J Trop Med Hyg 2010;82(6):1113–17.
4. Currie BJ, Ward L, Cheng AC. The epidemiology and clinical spectrum of melioidosis: 540 cases from the 20 year Darwin prospective study. PLoS Negl Trop Dis 2010;4(11):e900.
5. Chetchotisakd P, Chierakul W, Chaowagul W, et al. Trimethoprim-sulphamethoxazole versus trimethoprim-sulphameth-oxazole and doxycycline as oral eradicative treatment for melioidosis (MERTH): a multicentre, double-blind, non-inferiority, randomised controlled trial. Lancet 2013;doi:10.1016/S0140-6736(13)61951-0.

A 53-YEAR-OLD MAN FROM MALAWI WITH A CHRONIC COUGH

33

Camilla Rothe

Clinical Presentation

HISTORY

A 53-year-old Malawian man presents to a local hospital because of a productive cough for three months. He also reports night sweats and that he has lost some weight, but he is unable to quantify this.

Two months earlier he presented to a health centre with the same complaints. He was given presumptive antimalarials and amoxicillin for five days, but to no avail. The patient is not aware of any tuberculosis (TB) contacts. He is currently not on any medication and his past medical history is unremarkable. He is a farmer. He has never worked in a mine or in the construction industry. He is a non-smoker. He is married with five children; all are well.

CLINICAL FINDINGS

The patient is a 53-year-old man, slightly wasted. Temperature 38.8°C, blood pressure 100/80 mmHg, pulse 88 bpm, oxygen saturation 97% in ambient air. He appears mildly anaemic. On inspection of his mouth there is no oral thrush, no Kaposi's sarcoma and no oral hairy leukoplakia. His chest is clear and there are normal heart sounds without any murmurs. There is no lymphadenopathy; liver and spleen are not enlarged.

INVESTIGATIONS

The patient is sent for HIV voluntary counselling and testing. The HIV test result is reactive. His further laboratory results are shown in Table 33-1.

CHEST RADIOGRAPHY

His chest radiograph on admission shows prominent hili bilaterally but is otherwise normal (Figure 33-1).

TABLE 33-1 Laboratory Results on Admission		
Parameter	Patient	Reference
WBC (×10⁹/L)	3.2	4–10
Haemoglobin (g/dL)	9.8	13–15
MCV (fL)	90	80–98
Platelets (×10⁹/L)	305	150–350
CD4 count (cells/μL)	54	500–1200
Sputum for AFB	2× negative	Negative
Malaria RDT	Negative	Negative
Thick smear for *Plasmodium* spp.	Negative	Negative

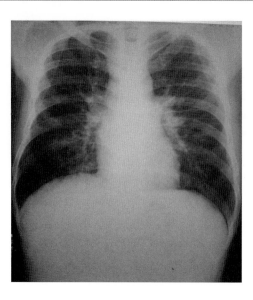

FIGURE 33-1 Chest radiograph on admission showing a prominent hilar region.

QUESTIONS

1. What is your suspected diagnosis?
2. How would you approach this patient?

Discussion

A 53-year-old Malawian man present with chronic cough and constitutional symptoms. A course of oral antibiotics did not bring any improvement. The patient is not aware of any TB contacts. On admission he is newly diagnosed with HIV and advanced immunosuppression. His sputum microscopy is negative for acid-fast bacilli (AFB). Chest radiography shows a prominent hilar region but is otherwise normal.

ANSWER TO QUESTION 1

What is Your Suspected Diagnosis?

In all HIV-positive patients with cough and weight loss who do not respond to antibiotics, tuberculosis is top of the list of differential diagnoses. In this case the most likely diagnosis is smear-negative TB.

TB in patients with advanced immunosuppression often presents with a clinical picture that is very different from immunocompetent individuals, and sputum smear-negative TB, which is uncommon in HIV-negative patients, is commonly seen in HIV-infected patients. The slightly prominent hilar region seen in the patient's chest radiograph is highly compatible with intrathoracic lymphadenopathy which is typical though not specific for TB. Physical examination of the chest is normal in about half of HIV-reactive patients with pulmonary TB.

The fact that the patient does not report any TB contact should not be overvalued. Firstly, TB in immunosuppression is often a consequence of reactivation and the primary infection may have been decades ago. Secondly, in resource-limited countries with high HIV prevalence, practically everyone is exposed to TB – this could occur though a ride on an overcrowded minibus or when congregating with friends and family in someone's small home in a high-density area.

Given that our patient is in an advanced stage of immunosuppression and has not taken any co-trimoxazole prophylaxis an alternative or possibly co-existing diagnosis to consider is *Pneumocystis jirovecii* pneumonia (PCP). A concomitant bacterial chest infection is possible but unlikely to explain the whole three months of illness.

Kaposi's sarcoma (KS) of the lung is another differential diagnosis to consider, but patients with pulmonary KS usually have manifestations of KS elsewhere (skin, oral mucosa). On chest radiography patchy infiltrations are commonly seen in the lower lung zones. Neither was the case in our patient, which makes this diagnosis unlikely.

Pulmonary malignancy or pulmonary sarcoidosis, which would be high on the list of differential diagnoses in industrialized countries, are much less likely than an infectious cause in the given setting.

ANSWER TO QUESTION 2

How Would You Approach This Patient?

Induced sputum could be examined for AFB. Novel real-time PCR-based tests such as XPert MTB/RIF are easy to use, more sensitive than microscopy and also help detect rifampicin resistance. Thanks to an endorsement by WHO and international donor support, XPert MTB/RIF is increasingly available even at remote hospitals in rural areas.

Mycobacterial cultures of the sputum should be done but results will take several weeks, too long to guide the clinician's acute decision.

If none of these investigations were available, it would still be justifiable to empirically start the patient on antituberculous treatment, since smear-negative TB is common and fatal if untreated.

The question of whether the patient should be started on anti-PCP treatment in addition to antituberculous therapy may be disputed amongst physicians. Since there are usually no diagnostic means available to diagnose PCP (the gold standard being bronchoscopy with lavage and microscopy) the infection cannot be ruled out.

PCP patients may present with normal oxygen saturations at rest but often desaturate on exercise test. This test may guide clinicians in their decision, but a normal exercise test cannot rule out PCP. If it is decided against treatment for PCP the patient should be started on a prophylactic dose of co-trimoxazole.

Additional antibiotic treatment should be considered in this febrile patient with advanced immunosuppression. Blood cultures should be taken in any febrile patient before starting antibiotic treatment. Apart from chest infections, Gram-negative sepsis secondary to non-typhoidal salmonellae needs to be considered.

THE CASE CONTINUED ...

Induced sputum results came back negative for AFBs and there was no sputum PCR available. His oxygen saturation on exercise test (walking down the corridor three times at a fast pace) was 98% as opposed to 97% at rest, and therefore negative.

The patient was treated for a possible bacterial chest infection, covering also for Gram-negative bacteria. He received ceftriaxone 2 g IV od and erythromycin 500 mg qid for five days. It was decided not to treat him for PCP and he received the prophylactic dose of co-trimoxazole (480 mg bid according to local national guidelines). Nonetheless, his fever persisted, even though the cough subjectively improved slightly.

TABLE 33-2 Clinical Presentation of TB in Patients With and Without Immunosuppression		
	HIV-negative or high CD4 count (>200/μL)	**Low CD4 count (≤200/μL)**
Cough and sputum production	Severe, productive	Often mild, small amounts of whitish sputum
Haemoptysis	Common	Rare
Chest radiography appearance	Cavities, upper lobe infiltrates and destruction	No cavities Infiltrates Hilar lymphadenopathy Miliary pattern May be completely normal
Sputum smear result	Often positive	Often negative
Extrapulmonary and disseminated TB*	≤20% of TB cases	Common, about 50%

*Disseminated = involving two or more non-contiguous organs concomitantly.
Source: *After Harries et al.,[3] Sharma et al.[4]*

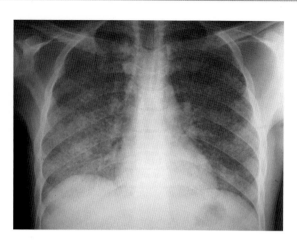

FIGURE 33-2 Chest radiograph of a patient with miliary TB.

On day 7 in hospital the patient was started on empirical treatment for smear-negative TB. After the first week of treatment, he started to feel better. His fever went down and the cough gradually settled. He was discharged home. Three weeks into TB treatment he was seen at the HIV clinic. He was doing well and had started antiretroviral therapy.

SUMMARY BOX

Tuberculosis in HIV-Infected Patients

Tuberculosis (TB) and HIV infection are the most important 'tropical' diseases in adults in many parts of sub-Saharan Africa. Co-infection with HIV and TB is common and poses a particular challenge to the clinician.[1]

Clinical presentation of TB changes with declining peripheral CD4 counts (Table 33-2).

Cavitating, smear-positive pulmonary TB, as seen classically in HIV-negative individuals, is uncommon in advanced immunosuppression.[1,2] Instead, patients more commonly present with sputum smear-negative TB. CXR may be completely normal and clinical symptoms are often discrete; patients may produce little sputum and haemoptysis is rare.

In HIV-reactive individuals there is also a higher percentage of extrapulmonary TB manifesting as pleural effusion, pericardial disease, extrathoracic lymph node TB, abdominal TB, TB meningitis and miliary disease (Figure 33-2). Severe anaemia is a common clinical clue to a co-infection with HIV/TB and reflects bone marrow involvement. Disseminated TB affecting two or more non-contiguous organs is also common.

Treatment of HIV/TB co-infected patients is also challenging. The rate of adverse events is higher and there are a number of pharmacokinetic interactions between rifampicin and antiretroviral drugs, mainly the non-nucleoside reverse transcriptase inhibitor (NNRTI) nevirapine and protease inhibitors.

Further Reading

1. Thwaites G. Tuberculosis. In: Farrar J, editor. Manson's tropical diseases. 23rd ed. London: Elsevier; 2013 [chapter 40].
2. Harries AD, Maher D, Nunn P. An approach to the problems of diagnosing and treating adult smear-negative pulmonary tuberculosis in high-HIV-prevalence settings in sub-Saharan Africa. Bull WHO 1998;76(6):651–62.
3. Harries AD, Maher D, Graham SM. HIV-related TB. In: WHO, editor. TB/HIV – A clinical manual. 2nd ed. Geneva: WHO; 2004. p. 36–8.
4. Sharma SK, Mohan A, Kadhiravan T. HIV-TB co-infection: epidemiology, diagnosis and management. Ind J Med Res 2005;121(4):550–67.

TABLE 35-1 Laboratory Results on Admission		
Parameter	**Patient**	**Reference**
WBC ($\times 10^9$/L)	3.7	4–10
Haemoglobin (g/dL)	10.2	12–16
MCV (fL)	92	80–98
Platelets ($\times 10^9$/L)	91	150–350
Fasting blood glucose (mmol/L)	5.43	5.0–6.7
Malaria RDT	Negative	Negative

TABLE 35-2 CSF Results on Admission		
Parameter	**Patient**	**Reference**
Leukocytes (cells/µL)	18	0–5
Protein (g/L)	0.8	0.15–0.40
Glucose (mmol/L)	1.97	2.22–3.88
India Ink	Negative	Negative
Culture	*C. neoformans*	Negative

Discussion

The patient presents with a chronic headache and 'blurred vision'. She is wasted and has a unilateral abducens nerve palsy. She is afebrile and has no neck stiffness. The full blood count shows normocytic anaemia and thrombocytopenia.

ANSWER TO QUESTION 1

What Are Your Differential Diagnoses?

The patient's clinical presentation suggests chronic meningitis. The two most important differential diagnoses are cryptococcal meningitis and tuberculous meningitis. Also, partially treated bacterial meningitis is a possibility, but the gradual onset of symptoms makes this less likely.

Chronic meningitis is commonly associated with immunosuppression. The patient lives in a part of the world with a high HIV prevalence. Her laboratory findings (anaemia, thrombocytopenia) are also common in untreated HIV infection.

Even though malaria may present with nonspecific symptoms and both thrombocytopenia and anaemia are commonly seen in malaria patients, the absence of fever, the negative rapid diagnostic test (RDT) and the history of taking artemisinin combination therapy make it an unlikely differential diagnosis. Also, malaria usually does not cause cranial nerve palsies.

ANSWER TO QUESTION 2

What Investigations Would You Like to Do?

AN HIV test is crucial and a lumbar puncture should be done without delay. Cerebrospinal fluid (CSF) opening pressure should be measured and documented. Routine CSF examination should include India Ink stain and bacterial and fungal cultures. If possible, cryptococcal antigen (CrAg) should be tested in blood and CSF.

THE CASE CONTINUED ...

A lumbar puncture was done on admission. The CSF looked clear, but the opening pressure was noted to be 50 cmH$_2$O (10–18 cmH$_2$O). The CSF results are shown in Table 35-2.

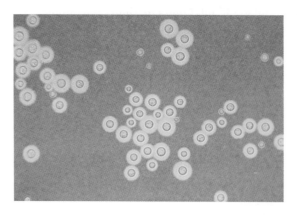

FIGURE 35-2 Photomicrograph of *Crytococcus neoformans* (India Ink stain). (*Source: www.cdc.gov; www.cdc.gov/fungal/cryptococcosis-neoformans/*)

A diagnosis of cryptoccocal meningitis was made based upon the positive fungal culture result. India Ink was negative, but sensitivity is only at around 50–70%.[1] CrAg, which is >95% sensitive, was not available.

The HIV serology came back reactive. The CD4 count was 22/μL. The patient was started on oral fluconazole 1200 mg (see Summary Box) and on co-trimoxazole prophylaxis. She received repeated therapeutic lumbar punctures until the headache settled.

Four weeks into her antifungal treatment antiretroviral therapy was started, she went back to her village and died after six weeks of an unknown cause.

SUMMARY BOX

Cryptococcal Meningitis

Cryptococcal meningitis (CM) occurs worldwide. Ninety-five per cent of CM cases in developing countries are HIV-associated. CM is the most common cause of adult meningitis in sub-Saharan Africa and parts of Asia where HIV prevalence is high.[2]

Cryptococcal meningitis is caused by the encapsulated environmental yeast *Cryptococcus neoformans*.[3] It is an opportunistic infection which occurs at advanced stages of immunosuppression, mostly at CD4 counts below 100/μL. Patients usually present with a subacute headache of several days to weeks duration. Other common clinical findings are cranial nerve palsies (N VI), confusion and impaired consciousness. CM is clinically indistinguishable from tuberculous meningitis (TbM), although fever and neck stiffness are more common in TbM.

CSF opening pressure is often markedly elevated. Further CSF findings are often nonspecific, and the CSF may even be normal. Diagnosis of CM is made by demonstrating the fungus in the CSF. This is done by culture, staining techniques (e.g. India Ink, Figure 35-2.) or by using a cryptococcal antigen-detection test (CrAg).

Recommended treatment is an induction therapy of combined amphotericin B plus flucytosine for the initial two weeks,[4] followed by oral fluconazole 400 mg daily for at least eight weeks and fluconazole maintenance therapy 200 mg daily until immunoreconstitution.

The reality in many resource-limited settings is different, and often oral fluconazole is the only available drug.[5] Fluconazole is fungistatic, which may be effective as a secondary prophylaxis, but is less useful as induction therapy when potent fungicidal drugs are needed to rapidly bring down the fungal burden.

Many patients with CM suffer from severe headache which does not respond to conventional analgesics. The headache is due to raised intracranial pressure (ICP) and therapeutic lumbar punctures bring immediate pain relief. LPs may have to be repeated on a daily basis until sustained pain control has been achieved and the ICP has come down.

HIV-positive patients with CM should start antiretroviral therapy, whereby the optimum timing is not yet clear. Prognosis of CM in resource-limited settings is poor and 10-week mortality on fluconazole monotherapy exceeds 60%.

Further Reading

1. Heckmann JE, Bhigjee AI. Tropical neurology. In: Farrar J, editor. Manson's Tropical Diseases. 23rd ed. London: Elsevier; 2013 [chapter 71].
2. Wood R. Clinical features and management of HIV/AIDS. In: Farrar J, editor. Manson's Tropical Diseases. 23rd ed. London: Elsevier; 2013 [chapter 10].
3. Hay RJ. Fungal Infections. In: Farrar J, editor. Manson's Tropical Diseases. 23rd ed. London: Elsevier; 2013 [chapter 38].
4. Perfect JR, Dismukes WE, Dromer F, et al. Clinical practice guidelines for the management of cryptococcal disease: 2010 update by the Infectious Diseases Society of America. Clin Infect Dis 2010;50(3):291–322.
5. Sloan DJ, Dedicoat MJ, Lalloo DG. Treatment of cryptococcal meningitis in resource limited settings. Curr Opin Infect Dis 2009;22(5):455–63.

A 25-YEAR-OLD BUDDHIST MONK FROM MYANMAR WITH UNILATERAL SCROTAL SWELLING

36

Kentaro Ishida / Camilla Rothe

Clinical Presentation

HISTORY

A 25-year-old Buddhist monk presents to a district hospital in Myanmar with a three-year history of left-sided scrotal swelling. The swelling is non-tender and has gradually increased in size. There is no history of fever. He has attempted to treat the swelling with traditional herbal medicine, but to no avail.

The patient comes from the central part of Myanmar. He reports that scrotal swelling is not an uncommon problem in his home region.

CLINICAL FINDINGS

The patient is a 25-year-old man in fair general condition. His vital signs are normal and he is afebrile. There is left-sided scrotal swelling, which cannot be reduced (Figure 36-1). There are no palpable inguinal lymph nodes.

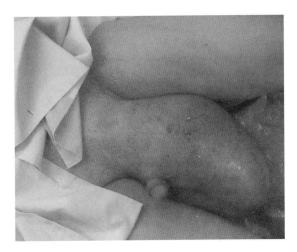

FIGURE 36-1 Massive left-sided scrotal swelling. The swelling is non-tender and non-reducible.

QUESTIONS

1. What is the differential diagnosis?
2. What investigations would you like to do?

Discussion

A young Burmese monk presents with progressive left-sided scrotal swelling. On examination, the swelling is non-tender and non-reducible. He does not have any other symptoms or signs.

TABLE 36-1 Direct Effect of Most Commonly Used Drugs on Different Stages of *W. bancrofti* and *Brugia* spp[2]

	Microfilaria	Adult
Diethylcarbamazine (DEC)	++	+
Ivermectin	++	−
Albendazole	−	+
Doxycycline	−	++

Source: ++ = *most eliminated*; + = *few/some eliminated*; − = *no effect*.

ANSWER QUESTION 1

What is Differential Diagnosis?

The most common differentials to consider in a chronic, unilateral, non-tender scrotal swelling are inguinal hernia and hydrocele. A testicular tumour also needs to be taken into consideration. Unlike hydroceles, hernias can often be reduced. Hydroceles may be verified by transillumination with a penlight.

The patient reports that scrotal swelling is common in the region where he comes from. This may suggest a possible infectious aetiology. The most important infectious disease to consider in this patient is lymphatic filariasis caused by *Wuchereria bancrofti*. Hydrocele is the most common clinical abnormality in men with bancroftian filariasis.

Also, urogenital schistosomiasis (*S. haematobium)* may lead to scrotal swelling, but it is not endemic in South-east Asia. Testicular tuberculosis is another infectious disease that may manifest with unilateral scrotal swelling. However, the long duration of the swelling in the absence of other signs and symptoms make this unlikely and it would not explain the large number of cases seen in his home region.

ANSWER QUESTION 2

What Investigations Would You Like to Do?

Ultrasound can help distinguish a testicular tumour from a hydrocele or hernia. Also, in case of lymphatic filariasis, adult worms may be seen on ultrasonography.

The traditional diagnostic gold standard for lymphatic filariasis is the proof of microfilariae in the blood. Samples should be collected when microfilaraemia is highest. For the majority of filarial species, this is between 9 pm and 3 am due to the nocturnal biting activity of most vectors. Microfilarial PCR assays have a sensitivity and specificity comparable to microscopy with an experienced microscopist, but are usually not available in a district hospital setting.

Circulating filarial antigen (CFA) tests detect antigens released by adult *W. bancrofti*. They are available as dipstick tests and can use fingerprick blood. Since there is no periodicity of adult-worm antigens, CFA tests can be taken at any time. Their sensitivity and specificity is high. CFA tests are also the preferred method for diagnosis of bancroftian filariasis within national control programmes. Antifilarial antibody tests may be of value in patients from non-endemic countries, however, in endemic settings they lack sensitivity and specificity.

THE CASE CONTINUED ...

Hydrocele was confirmed on ultrasound. The patient underwent hydrocelectomy and 3 L of clear fluid could be drained during the operation. He also received antifilarial treatment. He lived in a remote area and was lost to follow-up afterwards.

SUMMARY BOX

Lymphatic Filariasis

Lymphatic filariasis (LF) is caused by filarial nematodes (*Wuchereria bancrofti*, *Brugia malayi* and *B. timori*). LF is transmitted by a variety of mosquito species. It is endemic in South and South-east Asia, sub-Saharan Africa and parts of South America and the Caribbean. More than 100 million people worldwide are estimated to be infected with filarial parasites.[1,2]

Adult worms reside in the lymphatic vessels of the human host. They shed microfilariae which are ingested by female mosquitoes during blood-meals.

The most common features of bancroftian filariasis are hydrocele, acute adenolymphangitis and lymphoedema.

Hydrocele results from the accumulation of fluid in the tunica vaginalis surrounding the testes. Most cases are unilateral. In endemic areas hydroceles start to develop in early adulthood. Prevalence rates rise steadily with age. Rupture of dilated abdominal lymphatic vessels into the urinary system may lead to chyluria. Brugian filariasis is milder than infection with *W. bancrofti* and urogenital complications do not occur.

Acute adenolymphangitis (ADLA) occurs in episodic events that start with fever, chills and severe malaise. Regional lymph nodes are tender and enlarged and the affected limb may become swollen and hot, and the skin may peel off. Repeated episodes of ADLA can lead to lymphoedema.

Chronic lymphoedema most commonly affects the lower leg, but may also involve the arms, breasts and genitals.

The most advanced stage of chronic lymphoedema (stage III) is also referred to as 'elephantiasis'. Chronic ulceration with bacterial and fungal superinfection is a common problem.

Albendazole 400 mg STAT with either diethylcarbamazine (DEC; 6 mg/kg) or ivermectin (200 µg/kg) reduces microfilaraemia to very low levels (Table 36-1). DEC should not be given in areas co-endemic for onchocerciasis or loiasis due to potentially severe side-effects. Treatment in mass drug administration programmes (MDA) is recommended annually; whereas individual patients should get treatment every six months until microfilariae and CFA tests are negative, or life-long, if transmission goes on.

Doxycycline kills endosymbiontic *Wolbachia* bacteria which adult worms require for viability and reproduction. Several weeks of treatment are required and doxycycline is contraindicated in pregnancy and in children under the age of 9 years, which make it an unsuitable option for mass treatment. Its role may be in individual treatment of LF patients who do not have any of the contraindications.

For management of lymphoedema, meticulous hygiene is crucial, such as daily washing with water and soap and careful drying of the affected limb.[3] Bacterial and fungal infections should be treated early. Specialized shoes should be worn to prevent injury. Integration of lymphoedema care and leprosy or diabetic foot care programmes are being promoted.

Small hydroceles sometimes regress after anthelmintic treatment. Large hydroceles require surgery.[4]

Further Reading

1. Simonsen P, Fischer PU, Hoerauf A, et al. The Filariases. In: Farrar J, editor. Manson's Tropical Diseases. 23rd ed. London: Elsevier; 2013 [chapter 54].
2. Taylor MJ, Hoerauf A, Bockarie M. Lymphatic filariasis and onchocerciasis. Lancet 2010;376(9747):1175–85.
3. WHO. Lymphoedema and the chronic wound. The role of compression and other interventions. In: Macdonald JM, Geyer MJ, editors. Wound and Lymphoedema Management. Geneva: World Health Organization; 2010. p. 1–136.
4. Capuano GP, Capuano C. Surgical management of morbidity due to lymphatic filariasis: the usefulness of a standardized international clinical classification of hydroceles. Trop Biomed 2012;29(1):24–38.

37

A 29-YEAR-OLD WOMAN FROM MALAWI WITH CONFUSION, DIARRHOEA AND A SKIN RASH

Camilla Rothe

Clinical Presentation

HISTORY

A 29-year-old woman is brought to a hospital in Malawi by her relatives. She has been confused, restless and irritable for the past month. She also has watery diarrhoea, which started one week ago. She does not have a fever. It is January, which is the rainy season in that country.

Her past medical history has been uneventful. There have been no psychiatric disorders in the past. Her HIV status is unknown. She is not taking any medication. There are no known intoxications, no use of alcohol or recreational drugs.

The patient is married with four children. She is a housewife. Her husband works as a farmhand on a local chicken farm. The family come from a village where they live in a grass-thatched mud-hut and collect their water from a borehole. There is no electricity at home. They eat two meals a day, mainly maize porridge with a few vegetables. Only rarely can the family afford fish or meat.

CLINICAL FINDINGS

The patient is slim but not wasted. Glasgow Coma Scale 14/15 (confusion), the remaining vital signs are normal and she is afebrile. There is no neck stiffness. The patient's conjunctivae are pale. There is a noticeable skin rash around the patient's neck (Figure 37-1), on her forearms, hands and feet (Figure 37-2), where the skin appears hyperpigmented and dry. The skin changes are clearly demarcated. The

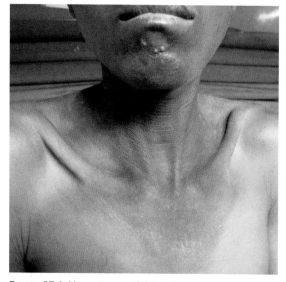

FIGURE 37-1 Hyperpigmented skin rash on sun-exposed skin.

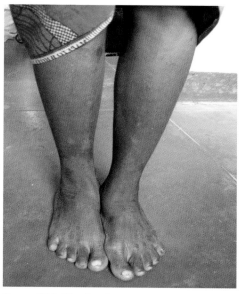

FIGURE 37-2 The skin changes involve both hands and feet. The skin appears dry and scaly.

rest of the physical examination is unremarkable. When asked, her relatives report that the rash had been present for the past two months.

1. What is the suspected diagnosis and what are your differential diagnoses?
2. How would you manage this patient?

Discussion

A young Malawian woman presents during the rainy season with a one-month history of confusion, acute watery diarrhoea and a rash that mainly seems to affect the sun-exposed areas of the skin. The family appear to be poor villagers; they live on an imbalanced diet.

ANSWER TO QUESTION 1

What is the Suspected Diagnosis and What Are Your Differential Diagnoses?

The patient presents with a triad of neuropsychiatric changes, watery diarrhoea and a photosensitive dermatitis. This clinical triad is typical of pellagra (vitamin B_3 deficiency). The rainy season during which the patient presents is not only the peak of malaria transmission, but is also the 'hungry season'. Stocks have been consumed, the new crop is not ready for harvesting yet and often large parts of the population go hungry. In our patient there is no hint towards a reason for her vitamin deficiency other than a poor diet (see Summary Box).

A combination of confusion, diarrhoea and skin changes in a sub-Saharan African setting should prompt any clinician to rule out HIV infection. Persistent confusion in the context of HIV is commonly seen in tuberculous meningitis, cryptococcal meningitis and progressive multifocal leukencephalopathy (PML), or may be caused by the human immunodeficiency virus itself (HIV-associated neurocognitive disorder). Both diarrhoea and skin changes of various etiologies commonly occur in HIV infection.

A further differential diagnosis to consider in a patient with photosensitive dermatitis, anaemia and neuropsychiatric changes is systemic lupus erythematosus.

ANSWER TO QUESTION 2

How Would You Manage This Patient?

A diagnostic HIV test should be carried out. The fact that the patient is currently unable to receive counselling and give her consent should not lead to a delay of the test since its result determines immediate further management. Once confusion has settled, the HIV test should be repeated to include a pre- and post counselling session. In case of a reactive HIV serology a lumbar puncture should be done to rule out tuberculous or cryptococcal meningitis.

A full blood count would help to assess the cause of the patient's clinical anaemia. If normocytic anaemia was found, creatinine should be checked, as chronic kidney disease is very commonly seen in the tropics. Patients often present late, and both confusion and dermatitis can be signs of uraemia.

In case of a microcytic, hypochromic anaemia patients should be treated with iron and possibly also receive folic acid substitution since a poor diet usually is not limited to just one nutritional component. ß-thalassaemia, commonly seen in tropical countries, also presents with microcytic anaemia and should be considered if there is no response to iron supplementation. In ß-thalassaemia the so-called Mentzer-index (MCV [fL] : Erythrocyte count [$\times 10^{12}$/L]) is typically below 13; in iron deficiency it is above 13.

Intestinal helminth infection can contribute to anaemia. Since reliable stool microscopy may not be feasible in a resource-constrained setting, pragmatic anthelmintic treatment appears justifiable. Vitamin B_3 (niacin) should be supplemented and it should be evaluated how the family's diet could be improved despite their poor socioeconomic circumstances. It is a slight irony in this case that the husband is working on a local chicken farm and still cannot afford a balanced diet that includes eggs and poultry for his family.

THE CASE CONTINUED ...

The HIV test came back non-reactive. The full blood count showed a microcytic anaemia with a haemoglobin of 6.7 g/dL and a Mentzer-index >13. The patient received an appropriate dose of vitamin B-complex, iron and folic acid supplementation and a single dose of albendazole. Her confusion settled within a week and the diarrhoea stopped. The patient and her family received dietary counselling. She was prescribed soothing applications for her skin lesions and was told to avoid sun exposure. She was discharged and asked to come back at three months for an outpatient follow-up visit including a repeat full blood count.

SUMMARY BOX

Pellagra

Pellagra is a nutritional disorder caused by the deficiency of niacin (vitamin B_3) or its precursor, the essential amino-acid tryptophan.[1] 'Pellagra' is derived from the Italian *pelle agra*, meaning 'rough skin'. It continues to be a problem in central and southern Africa where maize is the main staple food. Maize is poor in tryptophan, which is required for niacin synthesis. In some parts of Africa white maize is mainly consumed, which is nutritionally poorer than the yellow maize used as animal feed. Milling maize and removing its husks further deprives it of nutritious components. In many poor African countries, furthermore, diet may literally consist of just maize, whereas niacin-containing food items such as fresh fruits, vegetables, peanuts, fish, meat, milk and eggs are not affordable. Most nutritional disorders peak during the rainy season, including kwashiorkor and marasmus in children. Apart from a poor diet, pellagra may be caused by malabsorption, alcoholism, antituberculous treatment and other etiologies.[1]

Patients present with the three 'Ds' of dermatitis, diarrhoea and 'dementia'. The dermatitis often presents in a typical shape around the neck, which is referred to as 'Casal's necklace' after the Spanish physician who first described it in poor peasants in the eighteenth century. The skin tends to be dry, tender to touch and exposure to sunlight may be very painful.

'Dementia' stands for a large spectrum of possible neuropsychiatric symptoms including anxiety, depression, hallucinations, ataxia and spastic paraparesis. A fourth 'D', death, occurs if pellagra is left untreated. The diagnosis is made clinically.

Treatment is with niacin or nicotinamide. Recommended doses in adults range from 50 to 400 mg daily in the acute phase.[1,2] In severe cases, doses of up to 1,000 mg IV per day have been recommended.[1] Once acute symptoms have settled, continuation treatment is with 50–150 mg niacin daily for two weeks. Therapy should also include other B vitamins, zinc, magnesium and a diet rich in calories.[2] Skin lesions should be covered with soothing applications and the patient should avoid sun exposure until the lesions have resolved. Patients and their families require intense dietary counselling on how to improve their diet despite socioeconomic challenges.

Further Reading

1. Abrams S, Brabin BJ, Coulter JBS. Nutrition-associated disease. In: Farrar J, editor. Manson's Tropical Diseases. 23rd ed. London: Elsevier; 2013 [chapter 77].
2. Hegyi J, Schwartz RA, Hegyi V. Pellagra: dermatitis, dementia, and diarrhea. Int J Dermatol 2004;43(1):1–5.

A 24-YEAR-OLD FEMALE GLOBETROTTER FROM THE NETHERLANDS WITH STRANGE SENSATIONS IN THE RIGHT SIDE OF HER BODY

38

Juri Katchanov / Eberhard Siebert

Clinical Presentation

HISTORY

A 24-year-old Dutch yoga instructor presents to an emergency room in Berlin, Germany, with one episode of strange sensations in the right side of her body. This started in the right side of her face, marched to her right arm and then continued, to involve her right leg. She describes the feeling as 'pins and needles' lasting for about two minutes. She had a similar episode several months ago. At that time she did not consult a doctor.

Four years prior to this presentation, after finishing school she had left her home town in The Netherlands to go backpacking for two years. She travelled extensively through South America (Ecuador, Peru, Argentina) and South-east Asia (Thailand, Laos, Cambodia), staying in hostels or private accommodations. She describes herself as an 'eco-traveller', visiting the countryside and staying with local people. She has been a strict vegan for the past eight years. She would eat food from local vendors but never any animal products. Her main diet during her travelling consisted of fruits, vegetables, nuts and rice.

CLINICAL FINDINGS

On examination she looks well. Her body temperature is 36.7°C. Her neurological examination is completely unremarkable. The rest of her physical examination is also normal.

LABORATORY RESULTS

Her routine blood investigations, including C-reactive protein, are completely unremarkable. Her differential blood count and CSF examination are normal.

IMAGING

The MR imaging of her brain shows multiple cortical and subcortical cystic lesions in both hemispheres with gadolinium enhancement (Figure 38-1).

QUESTIONS

1. What is the clinical syndrome the patient presents with and what is the most likely diagnosis in the light of the imaging findings and the patient's travel history?
2. How would you treat this patient?

Discussion

A young Dutch woman presents with paraesthesias that spread over the right side of her body, lasting for about 2 minutes. Four years previously she went on an extensive backpacking trip around the world,

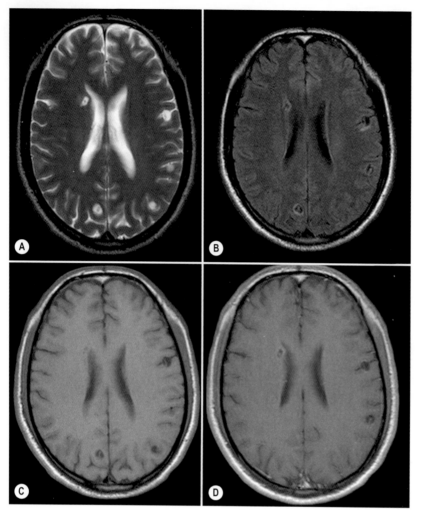

Figure 38-1 Cerebral MRI of the patient. T2-weighted (A), FLAIR (B), T1-weighted (C) and contrast-enhanced T1-weighted (D) images show multiple CSF isointense (cystic) lesions containing a scolex (central dot) in cortical and subcortical distribution. Some lesions show perifocal oedema and ring-enhancement after contrast administration (D).

visiting various places in South America and Asia. She lives on a vegan diet. Her physical examination including her neurostatus are completely normal. The basic blood and CSF results are normal and do not reveal any signs of inflammation. The MRI of the brain shows multiple cystic lesions in both hemispheres.

ANSWER TO QUESTION 1

What is the Clinical Syndrome?

The patient presents with a focal epileptic seizure. Her paraesthesias represent a so-called Jacksonian 'sensory march'. The neuroimaging reveals multiple cortical and subcortical lesions. The cortical lesions in the left hemisphere are likely to be responsible for the patient's epileptic disorder.

The lesions are cystic, some of them show gadolinium enhancement of the wall and surrounding oedema. Given the presentation (healthy-looking patient, no immunosuppression, no fever, one similar episode a while ago with no progression of symptoms) and her travel history to South America and South-east Asia the most likely diagnosis is neurocysticercosis with multiple cysts in the vesicular and colloidal stage. An enzyme-linked immunoelectrotransfer blot (EITB) for the detection of anticysticer-cal antibodies in serum and CSF should be done to confirm the diagnosis.

ANSWER TO QUESTION 2

How Would You Treat This Patient?

The patient should receive antiparasitic treatment, corticosteroids and antiepileptic drugs (see Summary Box and Table 38-1).

TABLE 38-1   Stage of Cysticercal Cyst and Treatment Recommendation

Neuroimaging	Stage	Biology	Anticysticercal Treatment	
Isointense/isodense to CSF, no contrast enhancement	Vesicular	Viable, non-immunogenic, can persist asymptomatically for years	Single cyst Multiple cysts >100 cysts	Albendazole ± steroids
Enhanced wall ('ring enhancement') on contrast imaging, surrounding oedema	Colloidal	Viable but degenerating, immunogenic	Single cyst Multiple cysts >100 cysts ('encephalitic')	Contraindication for anthelmintic treatment, steroids only
Thickened retracted cyst without oedema	Granulo-nodular	Degenerated	No anthelmintic treatment	
Calcification	Calcified	Final involuted stage		

Source: Baird et al.[4] and Carpio[5]

THE CASE CONTINUED ...

The EITB (enzyme-linked immunoelectrotransfer blot) came back positive for serum and CSF and a diagnosis of neurocysticercosis was made.

The patient was treated with albendazole 400 mg bd for one week and started on antiepileptic drugs. She declined treatment with steroids. She did not attend her three-month follow-up but returned as an outpatient one year later. She had remained seizure-free for one year. MR imaging of the brain showed regression of all cysts. A CT-scan on two-year follow-up showed two calcifications. Her antiepileptic treatment was stopped after a seizure-free period of three years.

SUMMARY BOX

Neurocysticercosis

Neurocysticercosis is a CNS infestation with the larval form of *Taenia solium* (the pork tapeworm).[1,2] It is widely prevalent in Africa, Asia and Latin America and is considered by WHO to be the most common preventable cause of epilepsy in the developing world.[3]

Humans acquire neurocysticercosis by eating food, e.g. salad or vegetables, contaminated with *T. solium* eggs. This explains why even individuals who do not eat pork meat for religious or ideological reasons can get neurocysticercosis.

Consumed ova release oncospheres that penetrate the intestinal wall to spread haematogenously throughout the host's body. In the CNS they become encysted affecting either the CNS parenchyma or, less commonly, the CSF space.

Symptoms and signs depend on the location of cysts. The most common clinical presentation is focal epileptic seizures. Cysts in the subarachnoidal space can cause hydrocephalus producing headache and altered mental state. Diagnosis is based on neuroimaging, serology and epidemiological evidence.

Only vesicular and colloidal cysts are amenable to anthelmintic treatment (Table 38-1). Albendazole can decrease the number of active lesions and reduce long-term seizure frequency. Corticosteroids should be considered in solitary cysts and are recommended in multiple cysts to reduce side-effects of antiparasitic therapy.

The duration of antiepileptic therapy depends on the course of the disease. Clinical and radiological follow-ups at three to six month intervals have been recommended.[5] If the patient has remained seizure-free and the cyst has resolved on neuroimaging, antiepileptic drugs might be withdrawn. In a patient with calcified cyst(s) it is probably prudent to continue antiepileptic treatment until the patient has been seizure-free for 1–2 years.

Further Reading

1. Heckmann JE, Bhigjee AI. Tropical neurology. In: Farrar J, editor. Manson's Tropical Diseases. 23rd ed. London: Elsevier; 2013 [chapter 71].
2. Baily G, Garcia HH. Other cestode infections: intestinal cestodes, cysticercosis, other larval cestode infections. In: Farrar J, editor. Manson's Tropical Diseases. 23rd ed. London: Elsevier; 2013 [chapter 57].
3. Garcia HH, Del Brutto OH. Neurocysticercosis: updated concepts about an old disease. Lancet Neurol 2005;4(10): 653–61.
4. Baird RA, Wiebe S, Zunt JR, et al. Evidence-based guideline: treatment of parenchymal neurocysticercosis: report of the Guideline Development Subcommittee of the American Academy of Neurology. Neurology 2013;80(15):1424–9.
5. Carpio A. Neurocysticercosis: an update. The Lancet Infect Dis 2002;2(12):751–62.

39

A 30-YEAR-OLD MALE TRADER FROM CHINA WITH PERSISTENT FEVER

Paul N. Newton / Valy Keoluangkhot / Mayfong Mayxay / Michael D. Green / Facundo M. Fernández

Clinical Presentation

HISTORY

A 30-year-old, male, Chinese, itinerant trader presents in Vientiane, Laos, with a seven-day history of fever, chills, headache and a dry cough. He developed slide-positive falciparum malaria whilst living in southern Laos and was treated with intravenous infusions and intramuscular artemether 80 mg for five days, which he had brought from China as standby therapy, but he did not improve. The fever persisted, jaundice developed and he was therefore transferred to Mahosot Hospital, Vientiane.

CLINICAL FINDINGS

On admission he was febrile (39.5°C), with normal blood pressure and Glasgow Coma Scale (GCS) score, but had nausea, dry cough, moderate dehydration, chest pain and abdominal tenderness. His chest was clear and no hepatosplenomegaly was detected.

INVESTIGATIONS

Giemsa-smear was negative for malaria parasites but a rapid diagnostic test (HRP-2) was positive for *Plasmodium falciparum*, consistent with recent falciparum malaria. Serum creatinine and glucose were normal. His further laboratory results are shown in Table 39-1.

TABLE 39-1	Laboratory Results on Admission	
Parameter	**Patient**	**Reference Range**
ALT (U/L)	301	<40
AST (U/L)	230	<37
ALP (U/L)	470	<120
Total bilirubin (μmol/L)	14	<14.5
Direct bilirubin (μmol/L)	6.4	<4.3

QUESTIONS

1. What are your most important differential diagnoses?
2. How would you approach this patient?

Discussion

A 30-year-old Chinese itinerant trader presents to a hospital in Laos with persistent fever after receiving a five-day course of antimalarial treatment with artemether for falciparum malaria. His blood smear is negative, but his rapid diagnostic test is positive for *P. falciparum*.

A 7-YEAR-OLD GIRL FROM WEST AFRICA WITH TWO SKIN ULCERS AND A CONTRACTURE OF HER RIGHT WRIST

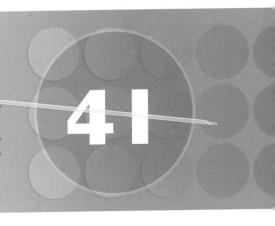

41

Moritz Vogel

Clinical Presentation

HISTORY

A grandmother presents her 7-year-old granddaughter to a district hospital in the tropical region of a West African country. She reports that following an insect bite approximately three months ago the girl had noticed an itchy papule on the back of her right hand, which increased in size over time. When the child complained of pain, a traditional healer was consulted who prescribed local herbal remedies. After some weeks the lesion ulcerated with increasing pain. Diclofenac and dexamethasone were prescribed at the local health post.

When a second lesion appeared on her right wrist, oral oxacillin was given. However, there was no improvement and the girl became increasingly unable to extend her wrist or to use her right hand. There is no history of major trauma or any systemic symptoms.

CLINICAL FINDINGS

A 7-year-old, anxious girl in good general condition holds her right wrist in a 45° flexion and 20° abduction position. Vital signs: pulse 108 bpm (normal 70–110), blood pressure 100/70 mmHg, temperature 37.9°C.

There are two skin ulcers: one is on the back of the right hand, measuring 3×3 cm, the second ulcer is on the medial side of her right wrist (0.5×1 cm). The larger ulcer is filled with necrotic tissue (Figure 41-1). The skin around the lesions shows hypo- and hyperpigmentation, lichenification and desquamation. On palpation there is an ill-defined induration surrounding the ulcers measuring 12×8 cm, which is itself encompassed by an oedema extending from the lower arm to the fingers. There is a 0.5×0.5 cm nodule above the medial right elbow. The flexion of the wrist is actively and passively limited to 45° ± 10°.

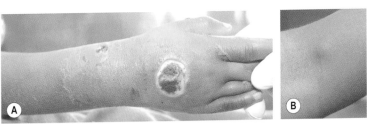

FIGURE 41-1 (A) Large skin ulcer on the back of the right hand filled with necrotic tissue; second smaller ulcer on the medial side of the wrist. (B) Small nodule above right elbow.

QUESTIONS

1. What is the most likely diagnosis and what is the differential diagnosis?
2. What is the appropriate clinical approach in the given context?

Discussion

A little West African girl presents with two progressive cutaneous ulcers linked by an area of alterated skin. The movement in the associated joint is restricted. The patient does not complain of generalized symptoms, but has a mildly elevated temperature.

ANSWER TO QUESTION 1

What is the Most Likely Diagnosis and What is the Differential Diagnosis?

Considering the geographical region of West Africa, the young age of the patient, the location of the lesion on the extremities, the absence of major trauma and the clinical picture most likely diagnosis is Buruli ulcer (BU). The history of an insect bite is an incidental finding, the mode of transmission of the causative organism, *Mycobacterium ulcerans*, remains unknown.

BU has traditionally been described as painless, but recent reports suggest that this may not always be the case. Pain and low grade fever as seen in this case may also be explained by bacterial superinfection. In areas endemic for Buruli ulcer the accuracy of clinical diagnosis in experienced hands is remarkably high.

A careful history and physical examination will provide guidance in differentiating numerous other infectious (bacterial, viral, fungal, parasitic) and non-infectious (trauma, envenoming, autoimmune, haematologic, neoplastic) causes of ulcers in tropical countries.

ANSWER TO QUESTION 2

What is the Appropriate Clinical Approach in the Given Context?

Considering the diagnostic and economic limitations in many tropical countries, a pragmatic approach to patient management is recommended. With limited resources, the cost for diagnostic or therapeutic procedures must be balanced with important supportive measures, such as improved nutrition.

Adequate wound care including pain relief according to WHO guidelines should be instituted immediately. The desired sterile, moist atmosphere of the wound can be achieved with saline-soaked gauze changed daily. As virtually all wounds are colonized with other bacteria when the patient first presents, povidone-iodine may be added initially. Anti-tetanus coverage must be secured.

Laboratory confirmation of BU by *M. ulcerans* PCR from swabs (or in case of closed lesions from fine needle aspiration) is possible. However, reliable laboratory capacity may not be available in every affected country.

The indication for surgical debridement depends on the clinical picture, but also on the availability of adequate anaesthetic and surgical care. Written documentation of pain control and picture documentation of wound progress is helpful in achieving or maintaining a high quality wound management standard.

BU-specific therapy should be commenced as soon as possible. If there are no systemic symptoms and PCR results can be expected within ten days, the toxicity of the currently recommended combination therapy of streptomycin (15 mg/kg/d) and rifampicin (10 mg/kg/d) may justify a delay until microbiological results have been obtained. If laboratory confirmation is unavailable or takes too long, treatment should be initiated and modified later if necessary.

THE CASE CONTINUED ...

PCR from a wound swab came back positive for *M. ulcerans* and the diagnosis of Buruli ulcer was confirmed. During the eight weeks of specific treatment and wound care the ulcer on the back of the hand healed almost completely, while the second smaller ulcer increased to approximately 8×10 cm in size (Figure 41-2).

Debridement and skin grafting were performed and the patient made an uneventful recovery. The restriction of movement was corrected by physiotherapy. The nodule at the medial side of the elbow ulcerated and healed with wound care alone.

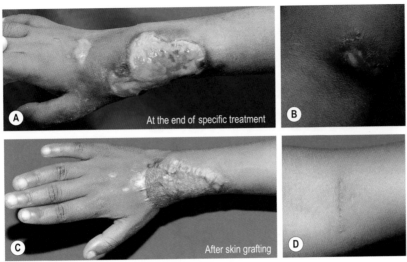

FIGURE 41-2 (A) At the end of specific treatment the ulcer on the back of the hand had healed almost completely. (C) Result after skin grafting. However, the second, smaller ulcer had increased in size and the nodule on the elbow had ulcerated (B). It healed spontaneously (D).

SUMMARY BOX

Mycobacterium ulcerans Disease (Buruli Ulcer)

Mycobacterium ulcerans disease (Buruli ulcer), a necrotizing infection mainly of the subcutaneous tissue, is the third most prevalent human mycobacteriosis after tuberculosis and leprosy.[1,2] The majority of patients with Buruli ulcer (BU) are children and adolescents living in rural communities of West Africa; however, cases have been reported from over 30 mostly (sub-) tropical countries and from the temperate regions of Australia, China and Japan. Endemic areas are associated with water bodies such as rivers and lakes. The mode of transmission remains unknown.

   M. ulcerans is characterized by its particular sensitivity to heat, its propensity to develop local and distant satellite lesions and its production of a macrolide toxin called mycolactone. This toxin causes local tissue destruction and protects the mycobacteria from the host's natural defenses via suppression of the local immune response.

   Clinically, *M. ulcerans* disease presents with skin lesions ranging from papules, nodules and plaques to the eponymous ulcers. The latter may involve the majority of a limb surface or trunk and can simultaneously occur at different body sites. All lesions are characterized by skin alterations including induration, hypo- and hyperpigmentation, lichenification and desquamation and may or may not be accompanied by an oedema. The ulcers are characterized by undermined edges and a 'cotton wool' appearance of the necrotic tissue at the base of the ulcer. Lesions are classically described as painless, but this has been questioned in recent reports. Diagnosis can be confirmed by PCR from a wound swab or from a fine needle aspiration, if available.

   Treatment of BU has been surgical for decades. Since 2004, WHO has recommended combination therapy with rifampicin (10 mg/kg/d) and streptomycin (15 mg/kg/d) for eight weeks, which achieves high specific cure rates.

   M. ulcerans is heat-sensitive and local heat application at temperatures >40°C for several weeks has also been shown to be curative. Regardless of the specific treatment, careful wound management, pain relief and skin grafting as well as physiotherapy for restricted movements remain indispensible cornerstones of Buruli ulcer treatment. Extensive necrosis of subcutaneous tissue at diagnosis may cause a significant increase in ulcer size under treatment. Once secondary bacterial infection has been ruled out, this must not be mistaken for treatment failure. Local or distant new lesions may become evident during or after treatment. This so called 'paradoxical reaction' is thought to be caused by a local immune reconstitution syndrome. The distinction between bacterial secondary infection, recurrence and paradoxical reactions remains challenging and should involve expert advice.[3–5]

Further Reading

1. Junghanss T, Johnson C, Pluschke G. *Mycobacterium ulcerans* disease. In: Farrar J, Hotez P, Junghanss T, Kang G, Lalloo D, White N editors. Manson's Tropical Diseases. 23rd ed. London: Elsevier; 2013 [chapter 42].

2. WHO. Buruli ulcer. Diagnosis of *Mycobacterium ulcerans* Disease. WHO/CDS/CPE/GBUI/2001.4. Geneva: World Health Organization; 2001. (under revision: http://www.who.int/buruli/information/publications/en/index.html)

3. WHO. Treatment of *Mycobaterium ulcerans* disease (Buruli ulcer): guidance for health workers. World Health Organization; 2012; http://www.who.int/iris/bitstream/10665/77771/1/9789241503402_eng.pdf.

4. WHO. Wound and lymphoedema management. In: Macdonald JM, Geyer MJ, editors. WHO/HTM/NTD/GBUI/2010.1. World Health Organization; 2010. Online. Available: http://whqlibdoc.who.int/publications/2010/9789241599139_eng.pdf.

5. WHO. Buruli Ulcer. In: Management of *Mycobacterium ulcerans* disease. A manual for health care providers Buntine and Crofts. World Health Organization; 2001. under revision: (http://www.who.int/buruli/information/publications/en/index.html)

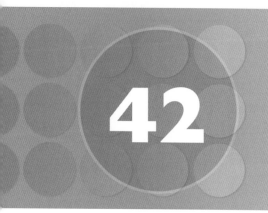

A 41-YEAR-OLD MALE TRAVELLER RETURNING FROM AUSTRALIA WITH ITCHY ERUPTIONS ON BOTH UPPER THIGHS

Camilla Rothe

Clinical Presentation

HISTORY

A 41-year-old male yoga teacher presents to a travel clinic in Europe because of itchy skin eruptions on both upper thighs for the past week.

He has just returned from a ten-day trip to northern Australia where he attended a yoga seminar. On his way to Australia he stopped over on a Thai island for a three-day beach holiday. Just after his arrival in Australia he developed three intensely itchy skin eruptions on both upper thighs. The itch is so intense that at times it keeps him awake at night.

There has been no fever, no cough or wheeze and he is otherwise completely well.

CLINICAL FINDINGS

On both upper thighs there are a total of three reddish, serpiginous tracks, about 2 mm in width (Figure 42-1). The inguinal lymph nodes are not enlarged. The chest is clear. The rest of the examination is unremarkable.

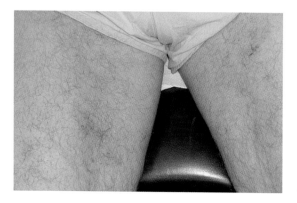

FIGURE 42-1 Three track-like skin eruptions on both upper thighs causing intense itching.

QUESTIONS

1. What is the clinical syndrome and what is the differential diagnosis?
2. What management would you recommend?

Discussion

A 41-year-old European man presents to a travel clinic with itchy serpiginous skin lesions. He has recently returned from a trip to Asia and Australia.

ANSWER TO QUESTION 1

What is the Clinical Syndrome and What is the Differential Diagnosis?

The clinical syndrome is a creeping eruption. A creeping eruption is defined as a linear or serpiginous, slightly elevated, erythematous track that moves forward in an irregular pattern. The most likely cause of the creeping eruption seen in this traveller is cutaneous larva migrans (CLM) caused by larvae of animal hookworms.

Creeping eruptions can also result from infection with larvae of *Strongyloides stercoralis* (larva currens, i.e. running larva), but this can easily be distinguished from CLM. *S. stercoralis* larvae move several centimetres an hour, i.e. considerably faster than larvae in cutaneous larva migrans. The eruptions in larva currens persist only for a few hours, whereby in CLM the track may stay for weeks.

Creeping eruptions can also be caused by adult nematodes such as *Gnathostoma* spp. and trematodes (*Fasciola* spp.). The larvae of parasitic flies have also been shown to cause creeping eruptions (migratory myiasis).

Hookworm-related cutaneous larva migrans is by far the commonest cause of creeping eruption seen in travel clinics worldwide. The patient was probably infected while lying on the beach or performing yoga exercises in the sand.

ANSWER TO QUESTION 2

What Management Would You Recommend?

The diagnosis of cutaneous larva migrans can be established clinically supported by the patient's travel history. There are no other investigations required. Antiparasitic treatment can be administered topically or systemically (see Summary Box).

THE CASE CONTINUED ...

The patient was prescribed a single-dose treatment of ivermectin (200 µg/kg). The drug had to be prescribed as 'off-label use' and purchased from an international pharmacy since it was licensed only for veterinary use in that particular country. The itchy eruptions settled within a few days of taking the drug.

Of note, access to ivermectin is difficult in many countries in the world. It is commonly licensed only for veterinary use, and in tropical regions where ivermectin-donation programmes for the control of onchocerciasis and lymphatic filariasis are in place it is equally difficult to regularly buy a human formulation of the drug.

SUMMARY BOX

Hookworm-Related Cutaneous Larva Migrans

Cutaneous larva migrans (CLM) is a creeping eruption resulting from accidental infestation of the human skin by larvae of dog and cat hookworms[1] (*Ancylostoma caninum*, *A. braziliense* and *Uncinaria stenocephala*). It is one of the most common dermatoses in returning travellers from tropical destinations.[2] Apart from its relevance in travel medicine it is endemic in resource-poor communities in the developing world, particularly in Central and South America, the Caribbean and South and South-east Asia.

CLM occurs in most warm and humid climates and where stray dogs and cats are common, or pets are not treated regularly with anthelmintics. The animals pass hookworm ova with the stool and the larval stages develop in sand or soil. CLM is usually acquired when walking barefoot, or sitting or lying on faecally contaminated ground.

Animal hookworm larvae enter the epidermis but are unable to cross the basement membrane and enter the human body. Confined to the skin they are unable to complete their life cycle as they would do in their animal host.

There usually is a pruritic papule at the site of larval entry. A raised erythematous track starts progressing in an irregular fashion. The onset of symptoms and the speed by which the creeping eruption progresses varies between different hookworm species,[3] but usually itching starts shortly after larval entry and the elevated track appears 1–5 days later.

The skin eruptions are most commonly found on the feet but may occur in any part of the body that came into contact with infested sand or soil. The itching is intense and may prevent affected people from sleeping. Very rarely, animal hookworms may invade the human body leading to pulmonary eosinophilia.[2,3]

Diagnosis is made clinically, supported by exposure history. Skin biopsy is not helpful since the larva is invariably in advance of its track. There are no reliable serological tests available and blood eosinophilia is present in the minority of cases.

Continued on following page

The treatment of choice is ivermectin (200μg/kg STAT). A single dose of ivermectin is more effective than a single dose of albendazole, but repeated doses of albendazole are a good alternative when ivermectin is contraindicated or not available. Albendazole 400 mg od should be administered for 3–7 days. Topical thiabendazole 10–15% tds for 5–10 days is also effective, but requires more compliance and can be difficult in multiple lesions.

Without treatment the lesion can persist for several months, and scratching may lead to bacterial superinfection, particularly in patients from resource-constrained communities.

For prevention at community level, cats and dogs should be dewormed and banned from beaches and playgrounds. In resource-limited settings this is usually not feasible.[3] Individual protection can be achieved by wearing appropriate footwear when walking on sand or soil in the tropics and using a sunchair on the beach since towels do not protect sufficiently.[3]

Further Reading

1. Brooker S, Bundy DAP. Soil-transmitted helminths (geohelminths). In: Farrar J, editor. Manson's Tropcial Diseases. 23rd ed. London: Elsevier; 2013 [chapter 55].
2. Vega-Lopez F, Ritchie S. Dermatological problems. In: Farrar J, editor. Manson's Tropical Diseases. 23rd ed. London: Elsevier; 2013 [chapter 68].
3. Heukelbach J, Feldmeier H. Epidemiological and clinical characteristics of hookworm-related cutaneous larva migrans. The Lancet Infect Dis 2008;8(5):302–9.

A 35-YEAR-OLD WOMAN FROM MALAWI WITH A PAINFUL OCULAR TUMOUR

43

Markus Schulze Schwering

Clinical Presentation

HISTORY

A 35-year-old woman presents to the outpatient department of a Malawian tertiary hospital. She has been referred by an ophthalmic clinical officer from a district hospital for exenteration of the left eye because of an ocular tumour.

The first symptoms started eight months ago when she noticed a whitish lesion growing on the conjunctiva of her left eye. She presented to a health centre and was prescribed nonspecified eye drops. However, over the following months the lesion grew bigger and turned reddish. She went to a traditional healer who prescribed herbal eye drops, which did not help either. The lesion grew constantly bigger and she finally lost her eyesight in the affected eye. Pain also increased, which made her present at her local district hospital.

The patient is known to be HIV-reactive. She has been on antiretroviral treatment for the past three years. The CD4-count is unknown.

CLINICAL FINDINGS

There is localized swelling of the left eyeball and orbit; lid closure is incomplete (Figures 43-1 and 43-2). The visual acuity in her right eye is 6/6, whereas the left eye has no light perception. Her left preauricular lymph nodes are swollen. She is afebrile and the rest of her physical examination is unremarkable.

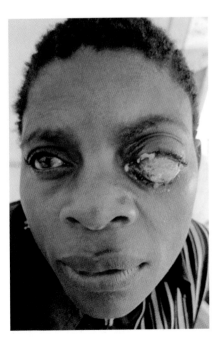

FIGURE 43-1 Left eye with marked axial proptosis, nasal upper lid with tetracycline eye ointment.

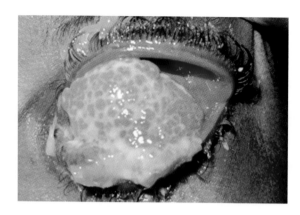

FIGURE 43-2 Papillomatous tumour obliterating the left eye.

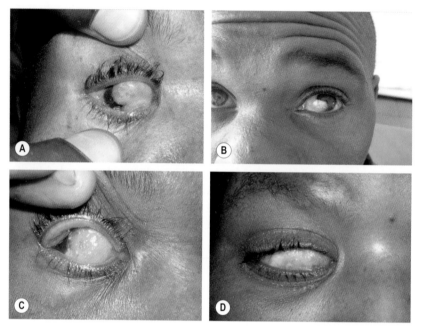

FIGURE 43-3 Squamous cell carcinoma of the conjunctiva (SCCC). This lesion is commonly seen in HIV patients in the tropics and should not be missed during routine clinical examination. *(Courtesy of Nicholas A.V. Beare)*

QUESTIONS

1. What is the suspected diagnosis?
2. How would you manage the patient?

Discussion

A HIV-reactive woman presents with a painful tumour of her left eye. It started as a whitish lesion on her conjunctiva several months ago. The lesion continued to grow and the affected eye became blind.

ANSWER TO QUESTION 1

What is the Suspected Diagnosis?

The lesion is most likely an advanced ocular surface squamous neoplasia (OSSN). OSSN are commonly seen in HIV-positive patients in sub-Saharan Africa. They start as discrete whitish conjunctival lesions (Figure 43-3) and may develop into large tumours if left untreated.

Early stages may be confused with pterygium, with an amelanotic naevus, or a lipoma. Malignant lesions such as amelanotic melanomas, lymphomas or adenocarcinomas may look similar as well.

ANSWER TO QUESTION 2

How Would You Manage the Patient?

The patient should be started on analgesic treatment with nonsteroidal antiinflammatory drugs. She should be counselled and booked for surgery. An extended exenteration of the left eyeball and orbit should be done. Control of the patient's HIV-infection is crucial, and her HIV-viral load should be checked.

Since the patient has lost her eyesight on the left side, the right eye should be carefully examined for possible growth of another OSSN that could be removed at an early stage. A fundoscopy should be performed in order to detect any abnormalities, especially an upcoming CMV infection.

THE CASE CONTINUED ...

The patient was admitted to hospital and counselled several times about the need for surgery. Yet she refused surgical intervention and was willing to accept only conservative treatment.

The patient's left orbit was covered with antibiotics and bandaged. When pain was sufficiently controlled the patient was discharged with the offer to come back any time. She was asked to report at her ART clinic for control of the viral load and possible switch of her antiretroviral therapy.

SUMMARY BOX

Ocular Surface Squamous Neoplasia

Ocular surface squamous neoplasias (OSSN) are commonly seen in HIV-reactive individuals in tropical countries.[1] Early diagnosis is crucial for successful treatment, and any clinician working in a tropical region with high HIV-prevalence should be able to recognize an OSSN.

The term OSSN is used to describe dysplastic lesions of the conjunctiva and cornea, ranging from conjunctival intraepithelial neoplasia (CIN) to invasive squamous cell carcinoma of the conjunctiva (SCCC). HIV infection and high exposure to UV light are considered the most important risk factors for OSSN. A five- to tenfold increase in incidence has been observed in parallel with the HIV epidemic. The current incidence of OSSN in sub-Saharan Africa is estimated to be 2.2 per 100 000 and it continues to rise[2] (USA: 0.3 per 100 000). The mechanism through which HIV infection favours development of OSSN is as yet unknown. Co-infection with human papilloma virus (HPV) has been implicated in the aetiology of OSSN, but the virus could only be detected in fewer than half of cases.

OSSN typically presents as a greyish, elevated, gelatinous mass surrounded by engorged conjunctival vessels. It often starts at the nasal side of the eye and spreads to involve the whole conjunctiva, lids, local tissue and lymph nodes. In the developing world, patients often present late with sometimes disfiguring lesions.

Early, non-invasive stages of OSSN can be treated with topical chemotherapeutic agents such as topical 5-flurouracil and mitomycin or subconjunctival interferon-α2b.[2,3] In many resource-constrained settings, topical medication is not available and treatment for all stages of OSSN is complete surgical excision. In more advanced disease, surgery may have to involve enucleation of the eye or exenteration of the orbit. Adjuvant treatment can decrease the recurrence rate which after simple excision is high (30–40 per cent). Possibilities for adjunctive treatment include topical chemotherapy, cryotherapy and intraoperative β-irradiation. None of these treatments has been subject to a randomized trial and availability in resource-constrained settings is limited.

Diagnosis of OSSN in an HIV-unknown individual should prompt the clinician to perform an HIV test. Since HIV seems to play a role in tumour development, HIV-reactive patients with OSSN should receive effective antiretroviral treatment (ART) to achieve virological control. Nevertheless, clinical trials to assess the importance of ART in the treatment of OSSN are awaited.

Further Reading

1. Beare NV, Bestawrous A. Ophthalmology in the tropics and sub-tropics. In: Farrar J, editor. Manson's Tropical Diseases. 23rd ed. London: Elsevier; 2013 [chapter 67].
2. Tiong T, Borooah S, Msosa J, et al. Clinicopathological review of ocular surface squamous neoplasia in Malawi. Br J Ophthalmol 2013;97(8):961–4.
3. Weinstein JE, Karp CL. Ocular surface neoplasias and human immunodeficiency virus infection. Curr Opin Infect Dis 2013;26(1):58–65.

A 7-YEAR-OLD GIRL FROM SOUTH SUDAN WITH UNDULATING FEVER

Karen Roodnat / Koert Ritmeijer

Clinical Presentation

HISTORY

A 7-year-old girl presents to a clinic in South Sudan with a four-week history of undulating fever. The fever occurs mainly in the afternoon hours accompanied by chills and sometimes convulsions. In between the febrile episodes she was initially fine and played normally. However, over time she has developed progressive anorexia, dry cough, chest pain, joint and back pain.

She has never been admitted to hospital but she has presented at another clinic recently where she received some unspecified tablets that did not bring any improvement.

CLINICAL FINDINGS

The girl is alert, pale, but not jaundiced. She is severely malnourished (Z-score <3). Her vital signs are: temperature 39.6°C, pulse 96 bpm, blood pressure 100/60 mmHg. Her chest sounds clear; normal heart sounds; soft abdomen with a splenomegaly of 4 cm below the left costal margin. There are multiple enlarged lymph nodes of about 1 cm in diameter in the cervical, axillary, inguinal and epitrochlear region. There are no skin lesions and no peripheral oedema.

LABORATORY RESULTS

The patient's blood test results are shown in Table 44-1.

Plasmodium falciparum rapid diagnostic test (RDT) and a blood film for malaria parasites are negative. *Brucella* spp. serology (IgG and IgM) is negative. Visceral leishmaniasis: rK39-antibody RDT is negative.

TABLE 44-1 Laboratory Results on Admission		
Parameter	Patient	Reference
WBC (x10⁹/L)	1.35	4–10
Haemoglobin (g/dL)	6.8	12–16
Platelets (x10⁹/L)	98	150–300

QUESTIONS

1. What are your most important differential diagnoses?
2. How would you approach this patient?

Discussion

In South Sudan, a young girl presents with a four-week history of fever, progressive anorexia, general body pains and a dry cough. On examination she is pale and severely malnourished. She has splenomegaly and generalized lymphadenopathy. The FBC shows pancytopenia. Serological rapid diagnostic tests for malaria, brucellosis and visceral leishmaniasis are negative.

ANSWER TO QUESTION 1

What Are Your Most Important Differential Diagnoses?

Chronic fever, splenomegaly and wasting in a child from South Sudan should raise the suspicion of visceral leishmaniasis or brucellosis. Tuberculosis and HIV infection both need to be ruled out as they can cause chronic fever, anorexia, weight loss, splenomegaly and generalized lymphadenopathy.

Malaria can cause fever, anaemia and splenomegaly, but two different negative tests make this unlikely. Also, the chronic fever is unusual; in a child one might expect a more acute course. Malaria does not cause any lymphadenopathy. Hyperreactive malarial splenomegaly syndrome (HMS) can cause gross splenomegaly and anaemia in regions hyperendemic for malaria, but HMS does not present with a fever, neither is lymphadenopathy part of the picture.

Typhoid fever can present with persistent fever and splenomegaly; a dry cough is also common. The duration of fever in this case may be slightly too long though and generalized lymphadenopathy is not a common feature of typhoid.

A splenic abscess could cause chronic fever and splenomegaly, but would not explain the generalized lymphadenopathy and the haematological changes unless the patient was acutely septic.

Chronic schistosomiasis due to *Schistosoma mansoni* infection can cause splenomegaly in the context of portal hypertension, but patients would not be febrile and lymphadenopathy is not part of the picture either.

Malignancies like leukaemia and lymphoma should be ruled out.

ANSWER TO QUESTION 2

How Would You Approach this Patient?

The little girl appears very sick and should be admitted to hospital. The list of differential diagnoses is long and there are many tests that would be requested if the same patient presented in an affluent setting.

In a resource-constrained place like South Sudan, a pragmatic clinical approach is necessary. The history should be taken as accurately as possible to narrow down the differential diagnosis. One should try to find out if the patient comes from an area where visceral leishmaniasis (VL) is endemic. For possible HIV infection it would be of great importance to find out if the parents and siblings are alive and well; and enquiries should be made if there are any close contacts who are suspected to have TB or who have a history of recent TB treatment.

The clinician has to cope with the investigations available, which may commonly not be in line with the internationally recommended standards. Gold standard for diagnosis of VL is the proof of the parasite in tissue specimens. However this is often not feasible under field conditions and serological tests are used instead. The rapid antigen test for VL (rK39) used in this case was negative (sensitivity of this test in South Sudan is 85–90%).

Since VL is high on the list of differential diagnoses a second serological test such as the Direct Agglutination Test (DAT) should be done and direct proof of the parasite should be attempted.

Sensitivity is highest for splenic aspirates (93–99%) followed by bone marrow (53–86%) and lymph node aspiration (53–65%), which can be further increased by culture and PCR. Splenic aspiration is complicated with life-threatening haemorrhages in 0.1% of procedures and therefore requires strict precautions, technical expertise and postinterventional monitoring.

Blood cultures if available would be helpful for diagnosis of typhoid fever, brucellosis and septicaemia.

THE CASE CONTINUED ...

The mother of the patient reported that the family came from an area where visceral leishmaniasis was known. It turned out that the uncle of the child had been treated for VL before. The girl's sister had recently been treated for TB.

The child's health continued to deteriorate. She had persistently high fever and became increasingly pale.

The DAT came back positive with a high titre (≥1:6.400), which supported the suspected diagnosis of visceral leishmaniasis.

Considering her critical condition, with severe malnutrition and progressive anaemia, the patient was started on liposomal amphotericin B and broad-spectrum antibiotics (ceftriaxone). The girl also received nutritional support with high-energy/high-protein ready-to-use therapeutic food (RUTF) and vitamin/mineral supplementation.

After five days the fever settled and the patient started to recover. Two weeks later the girl had gained some weight and was again able to walk and play.

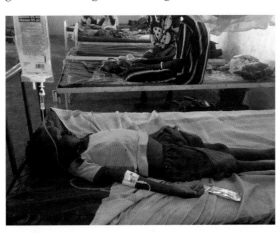

FIGURE 44-1 A child is receiving liposomal amphotericin B on a paediatric ward in South Sudan.

SUMMARY BOX

Visceral Leishmaniasis (Kala-Azar)

Visceral leishmaniasis (VL) is a vector-borne systemic disease caused by *Leishmania* protozans,[1,2] most commonly *L. donovani* and *L. infantum*. VL causes approximately 200 000–400 000 human cases and 20 000–40 000 deaths each year.[3] Ninety per cent of all cases occur in only six countries: India, Bangladesh, Sudan, South Sudan, Ethiopia and Brazil.

Transmission can be anthroponotic or zoonotic, differing by region and parasite strain. Humans most commonly acquire VL through the bite of an infected female sandfly, but other modes of transmission have been described.[1]

Leishmania promastigotes invade cells of the human reticuloendothelial system where they metamorphose into amastigotes and multiply. The incubation period varies greatly, from ten days to several years, but usually takes between two and six months.

The clinical presentation depends upon the infecting species, as well as on the host's genetic background and immune status. Most infections remain subclinical.

Clinical VL presents with symptoms and signs of a chronic systemic infection (fever, fatigue, anorexia, weight loss) and of parasite invasion of the mononuclear phagocyte system (enlarged lymph nodes, splenomegaly, hepatomegaly). In India, hyper-pigmentation has led to the name 'kala-azar' (Hindi for 'black sickness'). Potentially fatal complications include haemorrhage, congestive heart failure due to severe anaemia and bacterial superinfections.

In low-resourced settings, diagnostic options for VL are often limited. On FBC all three cell lines can be depleted. Demonstration of *Leishmania* amastigotes in samples from bone marrrow, spleen and lymph node is the classic confirmatory test for VL.[1] Under field conditions, direct proof of the parasite is often not feasible and several serological tests have been developed instead. The sensitivity and specificity of these tests generally vary and they should always be used in combination with a standardized case definition as suggested by WHO.[1]

The rK39 immunochromatographic test (ICT) and the direct agglutination test (DAT) were found to have the highest sensitivity and specificity. The rK39 ICTs are easy to perform, rapid (10–20 minutes), cheap and give easily reproducible results. The semi-quantitative DAT has a longer turnaround time of about 24 hours, and requires a laboratory with well-trained technicians.

Treatment of VL is complex: efficacy of the individual drugs varies geographically and depends upon the immune status of the patient. Parenteral drugs currently used are pentavalent antimonials, paromomycin and (liposomal) amphotericin B[4] (Figure 44-1). The oral drug in use is miltefosine. Combinations of antileishmanial drugs seem to help shorten therapy courses, reduce side-effects, improve treatment outcomes, delay resistance development and reduce treatment costs.

In HIV patients VL is even more difficult to treat as it does not respond well to the classic antileishmanial drugs and has a higher tendency to relapse.

Further Reading

1. Boelaert M, Sundar S. Leishmaniasis. In: Farrar J, editor. Manson's Tropical Diseases. 23rd ed. London: Elsevier; 2013 [chapter 47].
2. Murray HW, Berman JD, Davies CR, et al. Advances in leishmaniasis. Lancet 2005;366(9496):1561–77.
3. Alvar J, Velez ID, Bern C, et al. Leishmaniasis worldwide and global estimates of its incidence. PLoS ONE 2012;7(5):e35671.
4. WHO. Control of the Leishmaniases. WHO Technical Report Series 949. Geneva: World Health Organization; 2010.

A 2-MONTH-OLD GIRL FROM LAOS WITH DYSPNOEA, CYANOSIS AND IRRITABILITY

45

Mayfong Mayxay / Douangdao Soukaloun / Paul N. Newton

Clinical Presentation

HISTORY

You are working in the paediatric intensive care unit of a tertiary hospital in Vientiane, Laos. A 2-month-old baby girl presents with three days of irritability, poor breastfeeding, dyspnoea and grunting. Her mother is a 24-year-old rice farmer who describes that the baby suddenly became unwell but was not febrile nor coughing. The infant was born at term and had been very well until three days previously.

CLINICAL FINDINGS

The patient is an irritable infant, crying and grunting, with a temperature of 37.0°C, pulse 140 bpm (normal range 100–160), respiratory rate 40 breath cycles per minute (normal range 30–60). The blood pressure is not taken. The child is dyspnoeic and has central cyanosis, hepatomegaly and oedematous extremities. The rest of the physical examination appears normal, with clear chest and no heart murmurs.

QUESTIONS

1. What are your most important differential diagnoses?
2. What additional information do you need to obtain from the mother and what would be your quick response?

Discussion

A young Lao mother presents with her 2-month-old baby girl, who has been acutely unwell for the past three days. The child has been breastfeeding poorly and was noted to have grunting, which is a non-specific sign of severe systemic illness in infants. On examination, the child is irritable, cyanosed and shows signs of heart failure.

ANSWER TO QUESTION 1

What Are Your Most Important Differential Diagnoses?

The most important differential diagnoses to consider are congenital heart disease, respiratory diseases (e.g. bronchopneumonia, bronchiolitis and laryngitis), meningitis and infantile beriberi (thiamin or vitamin B_1 deficiency).

However, the absence of cough, wheezes, fever, tachypnoea and the normal chest examination suggests that respiratory diseases are unlikely. That the cyanosis has started well after birth, along with the sudden onset of symptoms and the absence of heart murmurs, suggests that congenital heart disease is unlikely. Absence of fever or bulging fontanellae make meningitis an improbable differential. The combination of dyspnoea, poor breastfeeding, abnormal cry, grunting and swollen extremities in a suitable endemic setting (South-east Asia) suggest infantile beriberi as the most likely diagnosis.

ANSWER TO QUESTION 2

What Additional Information Do You Need to Obtain from the Mother and What Would be Your Quick Response?

The most important information to be obtained from the mother is whether the child has been exclusively breastfed, whether the mother has practised food avoidance behaviour intra- and/or post-partum, and if the mother has any symptoms and signs suggestive of beriberi, such as paraesthesia and difficulty rising from a squatting position.

Prolonged food avoidance behaviour post-partum is common in lowland Lao culture. It is based upon the traditional belief that certain food items may harm the newborn. Most mothers eat milled glutinous rice but avoid eating vegetables and fruit, which results in low diet diversity for a few months after delivery.

Thiamin deficiency may be one result of such dietary restriction, and affected mothers excrete insufficient levels of vitamin B_1 in their breastmilk. This may lead to infantile beriberi. The cardiac form of the disease usually manifests during the second or third month of life. Infants present with dyspnoea, cyanosis, vomiting and irritability.

Children with infantile beriberi respond rapidly (i.e. within 30–60 min) to intravenous or intramuscular thiamin (50 mg), which should urgently be administered. The child should be closely monitored.

THE CASE CONTINUED ...

The mother reported that her child had been exclusively breastfed and that she had practised food avoidance since delivery. She had avoided eating beef, pork, vegetables and fruits. The mother reported that she herself had anorexia, weakness, a husky voice and limb paresthesia – symptoms of thiamin deficiency.

Intravenous thiamin (50 mg) was given immediately to the child after admission and she quickly and dramatically responded. Six hours later the baby was able to breastfeed normally and was discharged the following day. Blood samples were taken from the child and the mother. Analysis showed that both were thiamin-deficient.

The mother was given oral thiamin supplementation and advised to return to a well-balanced diet including thiamin-rich foods.

SUMMARY BOX

Infantile Beriberi

Infantile beriberi, or clinical thiamin (vitamin B_1) deficiency in infants, is a forgotten, fatal disease.[1] It mainly occurs in South and South-east Asia, where about 50–100 years ago it was recognized as a major public health problem.[2] It remains relatively common in Laos, probably because of prolonged intra- and post-partum maternal food avoidance behaviours.[3] There is also evidence that it is still of importance in Cambodia and Myanmar, and cases have been reported from refugee populations in Thailand.

Infantile beriberi occurs in exclusively breastfed babies of approximately three months of age whose mothers have thiamin deficiency resulting from inadequate thiamin intake.

It commonly manifests mainly as the 'wet' form of beriberi, characterized by heart failure with hepatomegaly and marked peripheral oedema. The disease typically presents as shock, often preceded by a hoarse cry, grunting, poor breastfeeding, irritability, dyspnoea and cyanosis. Clinically unapparent thiamin deficiency has also found to be common among sick infants admitted to hospital in Vientiane.[4]

Thiamin-deficient diet is made up largely of milled sticky rice that has had most of its vitamin B_1 removed as a result of the milling process. With the advent of mechanical rice milling in the late nineteenth century, which removed the main dietary source of thiamin in rice husk, beriberi became a major public health problem in Asia, responsible for considerable mortality. However, there has been very little recent epidemiological research, despite evidence that it remains focally important.

The pathophysiology of infantile beriberi remains unclear, but the cardinal problem is usually myocardial dysfunction. Thiamin deficiency may also present with a variety of other clinical syndromes, including encephalopathy, hypoglycemia and lactic acidosis.

Infantile beriberi is usually diagnosed clinically due to a lack of laboratories in endemic areas that can perform thiamin biochemical assays.[5] Treatment of infantile beriberi with thiamin is simple, inexpensive and highly effective. It should be administered parenterally to rapidly increase tissue thiamin levels. Thiamin supplementation should also be given to the mothers of infants with beriberi. Education about thiamin-rich foods and on the danger of food avoidance should be provided before discharge. Prevention is crucial, and better understanding of post-partum diets and thiamin supplementation for mothers is urgently needed.

Further Reading

1. Abrams S, Brabin BJ, Coulter JBS. Nutrition-associated disease. In: Farrar J, editor. Manson's Tropical Diseases. 23rd ed. London: Elsevier; 2013 [chapter 77].
2. Fehily L. The differential diagnosis of infantile beriberi. Trans R Soc Trop Med Hyg 1942;38(2):111–23.
3. Barennes H, Simmala C, Odermatt P, et al. Postpartum traditions and nutrition practices among urban Lao women and their infants in Vientiane, Lao PDR. Eur J Clin Nutr 2009;63(3):323–31.
4. Khounnorath S, Chamberlain K, Taylor AM, et al. Clinically unapparent infantile thiamin deficiency in Vientiane, Laos. PLoS Negl Trop Dis 2011;5(2):e969.
5. Soukaloun D, Lee SJ, Chamberlain K, et al. Erythrocyte transketolase activity, markers of cardiac dysfunction and the diagnosis of infantile beriberi. PLoS Negl Trop Dis 2011;5(2):e971.

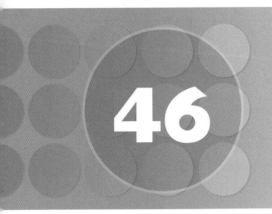

46

A 45-YEAR-OLD MAN FROM SRI LANKA WITH FEVER AND RIGHT HYPOCHONDRIAL PAIN

Ranjan Premaratna

Clinical Presentation

HISTORY

A 45-year-old Sri Lankan man presents to a local hospital with fever, chills, headache, body aches and severe right hypochondrial pain for the past week. He has also developed a dry cough during the past few days. He has vomited twice during his illness and has lost his appetite.

His abdominal pain is constant and dull in nature. It radiates to the right shoulder and is made worse when coughing and resting on the right side.

The patient has been well before the current illness. He admits to consuming locally brewed alcohol ('*toddy*', made of coconut flowers) daily for the last 10–15 years.

EXAMINATION

The patient looks generally ill, mildly dehydrated and is in pain. Temperature is 38.3°C, blood pressure 100/80 mmHg, pulse 102 bpm, respiratory rate 24 breath cycles per minute. There is no jaundice, no pallor and no lymphadenopathy. The abdominal examination reveals a tender hepatomegaly, however the tenderness is most prominent over the 6th to 9th intercostal spaces in the right mid-axillary line. The spleen is not enlarged. On auscultation there are few inspiratory crackles over the right lung base. The cardiovascular system and the nervous system are clinically normal.

INVESTIGATIONS

His laboratory results are shown in Table 46-1. A chest radiograph showed elevated right hemidia-phragm and patchy shadows in the right lower zone.

TABLE 46-1 Laboratory Results at Presentation		
Parameter	Patient	Reference
WBC (×10⁹/L)	14.7	4–10
Haemoglobin (g/dL)	12.3	12–16
Platelets (×10⁹/L)	224	150–350
AST (U/L)	54	13–33
ALT (U/L)	38	3–25
ALP (U/L)	446	40–130
Serum bilirubin total (μmol/L)	1.5	25.7–30.8
Serum bilirubin direct (μmol/L)	10.3	1.7–5.1
Blood urea nitrogen (mmol/L)	7	2.5–6.4
Serum creatinine (μmol/L)	124	71–106
C-reactive protein (mg/L)	48	<6

QUESTIONS

1. What is the likely diagnosis?
2. How would you manage this patient?

Discussion

A 45-year-old Sri Lankan man presents with fever, headache, body aches and constant right-sided abdominal pain for a week. He also has a dry cough. His past medical history is unremarkable, but he consumes local alcohol. He is febrile with tender hepatomegaly and intercostal tenderness on the right. There is no jaundice.

His blood results show very mildly elevated transaminases, an elevated alkaline phosphatase (ALP) and raised inflammatory markers.

ANSWER TO QUESTION 1

What is the Likely Diagnosis?

Tender hepatomegaly, intercostal tenderness and an elevated right hemidiaphragm in the context of fever point towards an infectious focus in the liver.

His transaminases are only slightly elevated; AST is higher than ALT, which could be explained merely by his regular alcohol consumption. In infectious hepatitis one would expect higher transaminase levels and clinical jaundice.

The most likely diagnosis in this man is a liver abscess, which could be amoebic or pyogenic. Given the epidemiological setting, the relatively young age of the patient and the absence of comorbidities such as diabetes or biliary disease, an amoebic liver abscess is more likely. Also, the alcoholic drink the patient consumes is locally known to be linked with amoebiasis, since the parasites commonly contaminate the clay containers used to collect *toddy*.

Another tropical infectious disease to consider in a febrile patient from Asia with any kind of organ abscess is melioidosis. Cases of meliodosis have been reported from Sri Lanka where the infection is rather rare; it is more commonly seen in other parts of Asia, such as Thailand, Lao PR, Vietnam and in northern Australia.

ANSWER TO QUESTION 2

How Would You Manage This Patient?

An ultrasound of the liver should be done. *Entamoeba histolytica* serology is highly sensitive and useful as a screening test; however, it may lack specificity in individuals from highly endemic tropical regions like the Indian subcontinent. Stool microscopy for *E. histolytica trophozoites* may be attempted but is less than 50% sensitive.

THE CASE CONTINUED ...

The ultrasound scan of his abdomen revealed a solitary hypoechoic lesion with an irregular wall measuring 7×6 cm in the right liver lobe. There was a small pleural effusion on the right.

Due to its large size the lesion was aspirated under ultrasound guidance, yielding brownish pus highly suspicious of an amoebic liver abscess.

The patient was treated with metronidazole for ten days and made a rapid and uneventful recovery.

SUMMARY BOX

Amoebic Liver Abscess

Amoebic liver abscess (ALA) is the most common extraintestinal form of invasive amoebiasis caused by *Entamoeba histolytica*.[1] The infection occurs worldwide, but is most common in tropical areas with overcrowding and poor sanitation.[2] Rates of ALA are three to 20 times higher in men between 18 and 50 years of age than in other populations.[3] Humans acquire the infection by ingestion of faecally contaminated food or water. Trophozoites of *E. histolytica* may penetrate the intestinal wall and haematogenously spread to the liver. Clinical manifestations include fever with chills, right hypochondrial pain, anorexia and weight loss, but most patients with ALA do not have a history of recent dysentery. A dry cough and fine crepitations over the right lung bases are common. Jaundice is unusual. Localized intercostal tenderness helps in the clinical diagnosis. ALA may rupture into the peritoneal cavity or through the skin or diaphragm. Haematogenous spread may cause metastatic abscesses in distant organs such as the brain.

Continued on following page

Leukocytosis, raised inflammatory parameters and an elevated alkaline phosphatase are the most common nonspecific laboratory findings.[4] Diagnosis is usually made by a combination of imaging studies and serology. Abdominal ultrasound scan is the most suitable imaging technique in resource-limited settings, but CT and MRI scans are also highly sensitive. None of the imaging techniques is specific for ALA. Plain radiography of the thorax may reveal elevation of the right hemidiaphragm.

Serology is highly sensitive but may lack specificity in individuals from endemic countries. Aspiration of a suspected ALA is not a routine investigation; it may occasionally be necessary to rule out a pyogenic abscess. The aspirated fluid is thick, odourless and brownish in colour; it is bacteriologically sterile and usually does not contain any amoebae. The term 'abscess' is a misnomer, as the 'pus' is in fact necrotic liver.[1]

Most patients rapidly respond to antibiotic treatment with metronidazole or tinidazole.

Metronidazole 750 mg tds PO or IV should be given for 7–10 days, tinidazole 2 g per day PO for 3–5 days. This should be followed by a luminal amoebicide such as diloxanide furoate, paromomycin or iodoquinol.

The role of therapeutic percutaneous aspiration or drainage is still controversial. It may be useful in large abscesses, ALA located in the left liver lobe and in abscesses that do not respond to nitroimidazole therapy within 72 hours when pyogenic infection is a concern.

Further Reading

1. Kelly P. Intestinal protozoa. In: Farrar J, editor. Manson's Tropical Diseases. 23rd ed. London: Elsevier; 2013 [chapter 49].
2. Hughes MA, Petri WA Jr. Amoebic liver abscess. Infect Dis Clin North Am 2000;14(3):565–82, viii.
3. Sharma N, Sharma A, Varma S, et al. Amoebic liver abscess in the medical emergency of a North Indian hospital. BMC Research Notes 2010;3:21.
4. Stanley SL. Amoebiasis. Lancet 2003;361:1025–34.

47

A 32-YEAR-OLD MAN FROM MALAWI WITH A PAINFULLY SWOLLEN NECK

Joep J. van Oosterhout

Clinical Presentation

HISTORY

A 32-year-old Malawian man presents to the first aid department of a local tertiary hospital with a six-week history of productive cough and chest pains, associated with weight loss, fevers and night sweats. He has also noticed that his neck has swollen and is painful. There are no other symptoms. He has never been admitted to hospital, but has been tested HIV-positive and was started on antiretroviral therapy (ART) with stavudine–lamivudine–nevirapine and co-trimoxazole prophylaxis two months earlier at a nearby health centre. His health passport (Figure 47-1) reveals that a recent CD4 count was 95 cells/mL and also that the patient has been treated for acid-fast bacilli (AFB) sputum smear-negative pulmonary tuberculosis 12 years ago.

CLINICAL FINDINGS

He looks moderately ill, is pale, sweating and has a temperature of 39.2°C, pulse 112 bpm, respiratory rate 28 breath cycles per minute and normal blood pressure. There are large, matted lymph glands in the neck. The rest of the examination is unremarkable.

INVESTIGATIONS

Full blood count: WBC 14.3×10^9/L (reference range: 4–10), haemoglobin 6.3 g/dL (13–15), MCV 66 fL (80–98), platelets 246×10^9/L (150–350).

Three sputum samples are negative for AFB. Fine needle aspiration of a neck gland yields pussy material. Microscopy for AFB is 2+ positive. There is no growth on blood culture.

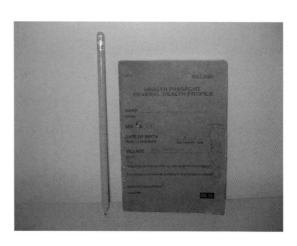

FIGURE 47-1 The patient's health passport.

INITIAL TREATMENT

The patient is admitted to hospital and started on TB re-treatment for tuberculous lymphadenitis with streptomycin, isoniazid, rifampicin, pyrazinamide and ethambutol, while continuing the same ART. Against expectation, he does not improve after three weeks. He still has fevers, night sweats, lack of appetite and the glands in the neck have further swollen and are now clearly fluctuant (Figure 47-2).

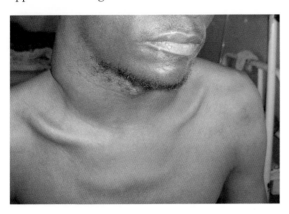

FIGURE 47-2 Increasing and fluctuant lymphadenitis in the neck.

QUESTIONS

1. What could be the reasons for the lack of clinical improvement?
2. Which investigations are indicated?

Discussion

A 32-year-old Malawian man who is known to be HIV-positive is admitted with a diagnosis of tuberculous lymphadenitis and immune reconstitution inflammatory syndrome (IRIS) of the unmasking type (see Summary Box). The tuberculosis (TB) diagnosis is based on microscopic findings. He unexpectedly deteriorates on antituberculous treatment.

ANSWER TO QUESTION 1

What Could be the Reasons for the Lack of Clinical Improvement?

Although the diagnosis of TB lymphadenitis is very likely when AFBs are identified in a lymph gland sample, atypical mycobacteria should also be considered, now that the initial response to TB treatment is unsatisfactory, especially given the deep immune suppression the patient had at the start of ART. Other reasons for a poor response to TB treatment are non-adherence, malabsorption and drug resistance. Given the frank fluctuation that is present, a bacterial lymphadenitis is probable, while a lymphoma seems much less likely.

ANSWER TO QUESTION 2

Which Investigations Are Indicated?

HIV viral load and a CD4 count should be done to determine the response to ART. A repeat fine needle aspiration (FNA) should be performed to check for AFBs. A Gram stain and bacterial culture should help rule out bacterial superinfection. Ideally, the aspirate should also be cultured to rule out infection with resistant *Mycobacterium tuberculosis* or atypical mycobacteria.

THE CASE CONTINUED ...

The patient denied missing any tablets, had no diarrhoea or other gastrointestinal symptoms, and had not left Malawi, where multi-drug resistance for TB is uncommon. IRIS of the paradoxical type was also considered to explain the lack of improvement (see Box), therefore corticosteroids were initiated.

Further investigations were done, with the following results: CD4 109 cells/mL; HIV-1 RNA < 400 copies/mL. Repeat FBC results were: WBC 7.8×10^9/L, haemoglobin 6.7 g/dL, MCV 84fL, platelets 428×10^9/L.

Because of the increasingly fluctuant swelling in the neck, a second fine needle aspiration was done, now showing frank yellowish pus. On microscopic examination, numerous coccoid bacteria and polymorphonuclear lymphocytes were observed. Unfortunately results from a bacterial culture were never received.

The diagnosis at this point was superimposed bacterial lymphadenitis, possibly iatrogenic due to the earlier aspiration, with *Staphylococcus aureus* being the most likely microorganism. The patient recovered well after incision and drainage, antibiotic treatment and a short course of corticosteroids while he continued on TB treatment and ART.

In the first full blood count, severe microcytic anaemia was present. Anaemia is extremely common in patients with advanced HIV immune suppression and TB co-infection; however the marked microcytosis is unusual. There was no good explanation for this finding since there was no source of blood loss in the history and the MCV had normalized in the second full blood count, which was against ß-thalassaemia as a cause of microcytic anaemia. The first full blood count also showed a leukocytosis when TB lymphadenitis was diagnosed. This finding is paradoxical because later, when the florid purulent bacterial infection was present, it had resolved. Multiple dynamic factors were apparently impacting on the white blood cell count in this patient, including HIV, TB, bacterial infection, immune reconstitution, corticosteroids, antiretroviral and antituberculous drugs and co-trimoxazole.

SUMMARY BOX

Immune Reconstitution Inflammatory Syndrome

HIV-associated immune reconstitution inflammatory syndrome (IRIS) is a deterioration of the clinical situation caused by increased inflammation due to improving immune competence resulting from successful ART.

The clinical manifestations are wide-ranging and depend on the underlying condition, which is mostly an opportunistic infection, but can also be a tumour, an autoimmune disease or another condition. In sub-Saharan Africa, tuberculosis and cryptococcal meningitis are the two most important IRIS presentations.[1] IRIS is very common, occurring in between 10 and 25% of patients who start ART. A widely accepted definition does not exist, although standardization has been attempted.[2] Definitions include measures of successful ART, exclusion of other causes of the clinical deterioration, such as toxicity, and a relationship in time between the symptoms and the start of ART.

IRIS is classified into two types. In the unmasking form, a condition is present but remains subclinical and undiagnosed due to severe immunosuppression before the start of ART and becomes clinically apparent within 6 months after ART initiation. In the paradoxical worsening form, a condition has been diagnosed and is being treated successfully, but clinical worsening occurs due to the increased inflammation following immune recovery after starting ART. Risk factors for IRIS include a low pre-ART CD4 count and haemoglobin level, a high pre-ART viral load, large pre-ART weight loss, large and rapid increase of the CD4 count and rapid reduction of the viral load on ART, and a short period between the start of treatment for an opportunistic infection and initiation of ART.[3]

Further Reading

1. Thwaites G. Tuberculosis. In: Farrar J, editor. Manson's Tropical Diseases. 23rd ed. London: Elsevier; 2013 [chapter 40].
2. Haddow LJ, Moosa MY, Easterbrook PJ. Validation of a published case definition for tuberculosis-associated immune reconstitution inflammatory syndrome. AIDS 2010;24(1):103–8.
3. Haddow LJ, Moosa MY, Mosam A, et al. Incidence, clinical spectrum, risk factors and impact of HIV-associated immune reconstitution inflammatory syndrome in South Africa. PLoS ONE 2012;7(11):e40623.

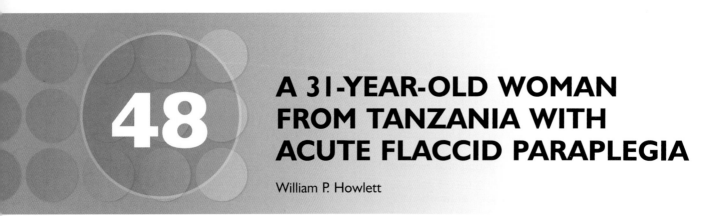

48

A 31-YEAR-OLD WOMAN FROM TANZANIA WITH ACUTE FLACCID PARAPLEGIA

William P. Howlett

Clinical Presentation

HISTORY

A 31-year-old woman is referred to hospital in Northern Tanzania with a loss of power and feeling in her legs. She describes being perfectly well up until two days earlier when she felt acute back pain which radiated band-like to the level of her umbilicus. The pain was severe, continuous, burning in nature and unrelieved by analgesics or position. Within 12 hours the pain had lessened but she developed numbness in her feet and legs ascending to the level of her waist, loss of power in her legs and loss of control of her bladder. There is a history of a febrile illness three weeks previously, treated as malaria. There is no past or family history of similar illness and no history of trauma. She is married with three children, the last born is 12 months old. She does not smoke or take alcohol and her HIV status during her last pregnancy was negative.

CLINICAL FINDINGS

Clinically she is well-nourished with normal vital signs. General examination is unremarkable; there is no spinal tenderness, deformity or gibbus. On neurological examination she is fully orientated and higher mental functions appear normal. Cranial nerves including fundoscopy and upper limbs are normal. She is unable to move her legs and examination of the lower limbs reveals a flaccid paraparesis with a sensory level at T10. On inspection her feet are in a slightly plantar-flexed position (Figure 48-1). Tone is reduced bilaterally, power is reduced (MRC grade 1/5) in all muscle groups. Reflexes are absent bilaterally and plantar reflexes are extensor. Sensation is reduced to light touch to the level of the umbilicus. Joint position sense is impaired in the feet and ankles and vibration absent to the anterior iliac crest bilaterally.

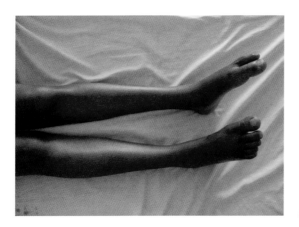

FIGURE 48-1 A patient with an acute-onset flaccid paraplegia. Note the plantar-flexion of her feet.

QUESTIONS

1. What is the clinical syndrome and where is the lesion?
2. What investigations would you plan to do?

Discussion

A 31-year-old woman from northern Tanzania presents with an acute-onset inability to walk. She had a febrile illness three weeks previously, but has otherwise been well.

ANSWER TO QUESTION 1

What is the Clinical Syndrome and Where is the Lesion?

The clinical syndromic diagnosis is acute flaccid paraparesis. The main neuroanatomical differential diagnoses of flaccid paraparesis are lesions of peripheral nerves, including their roots (polyneuropathies and polyradiculopathies), and acute lesions of the spinal cord (myelopathies). The sensory impairment up to the umbilicus (T10 level) and extensor plantar reflexes localize the site of the lesion to the spinal cord. The flaccidity and loss of reflexes can be explained by the early flaccid phase of acute spinal cord injury when spasticity appears days or weeks later (Table 48-1).

TABLE 48-1	**Flaccid versus Spastic Paraparesis**		
Clinical Presentation		**Neuroanatomical Diagnosis**	**Common Aetiologies in Tropical Countries**
Flaccid paraparesis	with bladder involvement and/or sensory level	Acute spinal cord lesion	e.g. inflammation of the spinal cord (= myelitis), ischaemia of the spinal cord (= spinal infarction)
		Acute cauda equina lesion	e. g. metastatic malignancy, schistosomiasis
	without bladder dysfunction, without sensory level	Polyradiculopathy	e.g. Guillain–Barré syndrome, tuberculous arachnoiditis
		Polyneuropathy	e.g. diabetic, HIV-related (incl. antiretrovirals, most commonly stavudine)
Spastic paraparesis		Chronic spinal cord lesion	e.g. compression of spinal cord due to Pott's disease, chronic viral infections such as HTLV-1 and HIV

ANSWER TO QUESTION 2

What Investigations Would You Plan to Do?

If available, the following investigations should be performed: full blood count, erythrocyte sedimentation rate (ESR), blood glucose, renal and liver function tests, HIV serology, VDRL test and schistosomiasis serology. The latter has to be interpreted with caution since it stays positive after past infection. Urine and stool analysis for ova of *Schistosoma spp.* should be done.

Lumbar puncture should be performed with measurement of opening pressure and testing cell differentiation, CSF protein, glucose, Gram and Ziehl–Neelsen stain and VDRL. Imaging should include radiographs of the chest and spine. Neuroimaging (e.g. spinal CT/MRI) is usually not available in sub-Saharan Africa.

THE CASE CONTINUED ...

The patient's full blood count, renal and liver function tests were normal. Results of further investigations are shown in Table 48-2. A spinal tap was done. The CSF-opening pressure was normal and looked clear. Further CSF results are shown in the Table 48-3. The chest and thoracolumbar spine X-rays were normal.

The main differential diagnosis of acute flaccid paraparesis that localizes in the spinal cord is acute spinal cord inflammation (acute transverse myelitis), and spinal cord ischaemia ('spinal stroke'). The CSF findings of increased lymphocytes and elevated protein level are suggestive of inflammation in the spinal cord. Hence, the clinico-laboratory diagnosis is that of acute transverse myelitis.

The management is based on principles of establishing and treating the cause and preventing complications. Treatment in this patient includes steroids and acyclovir directed against the main

TABLE 48-2 Laboratory Results on Admission

Parameter	Patient	Reference Range
ESR (mm/h)	19	≤10
Random blood glucose (mmol/L)	5.6	3.9–11.1
HIV serology	Negative	Negative
VDRL	Negative	Negative
Schistosomiasis serology	Negative	Negative
Urine for ova of *S. haematobium*	Negative	Negative
Stool for ova of *S. mansoni*	Negative	Negative

TABLE 48-3 CSF Results

Parameter	Patient	Normal Range
Leukocytes (cells/μL)	11 (90% lymphocytes)	0–5
Protein (g/L)	1.11	<0.45
Glucose (mmol/L)	3.9	2.8–3.8*
Gram stain	Negative	Negative
Ziehl–Neelsen stain	Negative	Negative
VDRL in the CSF	Negative	Negative

*½ to ⅔ of paired serum glucose sample.

TABLE 48-4 Pathophysiology of Acute Transverse Myelitis

	Pathophysiology	Treatment
'Idiopathic' (majority of the cases)	Presumably an autoimmune phenomenon	Corticosteroids against inflammation
	Might be a manifestation of an autoimmune demyelinating CNS disease (such as NMO and multiple sclerosis)	
Associated with infection	Direct invasion of the spinal cord by microorganisms	Causative treatment, e.g. acyclovir for VZV myelitis
	Autoimmune phenomenon as a result of infection elsewhere ('parainfectious')	Corticosteroids against inflammation
	Might be associated with vaccination against the microorganism	
Associated with a systemic autoimmune disorder	Autoimmune phenomenon	Corticosteroids against inflammation
	Often the autoimmune disorder (e.g. lupus or secondary vasculitis) in the patient is already known	

causes of acute transverse myelitis, e.g. autoimmune inflammation and viral infections (see Summary Box). Counseling of patient and family is very important, and family members/guardians should from the beginning be actively involved in physiotherapy and mobilization of the patient. General measures include strict two-hourly turning, frequent passive movements, urinary catheterization if there is a non-functioning bladder, and adequate analgesia according to the WHO analgesic ladder.

The patient was treated with corticosteroids and acyclovir. She partially improved and was discharged after three weeks. The power in her legs had slightly improved (MRC 2–3/5) and she had a urinary catheter *in situ*. She will be reviewed as an outpatient.

SUMMARY BOX

Acute Transverse Myelitis

Acute transverse myelitis (ATM) is an inflammation of the spinal cord characterized by an acute (hours) or subacute (days) onset, presenting typically with back pain, flaccid paraplegia, a sensory level on the trunk and urinary incontinence.[1–3] Females are more frequently affected, typically in their second and fourth decades. Evidence of inflammation within the spinal cord is shown by increased lymphocytes and elevated protein in the CSF. It can be associated with infections and autoimmune disorders. If the aetiology remains unknown, the ATM is termed idiopathic (Table 48-4). Idiopathic ATM is considered to be an autoimmune phenomenon. 'Idiopathic' ATM can be the first attack of an autoimmune demyelinating disease such as neuromyelitis optica (NMO), and rarely multiple sclerosis. However, multiple sclerosis is virtually unknown in tropical latitudes.

Treatment of idiopathic ATM in adults is largely empirical, with high doses of IV corticosteroids followed by oral prednisolone for 2–3 weeks. Empirical acyclovir is also recommended if varicella zoster virus (VZV) or herpes simplex virus (HSV) myelitis cannot be excluded. However, the majority of patients with ATM, 70–80%, remain disabled with flaccid paraparesis/paraplegia and incontinence.

Further Reading

1. Heckmann JE, Bhigjee AI. Tropical neurology. In: Farrar J, editor. Manson's Tropical Diseases. 23rd ed. London: Elsevier; 2013 [chapter 71].
2. Howlett WP. Paraplegia. Neurology in Africa. Kilimanjaro Christian Medical Centre and University of Bergen; 2012. Available at www.uib.no/cih/en/resources/neurology-in-africa.
3. Borchers AT, Gershwin ME. Transverse myelitis. Autoimmun Rev 2012;11(3):231–48.

49

A 33-YEAR-OLD MALE TRAVELLER TO INDIA WITH DIARRHOEA AND FLATULENCE FOR TWO WEEKS

Gagandeep Kang / Sudhir Babji

Clinical Presentation

HISTORY

A 33-year-old man from Finland who had been backpacking in India for the previous month presents to a private doctor in a small town with complaints of passage of loose stools (four or five episodes per day) for the past two weeks. He reports weight loss, anorexia, malaise, flatulence and abdominal cramping when passing stool. For the past three days he has had bloating and distension after intake of milk products with an urge to pass stool. He has mild nausea, but no fever. Stools were watery earlier but he went to a local pharmacy and was given ciprofloxacin which he took for five days, ending two days previously, and stools are now three or four per day, mushy, greasy and foul-smelling.

CLINICAL FINDINGS

A 33-year-old man, 180 cm, 72 kg (reports a 4 kg weight loss), mild nonspecific abdominal tenderness. No signs of dehydration. The rest of the examination is normal.

LABORATORY RESULTS

Stool for reducing substances: positive. Stool examination for enteric parasites: *Giardia* trophozoites are seen on fresh specimen. *Giardia* cysts are detected on formol-ether concentrated specimens (Figure 49-1).

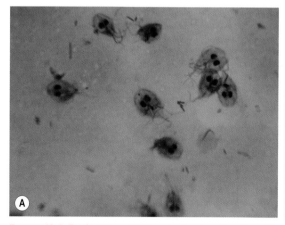
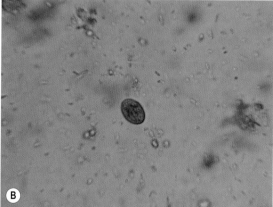

FIGURE 49-1 Fresh preparation showing trophozoites (A) and formol-ether concentration showing cysts (B) of *Giardia* spp.

QUESTIONS

1. What clinical features can be used to establish an aetiological diagnosis of infectious diarrhoea in the tropics?
2. What complications can result from an acute enteric infection?

Discussion

A 33-year-old Finnish traveller to India presents with passage of loose stools, four or five episodes a day for the past two weeks. The stools have become greasy and foul-smelling and he has bloating and distension after consumption of milk or milk products.

The presence of *Giardia* trophozoites and cysts in the stool sample is confirmatory of giardiasis. The presence of reducing substances in the stool indicates a carbohydrate malabsorption, most likely of post-infectious origin.

ANSWER TO QUESTION 1

What Clinical Features Can be Used to Establish an Aetiological Diagnosis of Infectious Diarrhoea in the Tropics?

In the absence of a laboratory, clinical features sometimes provide a clue to the cause of infectious diarrhoea (Table 49-1). Diarrhoea caused by small intestinal infection is typically high volume, watery and often associated with malabsorption and dehydration. Colonic involvement is more often associated with frequent small-volume stools, the presence of blood and a sensation of urgency.

Chronic diarrhoea or recurrent episodes of acute diarrhoea should prompt HIV testing.

ANSWER TO QUESTION 2

What Complications Can Result from an Acute Enteric Infection?

Common complications of acute enteric infections are shown in Table 49-2.

THE CASE CONTINUED ...

The patient was given tinidazole 2 g as a single oral dose. He was advised to restrict milk and high sugar products for a period of two weeks. He was counselled on food and water safety when travelling and was asked to return after three days. On review, he stated that his stool consistency had returned to normal and the frequency had decreased, he had no nausea and his anorexia had decreased. He had eaten a local dessert the previous day without realizing that it was made of reduced milk and had experienced some bloating and discomfort, but was otherwise feeling much better.

TABLE 49-1   Clinical Clues to Pathology and Possible Aetiological Agents of Diarrhoeal Disease

Clinical Observation	Pathophysiology	Possible Aetiology
Few, bulky or large watery stools	Small bowel, secretory	Enterotoxigenic *Escherichia coli* (ETEC), enteropathogenic *E. coli* (EPEC), *Salmonella*, *Vibrio parahaemolyticus*, *Giardia*, possibly *Shigella*
Large volume, watery diarrhoea	Small bowel, enterotoxin mediated	*Vibrio cholerae*, ETEC, *Cryptosporidium*
Many, small volume stools	Large bowel	*Shigella*, *Salmonella*, *Campylobacter*, *Yersinia enterocolitica*, *Clostridium perfringens*, *Entamoeba histolytica*
Tenesmus, faecal urgency, dysentery	Colitis	*E. histolytica*, enteroinvasive *E. coli* (EIEC), enterohaemorrhagic *E. coli* (EHEC), *Shigella*, *Campylobacter*, *Y. enterocolitica*, *Clostridium difficile*
Associated with vomiting	Gastroenteritis or toxin mediated	Calicivirus, rotavirus in children, *Bacillus cereus*, *Staphylococcus aureus* (food poisoning)
Associated with fever	Mucosal invasion or in children	*E. histolytica*, EIEC, EHEC, *Shigella*, *Salmonella*, *C. difficile*, *Campylobacter*, viral agents
Persistent diarrhoea (>2 weeks)	Secondary malabsorption, invasion	*Giardia*, *Cryptosporidium*, *E. histolytica*, *Aeromonas*. In immunosuppression: *Isospora belli*, *Cryptosporidium*, *Microsporidium*

TABLE 49-2 **Common Complications of Acute Enteric Infections**	
Complication	**Pathogen**
Carbohydrate intolerance or malabsorption	*Giardia lamblia/intestinalis*, rotavirus and other forms of viral gastroenteritis,
Fat malabsorption	*Giardia lamblia/intestinalis*
Haemolytic uraemic syndrome	Enterohaemorrhagic *Escherichia coli* (EHEC), *Shigella dysenteriae*
Guillain–Barré syndrome	*Campylobacter jejuni*
Reactive arthritis	*Campylobacter, Salmonella, Shigella, Yersinia* spp.
Enteritis necroticans	*Clostridium perfringens* type C
Liver abscess and other forms of extra-intestinal amoebiasis	*Entamoeba histolytica*
Chronic fatigue syndrome	*Giardia lamblia/intestinalis*, particularly in Scandinavia

SUMMARY BOX

Giardiasis

Giardiasis is caused by *Giardia lamblia* (also named *G. intestinalis*), a flagellate protozoan.[1] The parasite is present throughout the world, with several species found in animals. Not all infections result in symptoms, particularly in tropical countries where local populations with constant exposure rarely develop disease.

Symptomatic giardiasis is common in travellers to regions of South and South-east Asia, Africa (in particular North Africa), the Middle East and Latin America, where clean water supplies and standards of food hygiene are low.[2–4]

Giardia trophozoites are found in the small intestine of humans, and these non-invasive parasites appear to cause diarrhoea by blocking the absorptive surfaces of the gut and possibly by inducing fluid secretion. The trophozoites produce an environmentally resistant form, the cyst, which is passed in stool and enters the soil, water, food, or other surfaces after bowel movements. The most common method of infection is by drinking contaminated water. However, people may also become infected through hand-to-mouth transmission. This involves eating contaminated food or touching contaminated surfaces and unknowingly swallowing the parasite. The signs and symptoms of giardiasis usually occur within 7–14 days of exposure. Symptoms include diarrhoea, pale greasy stools, stomach cramps, gas, nausea, vomiting, bloating, weight loss and weakness. The symptoms usually last for 1–2 weeks, but may last as long as six weeks. Giardiasis can cause malabsorption of vitamin A, vitamin B_{12}, iron, fat and carbohydrates in up to 20–40% of the patients. Malabsorption can sometimes be prolonged and take several weeks to disappear. Chronic and multiple infections in young children have been shown to cause long-term effects on growth leading to stunting. The most common treatment is administration of drugs of the nitroimidazole group, with tinidazole being the drug of choice followed by metronidazole. Tinidazole is effective as a single dose and metronidazole is given tds for 5–7 days. Other drugs used are nitazoxanide, furazolidone and quinacrine. In rare cases of failure of a single drug, combination drug therapy is administered.

Further Reading

1. Kelly P. Intestinal protozoa. In: Farrar J, editor. Manson's Tropical Diseases. 23rd ed. London: Elsevier; 2013 [chapter 49].
2. Ross AG, Olds GR, Cripps AW, et al. Enteropathogens and chronic illness in returning travelers. N Engl J Med 2013; 368(19):1817–25.
3. Kaiser L, Surawicz CM. Infectious causes of chronic diarrhoea. Best Pract Res Clin Gastroenterol 2012;26(5):563–71.
4. Wright SG. Protozoan infections of the gastrointestinal tract. Infect Dis Clin North Am 2012;26(2):323–39.

A 34-YEAR-OLD HIV-REACTIVE WOMAN FROM MALAWI WITH SLOWLY PROGRESSIVE HALF-SIDED WEAKNESS

51

Juri Katchanov

Clinical Presentation

HISTORY

A 34-year-old woman presents to a neurology outpatient clinic in Malawi, with slowly progressive weakness of the left arm and leg.

Her problems started approximately three months earlier when she first noticed a limp in her left leg. The weakness progressed, and over the following weeks she also realized that her left arm was becoming affected.

The patient is a poor historian and often has difficulties describing the onset and timing of sequential events, but from her story it appears likely that the problems started insidiously and have been slowly progressing since. She denies any head trauma, headache, recent episodes of fever, nausea, visual impairment or loss of weight. The review of systems is unremarkable.

The patient was diagnosed with smear-positive pulmonary tuberculosis five months earlier. At that time she was also found to be HIV-reactive with a baseline CD4 count of 54/μL. She was started on antituberculous therapy, vitamin B$_6$, antiretrovirals and co-trimoxazole prophylaxis, all of which she is currently taking.

The patient works as a street vendor selling mobile phone vouchers. Despite her left-sided weakness she is still able to work sitting on a plastic chair and managing her vouchers and money with her right hand. She is divorced and does not have any children. She lives in an urban high-density area.

CLINICAL FINDINGS

She is afebrile and her vital signs and general examination are normal apart from slightly pale conjunctivae. On fundoscopy her fundi are normal without any signs of papilloedema or retinitis.

The neurological examination reveals a spastic hemiparesis on the left with hyperreflexia. The power in the left leg is 2/5 (active movement with gravity eliminated) and in her left arm 3/5 (active movement against gravity). There is a pronator drift on the left (Figure 51-1) indicating proximal weakness. Sensation of pain is reduced in her left leg and hand. The examination of her cranial nerves is normal.

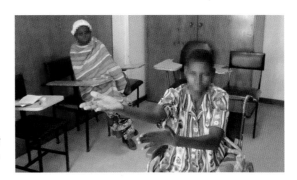

FIGURE 51-1 Pronator drift on the left side as a sign of left upper limb weakness. The patient was asked to stretch out both arms and close her eyes.

LABORATORY RESULTS

Full blood count: WBC 3.8×10^9/L (reference range: 4–10), haemoglobin 9.9 g/dL (12–14), platelets 140×10^9/L (150–350).

QUESTIONS

1. What is your differential diagnosis?
2. What is your diagnostic approach in the resource-limited setting?

Discussion

A 34-year-old HIV-reactive woman presents with a three-month history of progressive left-sided weakness of insidious onset. She was diagnosed with pulmonary tuberculosis (TB) and HIV five months prior to her presentation. She is on antiretroviral therapy (ART), co-trimoxazole prophylaxis and on antituberculous medication. On examination, there is a spastic hemiparesis on the left side with sensory involvement.

ANSWER TO QUESTION 1

What is Your Differential Diagnosis?

The combination of spastic hemiparesis with hyperreflexia and sensory impairment affecting one half of the body localizes the lesion into her brain.[1] The onset appears subacute and the progression is slow. This makes ischaemic and haemorrhagic lesions ('strokes') unlikely causes since they present (hyper-)acutely and usually do not progress. Most likely the patient has one or several focal brain lesion(s).

The differential diagnosis of focal brain lesions (FBLs) in HIV-infected individuals in tropical countries is broad. Patients may suffer from HIV-related brain diseases such as cerebral toxoplasmosis, progressive multifocal leukencephalopathy, CNS-lymphoma, cryptococcoma and CMV encephalitis. *Mycobacterium tuberculosis* infection of the brain parenchyma can present as tuberculoma or tuberculous abscess and can occur with or without immunosuppression.

Furthermore, HIV-positive individuals may of course suffer from conditions primarily unrelated to their HIV-infection such as a brain tumour, brain metastases or a cerebral abscess.

Endemic 'tropical' diseases such as neurocysticercosis, neuroschistosomiasis or, in Latin America, reactivated Chagas' disease, can also present with focal brain lesions and should be considered according to the local epidemiological pattern.

In this particular case, the patient developed a focal brain lesion two months after starting ART. Central nervous system disorders are common after ART initiation.[2] It is thought that the recovering immune system may 'unmask' or 'paradoxically deteriorate' pre-existing CNS infections. This phenomenon is called immune reconstitution inflammatory syndrome (IRIS) and, depending on the type, is called 'unmasking' or 'paradoxical' IRIS.

Tuberculoma, progressive multifocal leukencephalopathy (PML) and cryptococcoma have been well documented in the context of IRIS. Toxoplasmosis has been described after ART initiation, even in patients on co-trimoxazole prophylaxis.

Of note, our patient was diagnosed with TB at the time of ART initiation and CNS tuberculosis can deteriorate after ART introduction as well as after commencement of TB treatment.

ANSWER TO QUESTION 2

What is Your Diagnostic Approach in the Resource-Limited Setting?

The diagnostic work-up of FBL in a resource-limited setting primarily depends on the availability of investigations. It often remains mainly clinical, guided by epidemiological evidence and by the degree of immunosuppression in HIV-positive patients. Clinicians may often find themselves restricted to the pragmatic approach of 'treating the treatable'.

If the patient is HIV-positive, a CD4 count should be done. Some FBL are very unlikely if the CD4 count is above 200/µL, e.g. CNS lymphoma, cryptococcoma or cerebral toxoplasmosis. Cerebral TB can occur at any CD4 count. PML mostly manifests in patients with advanced immunosuppression but has also been described in patients with higher CD4 counts.[3]

Serum anti-toxoplasma-IgG and cryptococcal antigen (CrAG) are helpful, but are usually not routinely available. Negative anti-toxoplasma serology makes toxoplasmosis a very unlikely diagnosis, whereas a positive serological result documents past contact with the pathogen but fails to prove its relevance for the current illness.[4]

Sensitivity of CSF examination in FBL is low, and both cryptococcoma and tuberculoma may present with a normal CSF. However, if ZN-stain, CrAg, India Ink or fungal cultures are available, these tests should be done and might help establish the diagnosis.

Chest radiography and abdominal ultrasound are useful as they may reveal tuberculous lesions, metastases or a primary neoplasm.

Cerebral imaging plays an important role in diagnosing FBL, however, availability is extremely limited in resource-constrained settings. CT may at times produce nonspecific results confirming the clinical diagnosis of an FBL but failing to assist the clinician in narrowing down the spectrum of differential diagnoses. MRI is more informative; however, it is practically unavailable as a routine investigation in tropical low- and middle-income countries.

Cystic lesions on CT are indicative of neurocysticercosis. Cerebral oedema with mass effect and contrast enhancement would favour cerebral abscess, tuberculoma, toxoplasmosis and CNS lymphoma, whereas PML classically shows no mass effect and no enhancement.[3] Meningeal enhancement is typical for tuberculosis.[4]

THE CASE CONTINUED ...

Routine CSF examination was normal, India Ink stain and fungal cultures were negative. The patient was started on empirical anti-toxoplasmosis treatment with high-dose co-trimoxazole. ART and antituberculous treatment were continued. Prednisolone 1 mg/kg bodyweight was added to cover for presumed IRIS. The patient was put on a waiting list for a cerebral MRI scan, which was available thanks to a local research project.

On four-week follow-up her clinical status was unchanged. At eight weeks there was further deterioration of power in her left hand. An MRI of her head was done which showed multifocal T2 hyperintense lesions exclusively affecting the white matter and more prominent in the right hemisphere (frontal and temporal lobes). Furthermore, there was a small area of demyelination in the left cerebellar peduncle. These radiological findings were deemed strongly suggestive of progressive multifocal leukencephalopathy (PML).

A presumed diagnosis of PML was made. The patient was referred to a local rehabilitation centre for walking aids. The local palliative care team was involved.

SUMMARY BOX

Progressive Multifocal Leukencephalopathy

Progressive multifocal leukencephalopathy (PML) is caused by a reactivation of the human JC-polyoma virus.[3] JC stands for 'John Cunningham', the first patient from whom the virus was isolated. JC virus is neurotropic, affecting oligodendrocytes.

PML always occurs as a result of virus reactivation due to immunosuppression. Primary infection usually takes place during childhood and the virus remains quiescent in the kidneys, bone marrow and lymphoid tissue.[3] Upon reactivation, a productive infection of brain oligodendrocytes results in demyelination. The presenting symptoms include muscle weakness, sensory deficits, hemianopia, cognitive dysfunction, aphasia, and coordination and gait difficulties.

On imaging, multiple lesions are located in the subcortical white matter and cerebellar peduncles. The lesions look hypodense on CT, and hyperintense on T2 MRI. There is no oedema, mass effect or contrast enhancement.

The only treatment showing some benefit in PML patients is ART. Prognosis before introduction of ART was poor and only 10% of PML patients survived for one year. However, in the ART era the one-year survival rate has increased to 50%.[3]

PML occurring within the first months of ART is often described as PML-immune reconstitution inflammatory syndrome (PML–IRIS). Of note, PML–IRIS possibly accounts for nearly 25% of all PML cases in HIV-reactive patients. One study showed a beneficial effect of steroids in the management of PML–IRIS. However, in a setting with high prevalence of HIV-associated opportunistic infections and tuberculosis, it is probably advisable to apply steroids only if other common CNS infections are excluded or covered for.

Further Reading

1. Heckmann JE, Bhigjee AI. Tropical neurology. In: Farrar J, editor. Manson's Tropical Diseases. 23rd ed. London: Elsevier; 2013 [chapter 71].

2. Asselman V, Thienemann F, Pepper DJ, et al. Central nervous system disorders after starting antiretroviral therapy in South Africa. AIDS 2010;24(18):2871–6.

3. Tan CS, Koralnik IJ. Progressive multifocal leukoencephalopathy and other disorders caused by JC virus: clinical features and pathogenesis. Lancet Neurol 2010;9(4):425–37.

4. Modi M, Mochan A, Modi G. Management of HIV-associated focal brain lesions in developing countries. QJM 2004;97(7):413–21.

A 56-YEAR-OLD MAN FROM PERU WITH PROLONGED FEVER AND SEVERE ANAEMIA

52

Ciro Maguiña / Carlos Seas / Frederique Jacquerioz

Clinical Presentation

HISTORY

A 56-year-old male Peruvian is admitted to a hospital in the capital, Lima, with a two-week history of fever, jaundice and confusion.

Daily fever started three months after leaving a rural area in the highlands of Northern Peru (altitude of 2400 m), where the patient spent three weeks on vacations. In the second week of illness the patient noticed dark urine and jaundice, and few days before admission his wife noticed confusion and somnolence. While in the rural area, the patient and his wife were bitten at night by tiny mosquitoes; no personal protection was used. Otherwise there has been no animal contact. The past medical history is unremarkable.

CLINICAL FINDINGS

His blood pressure is 90/60 mmHg, pulse 110 bpm and regular, temperature 39.2°C, respiratory rate 22 breath cycles per minute. The patient appears confused and disorientated without any focal neurological findings or meningeal signs (GCS 14/15). Skin and conjunctivae are markedly pale and there is scleral jaundice. Cardiovascular and pulmonary examination are normal. The liver is slightly enlarged but there is no splenomegaly.

LABORATORY RESULTS

Creatinine, electrolytes and alkaline phosphatase are normal. His further routine laboratory results are shown in Table 52-1. Coomb's test is negative. The CSF results are within normal range.

FURTHER INVESTIGATIONS

A CT of the brain is normal. Abdominal ultrasound reveals hepatomegaly, but no focal lesions.

TABLE 52-1	Blood Results on Admission	
Parameter	**Patient**	**Reference Range**
WBC (x10⁹/L)	14.9	4–10
Neutrophils (x10⁹/L)	13.1	1.8–7.2
Lymphocytes (x10⁹/L)	0.9	1.5–4
Band forms (%)	4	0–5
Haemoglobin (g/dL)	6	13–15
Reticulocytes (%)	8	0.5–1.5
Platelets (x10⁹/L)	454	150–350
LDH (U/L)	1500	<250
Total bilirubin (µmol/L)	239	<19
Direct bilirubin (µmol/L)	103	<5

1. What are your differential diagnoses?
2. How would you approach this patient?

Discussion

A Peruvian man presents with a history of prolonged fever, altered neurological status and evidence of haemolysis after a stay in a rural area in the highlands of Peru.

ANSWER TO QUESTION 1

What Are Your Differential Diagnoses?

The most important differential diagnoses in this patient are malaria and bartonellosis.

Plasmodium vivax is the only species of *Plasmodium* prevalent in the highland regions of Peru. Interestingly, the patient presents with several features of severe and complicated malaria, including severe anaemia, jaundice and impaired consciousness. However, *P. vivax* is less commonly associated with severe malaria than *P. falciparum*. Bartonellosis is another important diagnosis to consider given the recent travel history in the highlands of Peru, where sandflies, the vector of bartonellosis, are present. The patient also reported being bitten by tiny mosquitoes. Less common infections to include in the differential diagnosis are rickettsial diseases (both endemic and epidemic typhus are present in Peru), leptospirosis, typhoid fever, brucellosis and several viral diseases, including the agents of viral hepatitis and yellow fever. However, none of them produces significant haemolysis and some are not endemic in the highlands (yellow fever for instance). Non-infectious causes of haemolysis should also be considered, including autoimmune disorders and haematological conditions.

ANSWER TO QUESTION 2

How Would You Approach This Patient?

The first step in this patient is to rule out malaria by performing a thick and thin smear or by using rapid diagnostic tests. Based on the exposure history and the high suspicion of bartonellosis, a thin film should be performed to calculate the differential leukocyte count and to look for the presence of *Bartonella bacilliformis* in red blood cells.

THE CASE CONTINUED ...

The patient progressed to shock. He was transferred to the intensive care unit (ICU) and required treatment with vasopressors. Blood films were negative for malaria. However, the thin film revealed massive red blood cell infestation by pleomorphic cocco-bacillary structures compatible with *B. bacilliformis* (Figure 52-1). Blood cultures were negative for bacteria, including cultures in special media

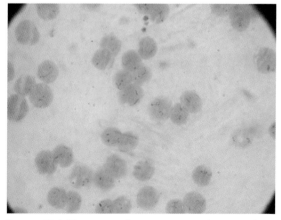

FIGURE 52-1 Thin smear showing massive infestation of red blood cells with cocco-bacillary structures (Wright stain).

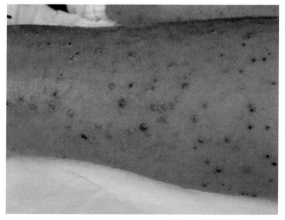

FIGURE 52-2 Multiple erythematous-violaceous papules of different sizes characteristic of the chronic phase (verruga peruana).

for *Bartonella*. The patient was started on a combination of intravenous ciprofloxacin and ceftriaxone for ten days. Altered mental status resolved after three days of antimicrobial treatment and fever subsided after five days. By day 4 the bacteria had disappeared from the blood smears. No further complications were observed during a three-month follow-up period.

SUMMARY BOX

Bartonellosis – Oroya Fever and Verruga Peruana

Bartonellosis, caused by *Bartonella bacilliformis*, is a vector-borne disease mainly found in the Andean valleys of Peru at an altitude between 500 and 3,200 metres, although transmission may occur at higher altitudes and in jungle areas as well.[1] Colombia and Ecuador have also reported sporadic cases. The disease is transmitted by female sandflies, mostly *Lutzomyia verrucarum* or *L. peruensis*, which characteristically bite indoors at night-time. Human beings are the only known reservoir. Most of the infections are asymptomatic or oligo-symptomatic. However, a minority of patients progress to severe disease ('Oroya fever') after a mean incubation period of 3–8 weeks (longer incubation periods up to nine months have been observed). Oroya fever is characterized by high temperatures, malaise, myalgias and severe haemolytic anaemia with jaundice, which results from intravascular destruction of red blood cells or by splenic removal of deformed infested erythrocytes.[2] Complications during this acute phase include heart failure, as well as pericardial and pleural effusions. CNS involvement, characterized by impaired consciousness, agitation and coma, occurs in approximately 20% of patients and is associated with higher mortality rates. Secondary immunosuppression has been reported during this phase and patients may present with opportunistic infections, e.g. salmonellosis, toxoplasmosis or *Pneumocystis jirovecii* pneumonia.[2] A distinctive cytokine pattern characterized by increased production of interleukin-10 and interferon gamma has been reported.

Following acute Oroya fever, within 1–2 months a chronic angioproliferative cutaneous stage ('verruga peruana') may occur in approximately 5% of treated patients and in an unknown percentage of untreated individuals. Occasionally, Veruga Peruana is seen without noticeable acute phase manifestations. It is mostly seen in children in endemic areas. Skin lesions are usually small (1–4 mm) red-violaceous painless papules located on the face or the extremities, and can be single or multiple (Figure 52-2). Nodular lesions can also be observed. The lesions resemble bacillary angiomatosis caused by *B. quintana* and *B. henselae*.

In the acute phase, diagnosis is made by proof of cocco-bacilli inside red blood cells. *B. bacilliformis* is a fastidious bacterium and culture requires a specific medium such as the Columbia agar incubated at 25–28°C for up to two weeks.

Two novel *Bartonella* species have been identified from Peru. *B. rochalimae* was identified in an American tourist with an acute febrile illness treated for presumed typhoid fever,[3] and *B. ancashi* was discovered in a Peruvian patient with multiple skin lesions.[4]

Recommended treatment of the acute phase includes ciprofloxacin alone or combined with ceftriaxone in severe cases. These antimicrobials also cover for *Salmonella* spp., the commonest opportunistic infection observed in these patients. Oral azithromycin is the drug of choice in the chronic phase. Alternatively, rifampicin can be used.[5]

Note: Oroya fever is also named Carrion's disease after a famous Peruvian medical student, Daniel Carrion, who in 1885 inoculated himself with blood from a patient's verruga peruana and developed acute bartonellosis (Oroya fever). He unfortunately died from the disease. However, his experiment demonstrated clearly that verruga peruana and Oroya fever were different clinical forms of the same infection.

Further Reading

1. Angelakis E, Raoult D. Bartonellosis, cat-scratch disease, trench fever, human Ehrlichiosis. In: Farrar J, editor. Manson's Tropical Diseases. 23rd ed. London: Elsevier; 2013 [chapter 30].
2. Maguiña C, Garcia PJ, Gotuzzo E, et al. Bartonellosis (Carrion's disease) in the modern era. Clin Infect Dis 2001;33(6):772–9.
3. Eremeeva ME, Gerns HL, Lydy SL, et al. Bacteremia, fever, and splenomegaly caused by a newly recognized bartonella species. N Engl J Med 2007;356(23):2381–7.
4. Blazes DL, Mullins K, Smoak BL, et al. Novel Bartonella agent as cause of verruga peruana. Emerg Infect Dis 2013;19(7):1111–14.
5. Maguina C, Guerra H, Ventosilla P. Bartonellosis. *Clin Dermatol* 2009;27(3):271–80.

A 24-YEAR-OLD WOMAN FROM UGANDA WITH FEVER AND SHOCK

Benjamin Jeffs

Clinical Presentation

HISTORY

A 24-year-old woman presents to a small hospital in rural Uganda because of a five-day history of a febrile illness. Apart from fever, the illness started with a sore throat and aching all over. She also developed some abdominal pain and diarrhoea. The patient has become increasingly unwell over the course of the past days. She is very weak and needs help to stand.

Her husband died of a severe febrile illness six days before she herself became ill. He had worked in a local gold mine and had previously been in good health. He had fallen ill about a week before his death. His wife had looked after him during his final illness and he had died at home.

CLINICAL FINDINGS

The patient looks very unwell. Her blood pressure is 85/65 mmHg, pulse rate 105 bpm, temperature 38°C. She has bilateral conjunctivitis. There is no rash and no lymphadenopathy. The heart sounds are normal and her chest is clear. Her abdominal examination is normal.

QUESTIONS

1. What are your differential diagnoses?
2. How would you approach the patient and what tests would you do?

Discussion

A young Ugandan woman presents to a rural hospital with a severe febrile illness. She is hypotensive and has bilateral conjunctivitis. Her husband has recently died after a short febrile illness.

ANSWER TO QUESTION I

What Are Your Differential Diagnoses?

The presentation is nonspecific and a wide range of acute infectious diseases are possible.

Both malaria and typhoid fever present with nonspecific symptoms and a septic picture, but neither would cause conjunctivitis.

A severe viral infection with an adenovirus or influenza would be possible but the patient appears slightly too unwell for this. Measles commonly presents with pronounced conjunctivitis, but at this stage one would see a rash.

The fact that the patient's husband has recently died of a similar severe febrile illness should raise the suspicion of a viral haemorrhagic fever (VHF). Marburg haemorrhagic fever (MHF) has been associated with mines.

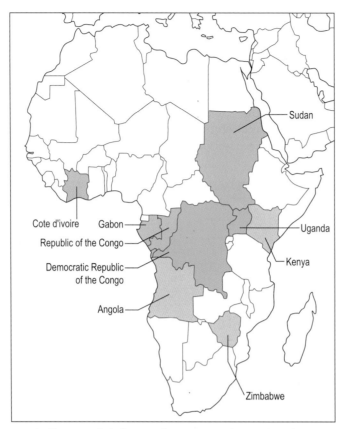

FIGURE 53-1 Endemic areas for filoviruses. Only filoviruses known to cause haemorrhagic fever are shown. Countries where Ebola and Marburg haemorrhagic fevers have been seen are indicated in green and blue, respectively, with countries in red indicating documentation of both diseases. Incidence and risk of disease may vary significantly within each country. Filoviruses are likely to occur outside these countries but have not yet been recognised. *(Reproduced from Farrar J, editor. Manson's Tropical Diseases. 23rd ed. London: Elsevier; 2013. Fig. 16.1. © Elsevier.)*

ANSWER TO QUESTION 2

How Would You Approach the Patient and What Tests Would You Do?

The patient should be treated with extreme caution due to the possibility of a viral haemorrhagic fever. Nosocomial spread of these diseases can cause hospital outbreaks with a high mortality. The patient should ideally be isolated in a side room. Blood tests should be kept to a minimum to reduce the risk to laboratory staff. Protective clothing such as gloves and a surgical gown are recommended during procedures. The risk of transmission of VHF viruses from a malaria slide is very low once the blood spot is dry, so it would be reasonable to do a malaria slide or a rapid diagnostic test. However the prevalence of *Plasmodium falciparum* parasitaemia in Uganda is high and a positive slide would not rule out VHF.

To protect laboratory staff all biochemical and haematological tests should be done using a near patient tester if possible.

The public health authorities should be alerted to the possibility of a case of viral haemorrhagic fever. Ideally testing for this should be organized, but samples are likely to need special shipping arrangements to be taken to a specialized laboratory.

THE CASE CONTINUED ...

A presumed diagnosis of Marburg haemorrhagic fever was made. The malaria slide showed a low level of parasitaemia with *P. falciparum*. A sample for Marburg and Ebola PCR was sent in a sealed plastic container. The patient was isolated in a side room and all patient contact was carried out while wearing gloves. She was treated with IV artesunate and then artemether/lumefantrine. She was given empirical IV ceftriaxone to cover for possible sepsis and was resuscitated with IV fluids.

Over the next few days the patient remained very unwell, then she started to improve. Once she had recovered she was kept in isolation for a further two days and was then allowed to return home. The day after her discharge a positive MHF PCR-result came back. Had this been known while she was in hospital, stricter infection control procedures, including double gloves, a mask, goggles and a disposable (waterproof) surgical gown, would have been appropriate.

Her family members, close friends and medical staff were interviewed; anyone who had had physical contact with her or her body fluids was told to monitor their temperature for 21 days from the time of contact which is the maximum incubation period for MHF. Anyone who developed a fever or became unwell during this period was isolated.

SUMMARY BOX

Filoviral Diseases

Marburg haemorrhagic fever (MHF) and Ebola haemorrhagic fever (EHF) are both caused by filoviruses.[1] They are clinically indistinguishable and cause severe illnesses with a high mortality rate. Symptoms are nonspecific and patients may present with fever, sore throat, general body ache, retrosternal chest pain and abdominal symptoms. Conjunctivitis is common. The most frequent cause of death is shock. Less than half of those who die develop haemorrhages due to disseminated intravascular coagulation.[2]

Since symptoms are nonspecific and testing is difficult in most of Africa, filoviral haemorrhagic fevers (FHF) are normally recognized only if a cluster of cases occurs. In particular, an outbreak in an endemic area in which health workers die should raise the suspicion towards FHF.

EHF and MHF have both been detected over wide areas of sub-Saharan Africa, with EHF being commonest in moist areas of West Africa (Figure 53-1). Both are zoonoses of bats. Many cases of MHF have been linked to entering or working in caves or mines, whereas cases of EHF are associated with butchering and eating apes or monkeys. These primates are dead-end hosts for the disease and catch the virus from eating in trees that are visited by fruit bats.

Filoviruses can spread between people through direct physical contact or contact with infected body fluids. Large nosocomial outbreaks involving the death of large numbers of medical staff have been recorded. Therefore strict infection control measures should be followed while caring for anyone with a suspected viral haemorrhagic fever.[3] There is no specific treatment for filoviral diseases but supportive therapy is likely to be beneficial. If the diagnosis is unconfirmed, empirical treatment should be given for other possible differential diagnoses.

Further Reading

1. Blumberg L, Enria D, Bausch DG. Viral haemorrhagic fevers. In: Farrar J, editor. Manson's Tropical Diseases. 23rd ed. London: Elsevier; 2013 [chapter 16].
2. Jeffs B, Roddy P, Weatherill D, et al. The Médecins Sans Frontières intervention in the Marburg hemorrhagic fever epidemic, Uige, Angola, 2005. I. Lessons learned in the hospital. J Infect Dis 2007;196(Suppl. 2):S154–61.
3. World Health Organization. Interim Infection Control Guidelines for Care of Patients with Suspected or Confirmed Filovirus (Ebola, Marburg) Haemorrhagic Fever. Geneva: WHO; 2008.

A 52-YEAR-OLD MALE SAFARI TOURIST RETURNING FROM SOUTH AFRICA WITH FEVER AND A SKIN LESION

54

Camilla Rothe

Clinical Presentation

HISTORY

A 52-year-old man presents to a tropical medicine clinic in Germany with fever for the past two days. He is also complaining of night sweats and a frontal headache. There are no joint pains and he has not noticed a rash.

Ten days ago he returned from a two-week holiday trip to South Africa. He visited Cape Town and travelled the Garden Route and through KwaZulu–Natal. He went on safari in Kruger Park and several other game reserves. He did not take any antimalarial chemoprophylaxis. His past medical history is unremarkable.

CLINICAL FINDINGS

Fair general condition. Tympanic temperature 37.5°C (after taking 1 g of paracetamol), pulse 80 bpm, blood pressure 130/70 mmHg.

No jaundice; neck supple. Enlarged lymph nodes in the left groin. You notice a small sticking plaster on the left upper thigh of the patient. He tells you that he has noted a skin lesion that he meant to show to a medical practitioner for advice. You ask the patient to take off the plaster (see Figure 54-1).

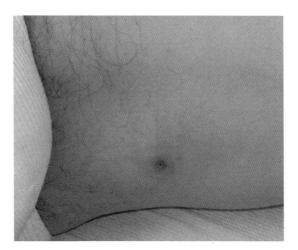

FIGURE 54-1 Small necrotic skin lesion (about 0.7 cm in diameter) with surrounding inflammation and lymphangiitis on the left upper thigh of the patient.

QUESTIONS

1. What is the diagnosis?
2. How would you manage this patient?

Discussion

A 52-year-old German man presents with a short history of fever after a trip to South Africa. On examination there is a small necrotic skin lesion on his upper thigh with adjoining lymphangiitis and lymphadenitis.

ANSWER TO QUESTION 1

What is the Diagnosis?

The skin lesion is a typical eschar. Given the travel history, the clinical diagnosis is African tick-bite fever. This rickettsial disease is a common cause of fever in safari tourists returning from Southern Africa.

ANSWER TO QUESTION 2

How Would You Manage This Patient?

The patient has travelled to KwaZulu–Natal, which is a malaria-endemic region, and he has not taken any antimalarial chemoprophylaxis. In any febrile traveller returning from a malaria-endemic region, malaria has to be ruled out, even if other diagnoses seem obvious.

The diagnosis of African tick-bite fever is primarily clinical. Serologies are not routinely taken and may be more of academic value in this case. African tick-bite fever is usually a mild, self-limiting disease. Doxycycline can be given to speed up recovery.

THE CASE CONTINUED ...

The malaria rapid diagnostic test, as well as thick and thin slide for malaria, came back negative. The patient was prescribed doxycycline at 100 mg bid PO for one week. The fever settled within the next few days and the lymphadenopathy subsided. The eschar eventually healed after about two weeks.

SUMMARY BOX

African Tick-Bite Fever

African tick-bite fever (ATBF) belongs to the spotted fever group of rickettsioses, a large group of infections which are mainly transmitted by ticks. ATBF is caused by *Rickettsia africae* and transmitted by cattle ticks of the genus *Amblyomma*, which act both as reservoir and as vector.

Further reservoir hosts are wild and domestic animals, such as cattle, buffalos, rhinos, and hippos. ATBF is endemic in most of rural sub-Saharan Africa and in the West Indies.[1]

ATBF commonly occurs in game hunters, safari tourists, cross-country runners and campers in veld areas or grasslands. ATBF is one of the most common causes of febrile presentations in international travellers to sub-Saharan Africa and it is the most common rickettsial infection encountered in travel medicine. By contrast, fairly little is known about incidence and risk factors of ATBF in local indigenous populations.[2]

The incubation period following the bite of an infected tick is about 6–10 days. Patients develop fever and flu-like symptoms such as myalgias and headache. There may be a characteristic inoculation eschar at the site of the bite with local lymphadenopathy. Multiple eschars are not uncommon, as *Amblyomma* ticks are known to aggressively attack their potential hosts. Despite the fact that African tick-bite fever belongs to the group of 'spotted fevers', a rash is seen in less than half of cases. ATBF is usually a mild illness and no deaths or severe complications have been reported so far.[1]

Diagnosis of ATBF is usually made clinically, but in febrile individuals living in or returning from tropical areas malaria should still always be ruled out.

Serology is the most commonly applied microbiological method for all spotted fevers, but it can usually only provide a retrospective diagnosis. The immunofluorescence assay (IFA) is currently considered gold standard. Diagnosis is confirmed if seroconversion and a fourfold increase in specific antibodies on paired admission and convalescent sample has been documented.

Treatment may not be necessary in mild cases. Doxycycline 100 mg bid PO may be given for 3–7 days. In pregnant women and in children macrolides or chloramphenicol are also effective.

Preventive measures include appropriate clothing, which should be impregnated with pyrethroids and topical insect repellents such as DEET. Whether tetracyclines can be used as chemoprophylaxis against ATBF is still a matter of dispute.[3]

Diagnosis is confirmed by visualization of *P. brasiliensis* (yeast form) on wet preparation of specimen and/or isolation in fungal culture. The yeast is easily observed on KOH preparation but its isolation in culture is difficult and takes 20–30 days.

Treatment includes azoles for mild and moderate cases. Itraconazole (200 mg/day for 12 months) is considered the drug of choice. Voriconazole and co-trimoxazole are alternatives; the latter is commonly used in Brazil. Amphotericin B deoxycholate (cumulative dose of 1–2 g) is indicated for severe and extensive disease. However the drug is not curative and should be followed by an azole or co-trimoxazole to complete 12 months' treatment.

Recently, case reports of severe and unusual extrapulmonary manifestations of paracoccidioidomycosis have been described in HTLV-1 infected patients and the two conditions might be associated.[3]

Further Reading

1. Hay RJ. Fungal infections. In: Farrar J, editor. Manson's Tropical Diseases. 23rd ed. London: Elsevier; 2013 [chapter 38].
2. Morejon KM, Machado AA, Martinez R. Paracoccidioidomycosis in patients infected with and not infected with human immunodeficiency virus: a case-control study. Am J Trop Med Hyg 2009;80(3):359–66.
3. Leon M, Alave J, Bustamante B, et al. Human T lymphotropic virus 1 and paracoccidioidomycosis: a probable association in Latin America. Clin Infect Dis 2010;51(2):250–1.

56 A 21-YEAR-OLD PREGNANT WOMAN FROM THE GAMBIA WITH A RASH

David Mabey

Clinical Presentation

HISTORY

A 21-year-old woman comes to your clinic in The Gambia complaining of a generalized, non-itchy rash that she has had for five days. She is otherwise well, and has no significant past medical history. She is 32 weeks pregnant. This is her first pregnancy.

CLINICAL FINDINGS

She has a generalized rash (Figure 56-1). Her mouth is normal, and there is no lymphadenopathy. She is not anaemic or jaundiced, and general examination is unremarkable.

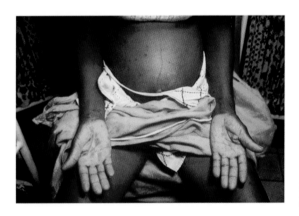

FIGURE 56-1 Generalized, non-itchy macular rash in a pregnant Gambian woman.

QUESTIONS

1. What is the most likely diagnosis, and how might this affect the outcome of her pregnancy?
2. How would you manage the patient?

Discussion

A 21-year-old pregnant Gambian woman presents because of a generalized macular rash involving the palms of both hands. The rash is non-itchy and she is otherwise fine.

ANSWER TO QUESTION I

What is the Most Likely Diagnosis, and How Might This Affect the Outcome of Her Pregnancy?

A generalized, non-itchy rash affecting the palms of the hands is syphilis until proven otherwise.[1] Syphilis in pregnancy has a serious impact on pregnancy outcome. A study in Tanzania showed that, among women with latent syphilis and a rapid plasma reagin (RPR) titre of ≥1:8, 25% delivered a stillborn baby, and 33% a low birth-weight baby.[2]

The baby may be born with signs of congenital syphilis, including a generalized bullous rash, jaundice and hepatosplenomegaly. In this case the prognosis is bad, with 50% mortality even with treatment. Alternatively, the baby may appear normal at birth, and present at the age of 3–4 months with failure to thrive and signs of congenital syphilis, usually including a generalized rash which affects the palms of the hands and soles of the feet (Figure 56-2). Other common signs include hepatosplenomegaly, painful periostitis involving the long bones, and a persistent nasal discharge, which may be bloodstained (the 'syphilitic snuffles').

ANSWER TO QUESTION 2

How Would You Manage the Patient?

Intramuscular benzathine penicillin is the treatment of choice for syphilis. A single dose of 2.4 million units is recommended for primary, secondary and early latent syphilis (of less than two years' duration). A single dose, given before 28 weeks' gestation, has been shown to prevent adverse outcomes due to syphilis.[3] As this patient has not been treated before 28 weeks, her infant should receive a course of treatment for congenital syphilis (IM procaine penicillin 50 000 units/kg daily for 10–14 days) or, if the infant's CSF is normal, a single IM dose of benzathine penicillin 50 000 units.

THE CASE CONTINUED ...

The patient was treated with a single IM dose of benzathine penicillin and she made an uneventful recovery. She delivered a normal infant at term.

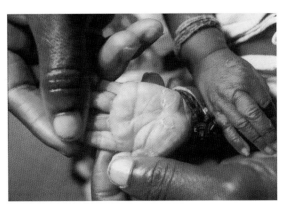

FIGURE 56-2 Congenital syphilis in a 3-month-old infant: desquamating lesion of the palms.

SUMMARY BOX

Syphilis in Pregnancy

Primary syphilis causes an ulcer, or chancre, at the site of inoculation, which is usually painless. Women are often unaware of the lesion as it may be on the cervix or vaginal wall. The secondary stage usually occurs 6–8 weeks later, causing a generalized rash that often affects the palms of the hands, and usually does not itch. There may be other manifestations, including jaundice or ocular involvement (uveitis). The clinical signs resolve over a few weeks in the absence of treatment, after which the patient enters the latent stage. A small minority develop tertiary lesions involving the cardiovascular or nervous system many years later. Progression may be more rapid in HIV-positive patients. Women with secondary syphilis, who have a disseminated infection, are most likely to affect their fetus, but the infection can cross the placenta in pregnant women with latent syphilis.

According to current WHO estimates, syphilis in pregnancy causes more than 500 000 adverse pregnancy outcomes per year, including more than 200 000 stillbirths and 100 000 neonatal deaths.[4] These could be prevented if all pregnant women were screened for syphilis, and treated with a single dose of penicillin if they test positive, before 28 weeks' gestation.

Serological tests for syphilis are either treponemal (e.g. TPHA, TPPA), or non-treponemal (e.g. RPR or VDRL). Treponemal tests remain positive for life, whereas non-treponemal tests usually revert to negative after successful treatment, so can be used as a test of cure. They may give false-positive results due to other infections (e.g. malaria), or autoimmune diseases. Until recently it has not been possible to screen women attending antenatal clinics that do not have access to a laboratory. However, treponemal point-of-care tests are now available at an affordable price (<$1) which can give a result in 15 minutes and require neither electricity nor laboratory equipment.

Further Reading

1. Richens J, Mayaud P, Mabey DCW. Sexually transmitted infections (excluding HIV). In: Farrar J, editor. Manson's Tropical Diseases. 23rd ed. London: Elsevier; 2013. [chapter 23].
2. Watson-Jones D, Changalucha J, Gumodoka B, et al. Syphilis in pregnancy in Tanzania. I. Impact of maternal syphilis on outcome of pregnancy. J Infect Dis 2002;186(7):940–7.
3. Watson-Jones D, Gumodoka B, Weiss H, et al. Syphilis in pregnancy in Tanzania. II. The effectiveness of antenatal syphilis screening and single-dose benzathine penicillin treatment for the prevention of adverse pregnancy outcomes. J Infect Dis 2002;186(7):948–57.
4. Newman L, Kamb M, Hawkes S, et al. Global estimates of syphilis in pregnancy and associated adverse outcomes: analysis of multinational antenatal surveillance data. PLoS Med 2013;10(2):e1001396.

A 37-YEAR-OLD WOMAN FROM MALAWI WITH HAEMATEMESIS

57

Camilla Rothe

Clinical Presentation

HISTORY

A 37-year-old woman from the Lower Shire Valley in Southern Malawi is referred from a clinic on one of the local sugar plantations to the district hospital. She has vomited blood three times over the past 24 hours. The blood is bright red in colour. There is no epigastric pain and no previous history of vomiting. There is no history of fever and abnormal bleeding and her stool has been normal in colour. Before the onset of symptoms she was fine. She has not taken any regular painkillers and does not drink any alcohol.

Her past medical history is unremarkable. She lives and works on a large sugar plantation in the area. She is married with three children, all are well. An HIV test done three months previously was negative.

CLINICAL FINDINGS

The patient is a 37-year-old woman who is slim but not wasted. Conjunctivae are slightly pale, but there are no subconjunctival effusions and she is not jaundiced. Her blood pressure is 90/60 mmHg, pulse 110 bpm, temperature 36.8°C, respiratory rate 28 breath cycles per minute.

On examination of the abdomen there is no abdominal tenderness. The spleen is palpable at 10 cm below the left costal margin. The liver is slightly enlarged but there are no stigmata of chronic liver disease. There is no shifting dullness and no peripheral oedema. Her lymph nodes are not enlarged. The rest of the physical examination is normal.

LABORATORY RESULTS

Her laboratory results on admission are shown in Table 57-1.

TABLE 57-1 Laboratory Results on Admission		
Parameter	Patient	Reference Range
WBC (x10⁹/L)	2.8	4–10
Haemoglobin (g/dL)	8.3	12–14
MCV (fL)	88	80–99
Platelets (x10⁹/L)	130	150–400

QUESTIONS

1. What is the most likely cause of her haematemesis?
2. What further investigations would you like to do to establish the diagnosis?

225

Discussion

A Malawian woman presents with a first episode of haematemesis. She has neither taken NSAIDs, nor alcohol. On examination she is afebrile, slightly pale, shocked and has an enlarged spleen. Her abdomen is non-tender. Her full-blood count shows pancytopenia with normocytic anaemia.

ANSWER TO QUESTION 1

What is the Most Likely Cause of Her Haematemesis?

Splenomegaly and pancytopenia in this case point towards the presence of portal hypertension[1] and she is most likely to bleed from gastro-oesophageal varices. In one series from Malawi, the presence of splenomegaly in patients with upper gastrointestinal bleeding was the single most specific clinical criterion to distinguish between a variceal bleed and a haemorrhage of other origin.[2]

Furthermore, portal hypertension is the most common cause of upper gastrointestinal bleeding in parts of sub-Saharan Africa, accounting for more than 50% of bleeds in some series.[2,3] The reason for this remains only partly understood. The prevalence of chronic viral hepatitis or alcohol abuse is no higher in the affected regions than elsewhere in the tropical world.

However, Malawi and other countries in the region are highly endemic for schistosomiasis. Virtually all water bodies in the country are infested with both *Schistosoma mansoni* and *S. haematobium* and it is likely that a high prevalence of hepatosplenic schistosomiasis with periportal fibrosis may explain why portal hypertension is so common in the region.

Little is known about causes of liver cirrhosis other than hepatitis B and C and their contribution to the burden of disease (e.g. autoimmune hepatitis, primary biliary cirrhosis, primary sclerosing cholangitis, haemochromatosis or Wilson's disease).

Other aetiologies of gastrointestinal bleeding, such as peptic ulcer disease, erosive gastritis or a bleeding tumour are less likely and would not explain the rest of her symptoms and signs. Notably though, in sub-Saharan Africa oesophageal cancer is strikingly common in young adults in their third and fourth decade of life. Risk factors remain poorly understood. Progressive dysphagia rather than haematemesis is usually the presenting symptom.[3]

Patients with visceral leishmaniasis (VL) can present with splenomegaly and pancytopenia; haemorrhage may occur secondary to thrombocytopenia. However, in VL there is usually a history of fever, and the patient's platelet count is only slightly diminished, which cannot explain her bleed. VL, furthermore, is uncommon in Southern Africa, even though few sporadic cases have been described from the region.

ANSWER TO QUESTION 2

What Further Investigations Would You Like to Do to Establish the Diagnosis?

In a resource-restrained setting, very limited options may be available to establish more than just a syndromic diagnosis.

The patient should be taken for gastroduodenoscopy without delay to detect and treat the source of bleeding. In case of oesophageal varices, an experienced ultrasonographer with a reasonable ultrasound machine may be able to distinguish between liver cirrhosis and periportal 'pipestem fibrosis' as seen in hepatic schistosomiasis (Figure 57-1). Hepatitis B or C-serologies should be done; other serologies for chronic liver disease are usually unavailable.

Liver biopsy would be the most helpful tool to distinguish between cirrhosis and fibrosis. It is usually unavailable and it is risky in an environment where postinterventional monitoring is poor and possible complications such as intra-abdominal bleeds are likely to go undetected.

THE CASE CONTINUED ...

The patient received IV fluids and was taken to the nearest central hospital for endsoscopy. The presence of oesophageal varices was confirmed and banding was done. There was no other source of bleeding.

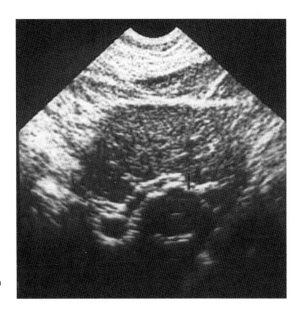

FIGURE 57-1 Ultrasound of the liver showing pipestem fibrosis *(Courtesy Prof. Joachim Richter).*

Hepatitis B and C serologies were negative. Stool for *S. mansoni* ova was negative. However, on ultrasound of the liver a pattern typical of pipe-stem fibrosis was described.

The patient received a single dose of praziquantel 40 mg/kg. She was discharged home.

SUMMARY BOX

Hepatosplenic Schistosomiasis

Hepatosplenic schistosomiasis is a complication of advanced infection with *Schistosoma mansoni*, *S. japonicum* and *S. mekongi*.

Only about 10% of people chronically infected with schistosomiasis develop late-stage disease. Risk factors for disease progression remain poorly understood. Apart from intensity and duration of infection, host genetic factors such as race and IFN-gamma polymorphism, variable degrees of semi-immunity and parasite strain differences may play a role.

Chronic infection with liver-pathogenic *Schistosoma* species results in periportal fibrosis and portal venous hypertension. One exception is *S. intercalatum* which occurs focally in Central and West Africa and causes granulomatous inflammation of the liver without portal hypertension.

Patients may present with symptoms of hypersplenism, such as abdominal discomfort and fatigue secondary to progressive anaemia. Ascites is uncommon due to the preserved hepatocellular function but may occur in advanced disease or in coexisting liver cirrhosis.

The classical clinical signs of liver cirrhosis (e.g. gynaecomastia, palmar erythema, alterations in hair distribution) are absent in pure schistosomiasis.

A common, primary presenting sign of hepatosplenic schistosomiasis is upper gastrointestinal (GI) bleeding from gastro-oesophageal varices. In some endemic countries in sub-Saharan Africa half or more of upper GI bleeds are caused by portal hypertension.[2,3]

The demonstration of *Schistosoma* eggs in the stool can be challenging in advanced disease since the adult flukes may have long since died and egg production may have stopped.

Experienced ultrasonographers may be able to detect the typical pattern of 'pipe-stem fibrosis'. The term refers to the macroscopic aspect of the liver which shows wide bands of fibrosis around portal tracts resembling the stems of a clay pipe. If available, liver biopsy may show ova of *Schistosoma* spp. along with proliferation of fibrous tissue in and around the portal tract.

Praziquantel may have an effect in treatment of early fibrosis, but has little role to play in advanced disease. Nevertheless, a single dose treatment with praziquantel 40 mg/kg is justified to reduce the worm burden. Bleeding varices should be endoscopically treated – which is often impossible in remote rural settings.

Non-selective beta-blockers used in liver cirrhosis to lower the portal-venous pressure and prevent further variceal haemorrhage do not seem to be beneficial in hepatosplenic schistosomiasis.

Further Reading

1. Bustindy AL, King CH. Schistosomiasis. In: Farrar J, editor. Manson's Tropical Diseases. 23rd ed. London: Elsevier; 2013 [chapter 52].
2. Harries AD, Wirima JJ. Upper gastrointestinal bleeding in Malawian adults and value of splenomegaly in predicting source of haemorrhage. East Afr Med J 1989;66(2):97–9.
3. Wolf LL, Ibrahim R, Miao C, et al. Esophagogastroduodenoscopy in a public referral hospital in Lilongwe, Malawi: spectrum of disease and associated risk factors. World J Surg 2012;36(5):1074–82.

58

A 25-YEAR-OLD WOMAN FROM EGYPT WITH SEVERE CHRONIC DIARRHOEA AND MALABSORPTION

Thomas Weitzel / Nadia El-Dib

Clinical Presentation

HISTORY

A 25-year-old woman from Bani Suwaif in Upper Egypt (115 km south of Cairo) presents to a hospital in Cairo complaining of severe diarrhoea for two months accompanied by weight loss of about 15 kg and amenorrhoea. The symptoms started with stomach rumbles and colicky abdominal pain; later on she suffered anorexia and vomiting. The diarrhoea is voluminous, not related to meals, and occurs both during the day and at night (five to ten times in 24 hours).

She received various antibiotics, including metronidazole, as well as antidiarrhoeal drugs, without any improvement. During the last month she has developed lower limb swelling and severe prostration.

CLINICAL FINDINGS

The patient appears generally unwell; she is pale and has angular stomatitis. Her temperature is 36.6°C, heart rate 100 bpm, blood pressure 100/60 mmHg, scaphoid abdomen with borborygmi, pitting oedema of the lower limbs, and decreased skin turgor.

LABORATORY RESULTS

Laboratory results are summarized in Table 58-1. D-xylose test shows evidence of malabsorption. On stool microscopy, numerous helminth ova are detected (Figure 58-1).

TABLE 58-1 Laboratory Results on Admission

Parameter	Patient	Reference
Potassium (mmol/L)	2.8	3.5–5
Sodium (mmol/L)	127	136–145
Calcium, total (mmol/L)	2.1	2.25–2.63
Albumin (g/L)	23	35–55
Haemoglobin (g/dL)	10.8	11.5–15.5
WBC (×10⁹/L)	6.6	3.8–11
Eosinophil count (×10⁹/L)	0.53	<0.45
Platelets (×10⁹/L)	350	150–350
Creatinine (µmol/L)	115	53–106

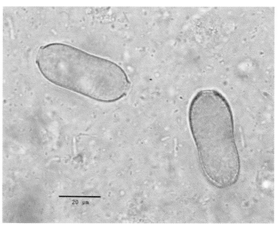

FIGURE 58-1 Helminth ova in a stool sample of a 25-year-old woman from Egypt with chronic diarrhoea.

228

1. Which helminth is causing the patient's clinical problems and why is it able to cause such severe infections?
2. Where does this parasite occur and how is it transmitted?

Discussion

A 25-year-old woman from Upper Egypt presents with severe chronic diarrhoea and colicky abdominal pains. She is afebrile but shows clinical signs of chronic malabsorption. Full blood count reveals mild eosinophilia, blood chemistry shows electrolyte derangement and hypoalbuminaemia. Stool samples yield helminth eggs.

ANSWER TO QUESTION 1

Which Helminth is Causing the Patient's Clinical Problems and Why is it Able to Cause Such Severe Infections?

The peanut-shaped eggs spotted on stool microscopy are typical ova of *Capillaria philippinesis*. The patient's complaints are very compatible with intestinal capillariasis and she resides in an endemic area. In contrast to most other intestinal helminths, *C. philippinesis* is able to multiply within the intestine of its final host causing long-lasting infection and severe clinical manifestations.

ANSWER TO QUESTION 2

Where Does this Parasite Occur and How is it Transmitted?

C. philippinensis is endemic in various East and South-east Asian countries such as The Philippines, Thailand, Laos, China, Korea, Japan and Taiwan. Furthermore, cases have been reported from Egypt, Iran and India. Sporadic cases may occur elsewhere. One indigenous case has recently been reported from Cuba and another patient acquired the infection most probably in Colombia. Capillariasis is transmitted through consumption of raw or undercooked fish.

THE CASE CONTINUED ...

The patient was admitted to hospital. Mebendazole was initiated at a dose of 400 mg bd and continued for three weeks. Oral and parenteral fluids and electrolytes were given for resuscitation, and she received a high protein diet and vitamins. During the first days of treatment, numerous adult helminths (length 3–5 mm) were found in further stool samples (Figure 58-2). The patient's general condition improved

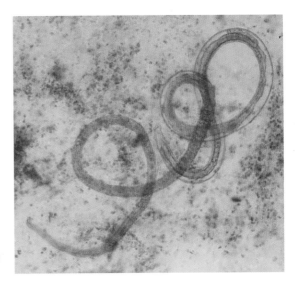

FIGURE 58-2 Adult *Capillaria philippinensis* in the patient's stool sample during treatment with mebendazole.

significantly within the first week and vomiting stopped. Diarrhoea subsided after two weeks of treatment.

SUMMARY BOX

Intestinal Capillariasis

Intestinal capillariasis is a zoonotic disease caused by *Capillaria philippinensis*, a tiny nematode usually infecting fish-eating birds which recently has been transferred to the genus *Paracapillaria*.[1] Humans are accidentally infected when eating raw or under-cooked small fresh- or brackish-water fish harbouring infective larval stages of the parasite.[2] Adult parasites invade the wall of the small intestine and live partially embedded in the mucosa of jejunum and ileum.[3] The unique life cycle includes an alteration of oviparous and larviparous females. Oviparous females shed thick-shelled eggs, which exit the body with the stool and, after being eaten by small fish, develop into the infective larvae. Larviparous females contain thin-shelled eggs, which mainly hatch *in utero* and permit an internal autoinfection and multiplication cycle, i.e. larvae develop into adults within the intestinal mucosa without leaving the host. This leads to a gradual increase of both worm burden and severity of clinical manifestations. With its autoinfection cycle, the parasite is one of the few intestinal helminths causing chronic and life-threatening infections. Patients present with colicky abdominal pain and intermittent or chronic diarrhoea, accompanied by anorexia, vomiting and dehydration. Without treatment, infection progresses to severe enteropathy with crypt atrophy and flattening of villi. Chronically infected patients suffer cachexia and pitting oedema of the lower limbs. Untreated, they may eventually die from severe protein loss, electrolyte imbalance and concomitant bacterial infections. Parasitological diagnosis relies on the demonstration of typical peanut-shaped eggs in stool samples, which have protruding polar plugs on both ends and measure $36–42 \times 20$ µm. Treatment is with mebendazole or albendazole for 20 or 10 days, respectively.

Further Reading

1. Jones MK, McCarthy JS. Medical helminthology. In: Farrar J, editor. Manson's Tropical Diseases. 23rd ed. London: Elsevier; 2013 [Appendix 3].
2. El-Dib N, Weitzel T. Capilariasis intestinal. In: Apt W, editor. Parasitología Humana. McGraw-Hill; 2013 [chapter 36].
3. Cross JH. Intestinal capillariasis. Clin Microbiol Rev 1992;5(2):120–9.

A 24-YEAR-OLD MAN FROM MALAWI WITH SKIN LESIONS AND BREATHLESSNESS

59

M. Jane Bates

Clinical Presentation

HISTORY

A 24-year-old Malawian businessman presents to your clinic having noticed dark spots on his arm and leg for the last month. These are progressing and he is now getting facial swelling.

On questioning, he also reports a three-month history of cough and worsening shortness of breath. He has no constitutional symptoms of weight loss, fevers or night sweats. His cough is productive of white sputum. He has no history of previous tuberculosis. He tested positive for HIV a week before coming to your clinic and has not yet started antiretroviral medication.

CLINICAL FINDINGS

The patient appears comfortable at rest with moderate facial oedema (Figure 59-1). His temperature is 36°C, respiratory rate 32 breath cycles per minute and pulse 102 bpm. Widespread dark plaques are noted on the skin and palate. On respiratory examination he has decreased air entry and dullness at the right lung base. He has swelling of his right leg from the foot to the knee, with prominent black plaques which are coalescing (Figure 59-2). The rest of the physical examination is normal.

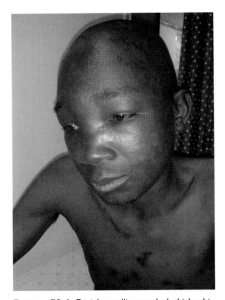

FIGURE 59-1 Facial swelling and darkish skin lesions on chest and nose of the patient.

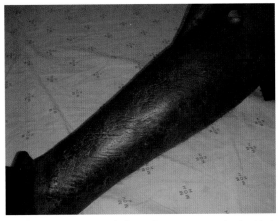

FIGURE 59-2 Swollen right leg with prominent coalescing black plaques.

1. What are your most important differential diagnoses?
2. How would you approach this patient?

Discussion

A young Malawian man presents with widespread darkish cutaneous and mucosal lesions. He also reports cough and shortness of breath for three months and there are some chest findings on examination of his right lung. He has recently been diagnosed as HIV-reactive.

ANSWER TO QUESTION 1

What Are Your Most Important Differential Diagnoses?

In a newly diagnosed HIV-infected patient with a chronic history of cough, the diagnosis of tuberculosis should always be considered and vigorous attempts made to exclude it. The skin lesions are typical for Kaposi's sarcoma (KS). The presence of palatal lesions increases your suspicion of pulmonary KS.

ANSWER TO QUESTION 2

How Would You Approach This Patient?

A CD4 count should be done to assess the degree of immunosuppression. Of note, KS can occur at any stage of HIV infection. The patient should be assessed for possible pulmonary tuberculosis, which should include a chest radiograph and sputum testing for acid-fast bacilli (AFB). If the patient is unable to produce any sputum, an induced sputum can be attempted. If available, a bronchoscopy remains the gold standard investigation for endobronchial Kaposi's sarcoma. Bronchoalveolar lavage can be used to further investigate for TB. Dual pathology of pulmonary KS and TB is not uncommon and it can be technically difficult to rule out TB with certainty as an underlying or concomitant cause of pulmonary pathology.

The main concern of the patient should be noted down as a baseline guide to assist with prioritizing interventions that promote quality of life. These concerns may be physical, psychological, social or spiritual in nature. General positive living advice, including safe sexual practice and partner and children testing for HIV, should also be addressed.

The patient should be started on antiretroviral therapy (ART) as soon as possible, since control of HIV is also the mainstay of treatment for KS. Kaposi's sarcoma is a WHO clinical stage 4 condition which qualifies the patient to start ART irrespective of the CD4 count.

Suitability for possible palliative chemotherapy includes consideration of major side-effects of available regimes, as well as taking time to explain the diagnosis to the patient. Information should be communicated in language understood by the patient, enabling the patient and his carers to explore issues, plan and develop realistic expectations from an early stage.

THE CASE CONTINUED ...

His main concern was shortness of breath. His wife was also HIV-reactive but not on ART and the patient requested a CD4 count test for her. His own CD4 count was 134 cells/µL, with Hb 10.2 g/dL and MCV 88.4 fL. Other parameters were normal.

His chest radiograph showed bilateral patchy opacifications in the lower and mid zones of the lungs (Figure 59-3). Such changes may be nonspecific but they are commonly seen in patients with pulmonary Kaposi's sarcoma.

Sputum tests were AFB-negative. A bronchoscopy was attempted but failed due to technical difficulties. The patient made no improvement with a short course of oral antibiotics. He was referred to start antiretroviral medication and palliative chemotherapy.

A presumptive course of antituberculous treatment may have been justifiable since smear-negative TB is very common in HIV-positive patients and it is difficult to rule out TB as a (concomitant) problem in this case.

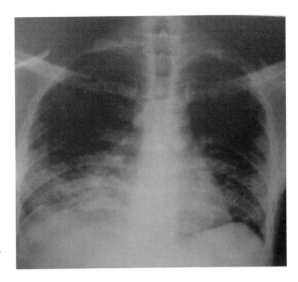

FIGURE 59-3 Chest radiograph showing bilateral patchy opacifications in the lower and mid lung zones.

SUMMARY BOX

Kaposi's Sarcoma

Kaposi's sarcoma (KS) remains the commonest malignancy worldwide for those infected with HIV. It is caused by human herpesvirus-8 (HHV-8), also known as Kaposi sarcoma-associated herpes virus (KSHV).[1] KS commonly affects the skin but may also involve lymph nodes, lungs and the gastrointestinal tract. Diagnosis is usually made by clinical appearance but biopsy may be necessary in atypical cases.

All patients with KS should be started on antiretroviral therapy. For those with more extensive cutaneous disease or visceral involvement, therapeutic options remain a challenge and outcomes remain poor. The goal of care needs careful consideration and discussion with the patient. Current evidence suggests that combining antiretroviral medication with chemotherapeutic agents such as doxorubicin, bleomycin or vincristin provides best tumour response, though optimal treatment strategies are not yet clear. More recently the role of molecularly targeted agents such as angiogenesis inhibitors has been discussed.

A number of chemotherapeutic agents may be contraindicated due to pre-existing comorbidities such as peripheral neuropathy.[2] Also, in resource-constrained settings chemotherapy may not be available at all.

In such cases a palliative approach is suitable, focusing on improving quality of life for the patients and their families. Holistic care and pain management should be attended to. Low-dose liquid morphine has an established role for symptom relief of breathlessness once all other causes have been excluded and/or treated optimally.[3] Implementation of non-drug measures, such as positioning and companionship to reduce distress and anxiety and to improve breathlessness, are also important.

Further Reading

1. Wood R. Clinical features and management of HIV/AIDS. In: Farrar J, editor. Manson's Tropical Diseases. 23rd ed. London: Elsevier; 2013 [chapter 10].
2. Francis H, Bates MJ, Kalilani L. A prospective study assessing tumour response, survival, and palliative care outcomes in patients with HIV-related Kaposi's sarcoma at Queen Elizabeth Central Hospital, Blantyre, Malawi. AIDS Res Treat 2012;2012:312564. doi:10.1155/2012/312564; Published online.
3. NICE (National Institute for Health and Care Excellence). Palliative cancer care – dyspnoea. Clin Knowl Summ 2012. Available from: <http://cks.nice.org.uk/palliative-cancer-care-dyspnoea> (accessed 14.01.2014).

60 A 6-YEAR-OLD BOY FROM MALAWI WITH PROPTOSIS OF THE LEFT EYE

Elizabeth M. Molyneux

Clinical Presentation

HISTORY

A 6-year-old Malawian boy from the lakeshore presents with a painless, proptosed left eye that his family first noticed three weeks ago. It has worsened rapidly though his vision is still normal. He denies any pain.

CLINICAL FINDINGS

On examination he is afebrile, the right eye is normal, the left eye is proptosed but non-pulsating. The pupil is round and clear and responds well to light. When he is asked to follow an object with his eyes the left eyeball hardly moves. He has no other swellings or abnormalities and though he is thin he is not malnourished.

QUESTIONS

1. What are the three most likely diagnoses?
2. What investigations would you do to confirm the diagnosis and direct your treatment plan?

Discussion

A young Malawian boy presents because of a progressive painless proptosis of his left eye for the past three weeks. His vision is not impaired. Apart from being proptosed, the eye on examination looks normal.

The boy resides in an area endemic for malaria and schistosomiasis.

ANSWER TO QUESTION 1

What Are the Three Most Likely Diagnoses?

This is a rapidly developing proptosis in a boy who lives in a malaria-endemic area; the most likely diagnosis is Burkitt's lymphoma.

The second possibility is that it is another type of B cell lymphoma; and the third possibility is rhabdomyosarcoma.

It is not a retinoblastoma, which starts in the eye and usually, but not always, presents at an earlier age. The process is painless, which excludes infection, and it is non-pulsating which makes the diagnosis of an arteriovenous malformation unlikely. Lacrymal gland tumours are more anteromedial than this mass.

ANSWER TO QUESTION 2

What Investigations Would You Do to Confirm the Diagnosis and Direct Your Treatment Plan?

There are three questions to ask: what is it, where is it and is it safe to treat?

What is it? A thorough history and physical examination will narrow the field. Is this a multifocal or localized lesion? Knowing the age will rule in some more likely diagnoses and rule out others. Are there any systemic or neurological signs and symptoms? A fine needle aspirate (FNA) or biopsy will confirm the diagnosis.

Where is it? Again the examination will assist. An abdominal ultrasound scan will demonstrate any intra-abdominal masses and organ involvement. A cytospun sample of cerebrospinal fluid (CSF) should be examined for malignant cells and a full blood count (FBC) and bone marrow aspirate (BMA) examined. A chest radiograph is useful if intrathoracic pathology is suspected.

Is it safe to treat? Anaemia (<7 g/dL) and thrombocytopenia (<50×10⁹/L) should be corrected before giving chemotherapy. A blood film and stool and urine samples should be examined to exclude or treat malaria or any other invasive parasitic infections such as schistosomiasis or strongyloidiasis. The abdominal ultrasound scan will demonstrate any renal involvement and forewarn of possible complications when treatment is given. Baseline renal function and liver function tests are useful but not essential. HIV status will not affect the treatment, but if positive, infections and anaemia should be anticipated during chemotherapy.

THE CASE CONTINUED ...

The boy was admitted and a full work-up was done as a matter of urgency (FNA, BMA, FBC, lumbar puncture (LP), HIV antibody test, stool and urine microscopy) and an abdominal scan was carried out. This was to enable treatment to start as soon as possible to prevent further proptosis and irreversible damage to the eye. Delay could mean the eye losing its blood supply and 'melting', leaving the boy sightless in that eye.

When the LP was done, intrathecal methotrexate and hydrocortisone were given as prophylaxis against CNS involvement. Oral allopurinol and hyper-hydration were commenced; chemotherapy was given the next day. The eye looked less proptosed within 48 hours and was back to normal within a week. He had four courses of chemotherapy in the next 30 days (Figure 60-1). A year later he was free of disease and pronounced cured.

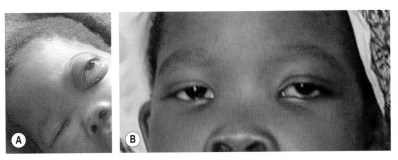

FIGURE 60-1   The boy before (A) and after (B) four courses of chemotherapy.

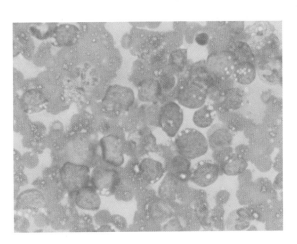

FIGURE 60-2   Histology of Burkitt's lymphoma (HE stain) showing monomorphic tumour cells of intermediate size, indistinct nuclei with coarse chromatin and vacuoles in the cytoplasm (×100 high-power field).

SUMMARY BOX

Burkitt's Lymphoma

Endemic Burkitt's lymphoma is a highly aggressive B cell non-Hodgkin's lymphoma. It is the fastest-growing tumour known in man and doubles its cells numbers every 24–48 hours (Figure 60-2). It is causally associated with the Epstein–Barr virus (EBV) and malaria, and has a chromosomal translocation that activates the c-myc oncogene. It is the most common childhood cancer (about 50%) in areas where malaria is holoendemic.[1,2] It is twice as common in boys as girls and the peak age of presentation is 6–7 years. Outcome with early diagnosis and intensive chemotherapy in children is excellent. In resource-constrained settings treatment intensity has to be balanced with good supportive care, the child's nutritional status and stage of the disease. This means that less aggressive treatment often has to be given with less successful outcomes. Nevertheless, with stage-adjusted therapies, designed by oncologists of the Paediatric Oncology in Developing Countries group (PODC), which is an arm of the International Society of Paediatric Oncology (SIOP), and by common consensus and studies done in low-income settings, 60% cure at one year can be achieved at a very low cost and manageable toxicity.[3]

Further Reading

1. Newton R, Wakeham K, Bray F. Cancer in the tropics. In: Farrar J, editor. Manson's Tropical Diseases. 23rd ed. London: Elsevier; 2013 [chapter 64].
2. Molyneux EM, Rochford R, Griffin B, et al. Burkitt's lymphoma. Lancet 2012;379(9822):1234–44.
3. Hesseling P, Israels T, Harif M, et al. Practical recommendations for the management of children with endemic Burkitt's lymphoma (BL) in a resource limited setting. Pediatr Blood Cancer 2013;60(3):357–62.

A 48-YEAR-OLD WOMAN FROM THAILAND WITH FEVER AND DISSEMINATED CUTANEOUS ABSCESSES, LYMPHADENOPATHY AND SWELLING OF HER LEFT ELBOW

61

Sabine Jordan

Clinical Presentation

HISTORY

A 46-year-old Thai woman is transferred to a German clinic for tropical diseases with a two-month history of recurrent cutaneous and subcutaneous abscesses, progressive lymphadenopathy and weight loss.

Despite various antibiotic therapies, clinical symptoms and inflammatory markers had deteriorated, resulting in hospital admission. Pus and blood cultures did not yield any growth, and histopathology of a lymph node biopsy showed nonspecific lymphadenitis. The symptoms started 6–8 weeks after her return from a family visit to northern Thailand; during her stay the patient had suffered from high fever, dry cough and fatigue.

CLINICAL FINDINGS

A 46-year-old female, 158 cm, 65 kg (BMI 26 kg/m^2), afebrile, blood pressure 130/80 mmHg, pulse 80 bpm.

Enlarged, tender cervical, nuchal, inguinal and axillary lymph nodes. Massive, tender swelling of the upper eyelids. Disseminated fluctuant cutaneous and subcutaneous abscesses with ambient erythema (Figure 61-1), discharge of pus on slight pressure. Painful swelling of the left elbow. The rest of the physical examination is normal.

IMAGING

A radiograph of the patient's left elbow is shown in Figure 61-2.

QUESTIONS

1. What are your most important differential diagnoses?
2. What investigations would you like to do?

Discussion

A 46-year-old woman from Thailand presents with a two-month history of recurrent and treatment-refractory cutaneous and subcutaneous abscesses, progressive lymphadenopathy and weight loss. Her

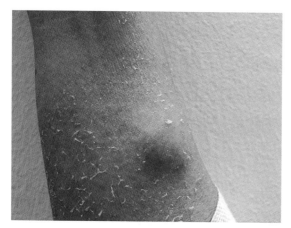

FIGURE 61-1 Subcutaneous abscess on the left forearm.

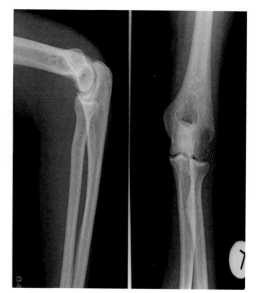

FIGURE 61-2 Radiograph of the left elbow, showing osteolytic lesions of the radial epicondylus, osteomyelitis and articular effusion.

TABLE 61-1 Laboratory Results on Admission		
Parameter	Patient	Reference
WCC (×10⁹/L)	30.8	3.8–11
Haemoglobin (g/dL)	8.2	12.3–15.3
MCV (fL)	88	80–94
Platelets (×10⁹/L)	592	150–400
CRP (mg/L)	267	<5
ESR (mm/h)	>110	<20

symptoms started 6–8 weeks after returning from a visit to northern Thailand. On examination, multiple cutaneous and subcutaneous abscesses and a generalized lymphadenopathy are noted. Laboratory findings show elevated systemic markers of inflammation (Table 61-1). A radiograph of the swollen elbow reveals osteomyelitis.

ANSWER TO QUESTION 1

What Are Your Most Important Differential Diagnoses?

The clinical picture and the laboratory and radiological findings are highly suspicious of a systemic infection. As previous antibiotic treatment courses were ineffective and microbiological tests were negative, fungal infections, such as histoplasmosis, and mycobacterial infections should be considered. Furthermore, bacterial infections with special requirements for cultivation and/or limited antibiotic susceptibility such as *Burkholderia pseudomallei*, *Brucella* spp., *Francisella tularensis* or *Actinomyces* spp. could have been misdiagnosed before.

Due to the extensive disease, underlying immunodeficiency, such as HIV-infection, diabetes mellitus, antibody deficiency or impaired granulocyte function, have to be ruled out.

If further microbiological investigations remain negative, rare autoimmune syndromes such as idiopathic nodular panniculitis (Weber–Christian disease) or aseptic abscesses syndrome have to be taken into account.

ANSWER TO QUESTION 2

What Investigations Would You Like to Do?

Further microbiological and histopathological investigations seem to be crucial in this case. Biopsies of skin, abscesses and lymph nodes should be sent for culture and histopathological studies. Testing should focus on fungal and mycobacterial infections. PCR (polymerase chain reaction) methods – where available – can help to accelerate the diagnosis, as isolation of the pathogen from culture might take several weeks. For histoplasmosis, serological antigen and antibody tests are available. These may also help to speed up the diagnostic process but negative results do not rule out infection; antibody testing lacks sensitivity in immunocompromised patients especially. Furthermore, the patient should be tested for HIV, and a fasting blood glucose level can help to rule out diabetes mellitus.

THE CASE CONTINUED ...

The clinically suspected diagnosis initially was melioidosis, which is a common cause of disseminated abscesses in patients from north-eastern Thailand. The patient received imipenem, which led to a slight improvement of her skin manifestations but inflammation parameters remained grossly elevated.

Various cultures from skin and lymph node biopsies remained sterile and so a submandibular lymph node was extirpated. Histologically, this lymph node showed fungal cells that were identified as *Histoplasma capsulatum* by PCR. This was later confirmed by culture. Serology for histoplasmosis remained negative.

In retrospect, the febrile illness the patient had suffered whilst in Thailand may have been acute pulmonary histoplasmosis (see Summary Box).

While on antifungal treatment with liposomal amphotericin B (3 mg/kg/d, total dose 3 g) the patient developed a generalized seizure. CSF analysis revealed a lymphocytic pleocytosis, which, despite the absence of direct pathogen detection, may have been a cerebral manifestation of histoplasmosis.

On treatment with liposomal amphotericin B the patient's clinical state and the laboratory findings improved dramatically. The patient was started on itraconazole maintenance therapy for a further six months.

No evidence of immunosuppression was found in the diagnostic work-up (HIV serology was negative, fasting blood sugar level was within normal range).

On follow-up the patient presented in a fair general condition. Some of the former abscess sites showed postinflammatory hyperpigmentation, enlarged lymph nodes were no longer present and the osteolytic lesions were partly recalcificated. Repeat histoplasma serology remained negative.

SUMMARY BOX

Histoplasmosis

Histoplasmosis is caused by *Histoplasma capsulatum*, a dimorphic fungus that remains in a mycelial form at ambient temperatures and grows as yeast at body temperature in mammals.[1,2] The fungus can be found in temperate climates throughout the world, predominantly in river valleys in parts of the USA, the West Indies, Central and South America, Africa, India, East Asia and Australia. The soil in areas endemic for histoplasmosis provides an acidic damp environment with high organic content that favours mycelial growth. Highly contaminated soil is found near areas inhabited by bats and birds. Birds cannot be infected by the fungus and do not transmit the disease; however, bird excretions contaminate the soil, thereby enriching the growth medium for the mycelium. In contrast, bats can become infected, and they transmit histoplasmosis through their droppings. Contaminated soil can be potentially infectious for years. Outbreaks of histoplasmosis have been associated with construction and renovation activities that disrupt soil contaminated with *Histoplasma* spp.

Inhalation of fungal spores may lead to acute pulmonary histoplasmosis; however, approximately 90% of individuals with acute infection remain asymptomatic. In patients with underlying lung pathology, chronic pulmonary disease can occur. Patients develop cavities that may enlarge and result in necrosis. Untreated histoplasmosis may lead to progressive pulmonary fibrosis that leads to recurrent infections and respiratory and cardiac failure.

In children, older individuals and immunocompromised patients, dissemination of the infection may occur. The symptoms of disseminated histoplasmosis typically include fever, malaise, anorexia and weight loss. Physical examination will often show hepatosplenomegaly and lymphadenopathy, and in some patients mucous membrane ulcerations as well as skin ulcers, nodules, or molluscum-like papules may be seen. Rarely, disseminated infection can also occur in immunocompetent patients.

Continued on following page

In disseminated disease, culture of tissue samples or body fluids and histopathology should be obtained. PCR can help to speed up the diagnostic process as isolation from fungal cultures takes up to three weeks. Serology lacks sensitivity, especially in immunocompromised patients. In these cases blood and urine antigen testing should be done.

In patients with disseminated infection initial treatment with liposomal amphotericin B (3–5 mg/kg daily) is highly effective. Itraconazole (200–400 mg daily) is favoured for maintenance therapy. The duration of treatment depends on the severity of infection and the immune status of the patient. IDSA (Infectious Diseases Society of America) guidelines recommend 6–18 months in total.[3]

Further Reading

1. Hay RJ. Fungal infections. In: Farrar J, editor. Manson's Tropical Diseases. 23rd ed. London: Elsevier; 2013.
2. Kauffman CA. Histoplasmosis: a clinical and laboratory update. Clin Microbiol Rev 2007;20:115–32.
3. Wheat LJ, Freifeld AG, Kleiman MB, et al. Clinical practice guidelines for the management of patients with histoplasmosis: 2007 update by the Infectious Diseases Society of America. Clin Infect Dis 2007;45:807–25.

A 28-YEAR-OLD MAN FROM GHANA WITH A CHRONIC ULCER ON HIS ANKLE

62

Fredericka Sey / Ivy Ekem

Clinical Presentation

HISTORY

A 28-year-old West African man presents to a clinic in Ghana complaining of a painful ulcer on his left ankle. The ulcer has been present for the past four months and is not healing (Figure 62-1). There is no history of prior trauma, however, he had a previous ulcer on his right ankle some years ago which took about a year to heal. He also complains of pain in his right thigh and in both knees.

CLINICAL FINDINGS

The patient is short for an adult; he is pale and has a tinge of jaundice. The ulcer is on his left ankle, next to the medial malleolus; the skin surrounding it is hyperpigmented. There is tenderness in both knee joints and in his right thigh. The rest of the physical examination is normal. Vital signs: Temperature 36.6°C, pulse 88 bpm, blood pressure 110/70 mmHg.

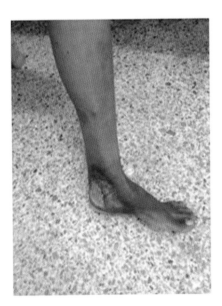

FIGURE 62-1 The patient's left leg showing an ulcer surrounded by hyperpigmented skin on the medial malleolus.

QUESTIONS

1. What is your differential diagnosis?
2. How would you confirm the diagnosis?

Discussion

A 28-year-old West African man presents with a chronic, painful ankle ulcer. He had a similar ulcer on the other foot a few years prior. He also complains of bone pains. He is short for an adult, pale and mildly jaundiced.

ANSWER TO QUESTION 1

What is Your Differential Diagnosis?

The chronic nature of the ulcer, its site and the surrounding hyperpigmentation make a venous ulcer likely. The patient's bone pain, jaundice and pallor could point to a haemolytic anaemia. Various hereditary haemolytic anaemias may be complicated by chronic leg ulceration, e.g. haemoglobinopathies (thalassaemia and sickle cell disease), spherocytosis and pyruvate kinase deficiency. In the West African context, sickle cell disease is the most likely diagnosis.

Further differentials would be tropical ulcer, diabetic ulcer, or chronic osteomyelitis with a discharging sinus. Buruli ulcer, caused by *Mycobacterium ulcerans*, is usually painless. Other mycobacterial infections can also present with chronic skin ulcers. Pyoderma gangrenosum and malignant diseases also need to be considered.

ANSWER TO QUESTION 2

How Would You Confirm the Diagnosis?

A full blood count and a peripheral blood film should be done. In sickle cell disease, during an acute crisis, abundant sickled red cells can be seen on a blood film. Other characteristic but nonspecific features include target cells, Howell–Jolly bodies, polychromasia and nucleated red cells. The presence of HbS can be demonstrated by using a simple sickle-slide or solubility test. Blood is mixed with sodium metabisulphite which will provoke sickling of cells containing HbS; this can be demonstrated on a slide. If resources allow, confirmation is by haemoglobin electrophoresis, liquid chromatography or isoelectric focusing.

Fasting blood sugar and wound swab for culture and sensitivity as well as a radiograph of the left leg should be done to rule out other differential diagnoses and osteomyelitis.

THE CASE CONTINUED ...

Blood was taken and the available results are shown in Table 62-1. The patient's blood film is shown in Figure 62-2. The sickling test was positive and haemoglobin electrophoresis showed a homozygous HbSS-type. The wound swab grew *Pseudomonas spp.* sensitive to levofloxacin. Radiography showed a periosteal reaction with slightly sclerotic bones.

The diagnosis made was sickle cell disease with a chronic ankle ulcer. The patient was managed with alternate daily wound dressing using normal saline irrigation and povidone-iodine. High white cell counts are commonly seen in sickle cell disease. They may be the result of bone marrow stimulation and do not necessarily indicate systemic infection. However, in view of the patient's generally poor condition and the *Pseudomonas* grown from his wound swab, it was decided to give him systemic antibiotic treatment.

Strict bed rest was difficult to enforce because the young man was self-employed and could not afford to take the required time off work. His recurrent bone pain was managed conservatively with good hydration, prompt treatment of infections and relief of other identifiable precipitants of crises.

TABLE 62-1 Laboratory Results		
Parameter	**Patient**	**Reference Range**
WBC (×10⁹/L)	17.6	4–10
Haemoglobin (g/dL)	6.9	13–15
Fasting blood glucose (mmol/L)	4.8	4.4–6.1

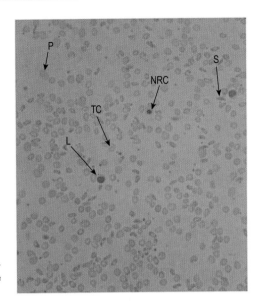

FIGURE 62-2 Patient's blood film: irreversibly sickled cells (S), poly-chromasia (P), target cells (TC), nucleated red cells (NRC) – note similarity with lymphocyte (L). Adequate platelets.

He received daily folic acid supplementation. Pain relief was achieved with paracetamol and tramadol.

However, on follow-up three years later, the ulcer was still not healed. Grafting is under consideration, when healthy granulation tissue is achieved.

SUMMARY BOX

Leg Ulcers in Sickle Cell Disease

Sickle cell disease (SCD) is a collection of autosomal-codominant genetic disorders characterized by the production of abnormal sickle haemoglobin S (HbS).[1] Homozygous HbSS leads to sickle cell anaemia, the most severe form of SCD. Sickle cell disease is the commonest hereditary haematological disorder.

HbS has the tendency to polymerize during hypoxia. This leads to a reduction of the flexibility of the erythrocyte and to the typical sickle shape of the affected cell. Sickled red blood cells lead to haemolysis and vaso-occlusion.

The disease is characterized by episodes of acute illness against a background of progressive organ damage. Any organ can be affected by SCD at any age, however certain features tend to predominate in certain age groups.[1]

Leg ulcers tend to manifest in adulthood.[2] Pathophysiology is complex and remains incompletely understood. Ulcers in SCD occur in areas with thin skin and little subcutaneous fat, most commonly on the ankles. They are notoriously difficult to treat. The ulcers are slow to heal and are characterized by unexplained relapses. They are commonly very painful and patients may occasionally require opioids for pain control.[3] Colonization with pathogenic bacteria is common. Periosteal reaction is usually seen in the underlying bones but osteomyelitis is uncommon.

Of the many treatments, the most certain to aid healing is complete bed rest with leg elevation. Oral zinc sulphate tablets (200 mg tid) have been shown to be helpful. Systemic antibiotic therapy is given in acute sepsis. The use of hydroxyurea in leg ulcers is controversial. Chronic transfusion regimens to maintain the haemoglobin level above 10 g/dL may help, when conservative therapy fails. Skin grafting for clean wounds is recommended, especially when the defect is large. The relapse rate is high, however.

Further Reading

1. Thachil J, Owusu-Ofori S, Bates I. Haematological diseases in the tropics. In: Farrar J, editor. Manson's Tropical Diseases. 23rd ed. London: Elsevier; 2013 [chapter 65].
2. Delaney KM, Axelrod KC, Buscetta A, et al. Leg ulcers in sickle cell disease: current patterns and practices. Hemoglobin 2013;37(4):325–32.
3. Halabi-Tawil M, Lionnet F, Girot R, et al. Sickle cell leg ulcers: a frequently disabling complication and a marker of severity. Br J Dermatol 2008;158(2):339–44.

A 38-YEAR-OLD EXPATRIATE MAN LIVING IN MALAWI WITH DIFFICULTIES PASSING URINE

63

Joep J. van Oosterhout

Clinical Presentation

HISTORY

A 38-year-old European expatriate presents at the medical outpatient clinic in a tertiary hospital in Malawi with progressive constipation and difficulties in passing urine for the past three weeks. He noticed that he had to use increasing abdominal pressure to pass urine and eventually became only able to pass small amounts at a time. This is associated with increasing lower abdominal discomfort, abnormal sensations in the groins and around the genitals and some erectile dysfunction. He has no weakness and there is no dysaesthesia and no loss of sensation in his legs. However, he mentions that walking did not feel normal, although he cannot fully explain what the abnormality is. He has no backache.

Over the past two months he has experienced unintentional weight loss of 8 kg and fatigue without fever or night sweats. He blames this on stressful circumstances at work. He has sexual contact with his wife only, to whom he has been married for several years.

One week prior to presentation he had noticed reddish discoloration of his urine. He had no painful micturition or fever at that time. He visited a local clinic and was prescribed four different types of medication, which he completed. There is no history of trauma and the rest of his previous medical history is unremarkable.

PHYSICAL EXAMINATION

He looks healthy and has normal vital signs. There are no abnormalities on general examination, except for a palpable bladder. The rectal examination reveals a low anal sphincter tone and the genital examination is normal. He has lively, symmetrical tendon reflexes in the legs without clonus or pathological plantar reflexes, and no abnormalities in the rest of the neurological examination.

QUESTIONS

1. Which important pieces of information are missing?
2. What are possible diagnoses and which investigations would you order?

Discussion

A 38-year-old European expatriate living in Malawi presents with constipation, bladder retention, an episode of probable haematuria, erectile dysfunction, genital paraesthesia, significant weight loss and fatigue. There are no abnormal neurological findings on examination, however most of the complaints are compatible with a conus syndrome due to a lesion within the conus medullaris or due to compression. The constitutional symptoms suggest an underlying chronic infection or malignancy.

ANSWER TO QUESTION 1

Which Important Pieces of Information Are Missing?

The important missing pieces of information are details of the recent visit to the local clinic and exposure to fresh water in Malawi. On physical examination, the anal reflex should have been tested.

ANSWER TO QUESTION 2

What Are Possible Diagnoses and Which Investigations Would You Order?

The most important differential diagnosis for a conus medullaris syndrome in a young, otherwise healthy man living in tropical Africa is schistosomiasis of the myelum. Other important infections to consider are spinal tuberculosis, a spinal abscess and neurosyphilis. A tumour or metastases impinging on the conus medullaris should be ruled out.

Urine microscopy for ova of *Schistosoma haematobium* should be ordered. A full blood count should be done, including a white cell differential count to look for eosinophilia. Creatinine and C-reactive protein should be tested.

Schistosomiasis serology would be useful in this expatriate. A VDRL and an HIV test should be done. An ultrasound of the abdomen assessing bladder volume before and after micturition and imaging of the spinal cord should be requested.

THE CASE CONTINUED ...

The patient was able to retrieve details of his urine microscopy from the local clinic. *Schistosoma haematobium* eggs had been identified in his urine and he had been treated with a full dose of praziquantel, a course of ciprofloxacin, buscopan and bisacodyl. He had swum regularly in Lake Malawi.

An abdominal ultrasound scan after attempted micturition showed a large bladder residue, without further abnormalities.

Full blood count showed a normal absolute WBC of 9×10^9/L with an eosinophilia of 21.8% (reference range: 1–6%) or 1.15×10^9/L (reference: $<0.45 \times 10^9$/L). ALT was slightly elevated. Creatinine and CRP were normal.

An HIV test and the VDRL were negative and microscopy of a stool and urine sample were normal. Serological tests for schistosomiasis were not available.

An MRI scan of the myelum was performed (Figure 63-1). An enhancing 1 cm large lesion was seen at the anterior aspect of the conus, with associated high T2 signal representing oedema extending from the lower end of the conus to the level of T9. In addition there was nodular thickening of the urine bladder wall at the base and the posterior aspect.

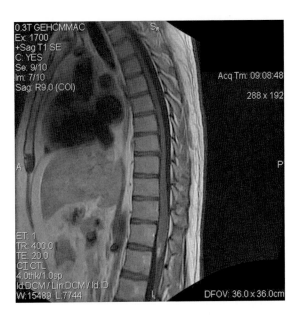

FIGURE 63-1 MRI scan myelum.

The diagnosis of an infection with *Schistosoma haematobium* was made as evidenced by the urine findings and supported by the eosinophilia and the abnormalities seen in the bladder wall on MRI scanning. This was complicated by neuroschistosomiasis (see Summary Box) with lesions in the conus medullaris of the myelum, causing a conus syndrome. A dual infection with *S. haematobium* and *S. mansoni* is possible, since *S. mansoni* is the more common pathogen causing spinal cord schistosomiasis, and both pathogens are endemic in Malawi. Theoretically, the myelum abnormalities could have been caused by other conditions, such as tuberculosis and metastatic cancer, for instance from a bladder carcinoma. While it has been argued that *S. haematobium* infection is a risk factor for bladder carcinoma, this is mainly observed in long-term heavy infections, which are uncommon in expatriates. Further tests to rule out such distinct possibilities are not readily available in Malawi and were not deemed necessary.

The patient required urinary catheterization for two weeks. He made a full recovery after a second course of praziquantel and a course of high-dose prednisolone, tapered off over two months. He was well after more than two years of follow-up.

SUMMARY BOX

Neuroschistosomiasis

Neuroschistosomiasis can occur in the brain and more frequently in the myelum.[1] Cerebral schistosomiasis can be asymptomatic or present with seizures, lateralizing signs and meningo-encephalitis. Myeloschistosomiasis (also known as spinal cord schistosomiasis, SCS) is more frequent in *S. mansoni* than in *S. haematobium* infections and often causes severe disability due to paraparesis and bladder dysfunction.[2] It is also the most important severe complication of schistosomiasis in travellers.[3]

Our understanding of the pathophysiology of neuroschistosomiasis is limited. For unknown reasons, ectopic worms lodge in the venous plexus around the CNS instead of their normal habitat. Laminectomy with biopsy of the nervous tissue is the only method that gives a definite diagnosis of SCS. However, this procedure should be avoided because of its risks. Diagnosis is based upon spinal imaging and proof of exposure to the parasite. Urine should be examined for *S. haematobium* eggs, for *S. mansoni*, stool microscopy may be attempted but lacks sensitivity which is much higher for rectal biopsies. Serological tests are useful in patients from non-endemic countries. Other causes of myelitis should be ruled out, which is often impossible in low-resourced settings where pragmatic treatment for myeloschistosomiasis may be justified.

Treatment of myeloschistosomiasis is with anti-schistosomal drugs (praziquantel) plus corticosteroids and is based on case series and expert opinion. The pathology is due to inflammation around *Schistosoma* eggs. Praziquantel kills adult flukes only and thereby stops further eggs being shed into the myelum. Most early improvement of the neurological presentation is expected from corticosteroids. The optimal dose and duration are not well known.[4] Up to six months of high-dose corticosteroids is recommended.

About 65% of patients with myeloschistosomiasis who are treated early recover completely or are left with negligible deficits that do not cause any functional limitations; the remaining patients are left with sequelae that vary from mild to severe.[2]

Further Reading

1. Bustinduy AL, King CH. Schistosomiasis. In: Farrar J, editor. Manson's Tropical Diseases. 23rd ed. London: Elsevier; 2013 [chapter 52].
2. Ferrari TC, Moreira PR. Neuroschistosomiasis: clinical symptoms and pathogenesis. Lancet Neurol 2011;10(9):853–64.
3. Gryseels B, Polman K, Clerinx J, et al. Human schistosomiasis. Lancet 2006;368(9541):1106–18.
4. Silva LC, Maciel PE, Ribas JG, et al. Treatment of schistosomal myeloradiculopathy with praziquantel and corticosteroids and evaluation by magnetic resonance imaging: a longitudinal study. Clin Infect Dis 2004;39(11):1618–24.

64

A 40-YEAR-OLD WOMAN FROM THAILAND AND HER BROTHER-IN-LAW WITH SEVERE HEADACHE

Camilla Rothe / Juri Katchanov

Clinical Presentation

HISTORY

A 40-year-old Thai woman presents to an outpatient clinic in Germany with a history of severe headache for the past eight days. The headache was of gradual onset and did not respond to any painkillers. There is no fever and no chills. She denies any visual problems, any weakness of her limbs or memory problems.

Ten days earlier she had returned from a four-week journey to north-east Thailand, where she visited friends and relatives. During her visit she ate traditional regional dishes, including freshwater fish, seafood, snails and frogs. She reports that her brother-in-law, with whom she had shared several traditional meals, has also fallen ill with a severe headache.

She presented to a municipal hospital three days earlier. A CT scan of her brain was performed and reported to be normal. Her blood count was also normal. A differential white cell count has not been done.

Her past medical history is unremarkable. The patient is married, she is a housewife and has lived in Germany for the past 13 years.

CLINICAL FINDINGS

On examination, she is afebrile, her neck is supple and Lasègue's sign (straight leg raise) is negative. Pupils are equal, round and react to light and accommodation, and there are no cranial nerve palsies. The remainder of the neurological examination, including the assessment of higher cortical functions such as language, memory and praxia, is unremarkable. There is no rash, no oral thrush and there are no subcutaneous swellings. Cardiopulmonary examination is normal. Liver and spleen are not enlarged and there is no lymphadenopathy.

LABORATORY RESULTS

Her laboratory results at presentation in the clinic are shown in Table 64-1.

QUESTIONS

1. What is your presumptive diagnosis?
2. Which investigation would you perform to substantiate your diagnosis?

Discussion

A 40-year-old Thai woman presents with a history of severe intractable headache after a stay in north-east Thailand where she enjoyed traditional regional dishes. Her brother-in-law in Thailand is suffering from the same severe headache. On examination, she is afebrile with no meningism and no focal neurological deficits. Her blood results reveal peripheral eosinophilia and elevated IgE levels. A CT scan of her brain done elsewhere showed no abnormalities.

TABLE 64-1 Laboratory Results at Presentation in the Clinic

Parameter (units)	Patient	Reference
WBC ($\times 10^9$/L)	12.3	4–10
Eosinophils ($\times 10^9$/L)	2.34	<0.5
Haemoglobin (mg/dL)	11.7	12–14
MCV (fL)	70	83–103
Platelets ($\times 10^9$/L)	330	150–350
ESR (mm/h)	20	≤10
IgE (U/mL)	944	<100
Creatinine (µmol/L)	62	<80
ALT (U/L)	28	<30
GGT (U/L)	35	<40
C-reactive protein (mg/L)	<5	<5

ANSWER TO QUESTION 1

What is Your Presumptive Diagnosis?

The most likely diagnosis is a food-borne parasitic infection of the meninges. The key points from the history which support a food-borne infection are: (1) temporal relationship with travelling to north-east Thailand, where food-borne nematodes are prevalent; (2) consumption of traditional Thai food, including raw or undercooked freshwater fish, seafood, snails and frogs; (3) the occurrence of similar symptoms in a relative who participated in the same meals ('outbreak').

Headache is a typical symptom of meningitis, so infestation of the meninges is very likely. The diagnosis of a parasitosis is strongly supported by the presence of considerable blood eosinophilia and elevated IgE levels in serum.

ANSWER TO QUESTION 2

Which Investigation Would You Perform to Substantiate Your Diagnosis?

Parasitic infection of the meninges typically results in eosinophilic meningitis. The next investigation to perform is a lumbar puncture to confirm meningitis and to look for a possibly eosinophilic profile of inflammation. Eosinophilic meningitis in an otherwise healthy person with positive history of exposure to helminths and features of an outbreak is almost always due to a parasitic infestation.

The main differential diagnoses are fungal meningitis with *Coccidioides immitis* (in North and Central America), lymphoma, eosinophilic leukaemia, sarcoid and idiopathic hypereosinophilic syndrome.

It is important to measure the CSF opening pressure. If it is elevated, serial spinal taps might relieve the symptoms.

THE CASE CONTINUED ...

A lumbar puncture was performed. The cerebrospinal fluid showed 1877 leukocytes/µL (reference value <5), with 42% eosinophils, 39% lymphocytes, 18% monocytes and 1% neutrophils (Figure 64-1). CSF protein levels were elevated at 1.59 g/L (reference value <0.45), glucose was 1.85 mmol/L (reference range: 2.2–3.9).

On microscopic examination of the CSF, no larvae could be detected. Ziehl–Neelsen stain as well as cryptococcal antigen were negative. There were no suspected malignant cells. CSF culture did not yield any bacterial or fungal growth. Urine and stool microscopy did not show any ova of *Schistosoma* spp. *Taenia solium* serology was negative, as were *Fasciola hepatica* and *Paragonimus* serologies. *Toxocara canis* serology was weakly positive but did not show any change of titre on follow-up. HIV serology was negative. The specimens were sent to Bangkok, where Western blotting confirmed the presence of specific antibodies against 31 kD *Angiostrongylus cantonensis* antigen.

The initial CSF opening pressure was elevated, at 34 cmH$_2$O (reference range 12–20). Lumbar puncture relieved the patient's headache and was therefore repeated twice, whereupon the patient felt

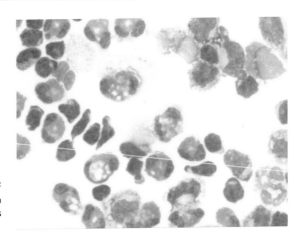

FIGURE 64-1 Romanowski–Giemsa stain of the CSF sample revealing large numbers of eosinophils with red (eosinophilic) cytoplasm. Courtesy Prof. Thomas Schneider.

TABLE 64-2 Main Causes and Characteristics of Parasitic Eosinophilic Meningitis

Pathogen	Incubation Period	Source of Infection	Geography	Clinical Features	Serology
Angiostrongylus cantonensis	2–35 days	Consumption of infected crustaceans, snails, prawns, crabs, frogs, and/or contaminated vegetables	South-east Asia, Pacific basin, Australia, Caribbean	Paraesthesia of trunk, limbs, or face	Western blot of antibodies against 31 kD antigen*
Gnathostoma spinigerum	Days to months	Consumption of infected poultry or fish	South-east Asia (mainly Thailand), emerging in sub-Saharan Africa	Migrating subcutaneous swellings, creeping eruption, sharp radicular pain at onset	Western blot of antibodies against 24 kD antigen*

*Serology can be negative in acute state and a paired convalescence sample should be taken after four weeks.

markedly better. No further specific treatment was prescribed. She received iron tablets for a mild microcytic anaemia. The patient was discharged significantly improved after a one-week hospital stay. At four-week follow-up she had fully recovered and her peripheral eosinophil count had returned to normal.

SUMMARY BOX

Eosinophilic Meningitis

Eosinophilic meningitis is defined as the presence of ten or more eosinophils per microlitre of CSF, or eosinophilia of at least 10% of the total CSF leukocyte count. Invasion of the central nervous system by the food-borne nematodes *Angiostrongylus cantonensis*, and less frequently, *Gnathostoma spinigerum*, are the most common causes (Table 64-2). Rarely, neurocysticercosis, neuroschistosomiasis, paragonimiasis, fascioliasis, toxocariasis, baylisascariasis and trichinellosis can be associated with eosinophilic meningitis;[1,2] however, the meningeal involvement is usually not prominent.

Angiostrongylus cantonensis, the rat lungworm, is the most common infectious cause of eosinophilic meningitis. Humans are infected by ingestion of *Angiostrongylus* larvae in intermediate hosts such as fresh water snails and slugs; or transport hosts, such as prawns, crabs and frogs; or salad and vegetables contaminated with slime of infected snails. Once ingested, the third stage larvae (L3) penetrate the intestinal wall, reach the portal vein and from there enter the systemic circulation. *A. cantonensis* is a truly neurotropic helminth. Humans are dead-end hosts, the larvae die in the human subarachnoid space causing an eosinophilic inflammatory response.

Angiostrongyliasis is usually mild and self-limiting and the prognosis is favorable. Symptoms tend to resolve within four weeks of onset. Treatment is directed at symptomatically easing headache with analgesics and serial lumbar punctures. The use of corticosteroids alone or in combination with albendazole may be beneficial in selected cases, but this is overall still disputed due to a lack of data from large randomized clinical trials.[3]

Further Reading

1. Heckmann JE, Bhigjee AI. Tropical neurology. In: Farrar J, editor. Manson's Tropical Diseases. 23rd ed. London: Elsevier; 2013 [chapter 71].
2. Graeff-Teixeira C, da Silva AC, Yoshimura K. Update on eosinophilic meningoencephalitis and its clinical relevance. Clin Microbiol Rev 2009;22(2):322–48.
3. Wang QP, Lai DH, Zhu XQ, et al. Human angiostrongyliasis. The Lancet Infect Dis 2008;8(10):621–30.

A 4-YEAR-OLD GIRL FROM BOLIVIA WITH A DARK NODULE ON HER TOE

65

Thomas Weitzel

Clinical Presentation

HISTORY

A 4-year-old girl presents with a history of several days of a slowly growing nodule on the fifth toe of her right foot that is moderately painful when wearing shoes. The family moved from Chile to the Cochabamba region in Bolivia about six months ago, where they live on a farm. Her 9-year-old brother has similar lesions on two toes.

CLINICAL FINDINGS

The patient is a 4-year-old girl in good general health. Close to the root of the fifth toe's nail of the right foot there is a dark-brown small nodule with a tiny central ulceration, surrounded by minimal inflammatory reaction (Figure 65-1). The parents report that when they had tried to squeeze the lesion, they observed white oval granules emerging from the nodule.

QUESTIONS

1. How would you diagnose this disease?
2. How would you treat the patient?

Discussion

A 4-year-old girl who lives on a farm in Bolivia presents with a slowly growing nodular lesion on her toe. Her brother has similar lesions on his feet.

ANSWER TO QUESTION 1

How Would You Diagnose This Disease?

The macroscopic presentation and localization of this lesion allows the clinical diagnosis of tungiasis. Physicians who are not familiar with the disease might send a sample for microscopic confirmation. Figure 65-2 shows parts of the parasite and an egg in a tissue sample. The female flea is usually destroyed during the process of removal, but parts of the body as well as eggs can still be found.

ANSWER TO QUESTION 2

How Would You Treat the Patient?

The parasite should be completely removed using a sterile needle and/or curette. The resulting round lesion must be disinfected and dressed. The patient's tetanus vaccination status should be checked and the wound should be observed and if necessary treated for superinfection.

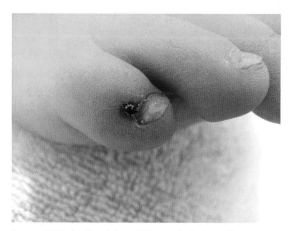

FIGURE 65-1 Small nodule on fifth toe of right foot. (Toenails with leftovers of glitter nail polish.)

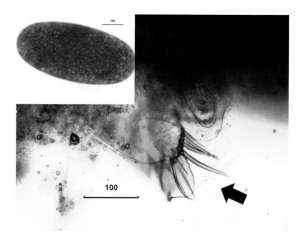

FIGURE 65-2 Microscopic examination of removed tissue containing parts of female flea (arrow) and typical eggs (size 600 × 280 μm).

THE CASE CONTINUED ...

The skin lesion healed within a week without complications.

SUMMARY BOX

Tungiasis

Tungiasis is caused by the female *Tunga penetrans* (syn. sand flea, jigger, bicho do pé), which burrows into the epidermis of humans and various animals before oviposition.[1,2] There the parasite engorges to a size of approximately 1 cm, causing a slowly growing nodular skin lesion. The flea is completely embedded into the skin, except for the tip of the posterior end, through which the respiration, defecation and oviposition occurs.

Typical localizations are the feet's periungual regions, interdigital spaces and soles. However, other body parts might be affected after contact with contaminated soil.

Clinically, the flea together with the surrounding inflammatory reaction initially presents as a pale nodule with a dark centre; later the lesion might turn brown with a dark crust. It often causes local itching or pain. Symptoms are usually mild in patients visiting endemic areas and start after several days in cases of first infestation. Individuals living in endemic regions might suffer massive and repeated infestations leading to superinfection with complications such as gangrene, bacteraemia or tetanus.

The parasite is endemic in Latin America from Mexico to Northern Argentina and the Caribbean. From there it was introduced into sub-Saharan Africa, probably about 150 years ago. Tungiasis belongs to the category of neglected and poverty-related infectious disease. In poor communities of endemic countries, constant re-infection causes severe morbidity including deformation and permanent disability.[3] Important zoonotic reservoirs for human infections include pigs, dogs and rats. In travellers, tungiasis is found in about 1% of those presenting with dermatological problems.

The diagnosis is usually based on the clinical presentation. In non-endemic regions, the parasite and its eggs may be demonstrated in tissue samples and histopathological sections. Treatment consists of removing the flea with a sterile needle or curette with or without local anaesthesia, disinfection and prevention or treatment of concomitant bacterial infections.[4]

To prevent the disease, contact with contaminated sand or soil should be avoided, e.g. by using solid footwear. The effect of commonly used repellents has not been studied. Another strategy is to daily inspect the feet and extract sand fleas in an early stage of penetration.

Further Reading

1. Vega-Lopez F, Ritchie S. Dermatological problems. In: Farrar J, editor. Manson's Tropical Diseases. 23rd ed. London: Elsevier; 2013 [chapter 68].
2. Mumcuoglu KY. Other ectoparasites: leeches, myiasis and sand fleas. In: Farrar J, editor. Manson's Tropical Diseases. 23rd ed. London: Elsevier; 2013 [chapter 60].
3. Feldmeier H, Sentongo E, Krantz I. Tungiasis (sand flea disease): a parasitic disease with particular challenges for public health. Eur J Clin Microbiol Infect Dis 2013;32(1):19–26.
4. Heukelbach J. Revision on tungiasis: treatment options and prevention. Exp Rev Anti-infect Ther 2006;4(1):151–7.

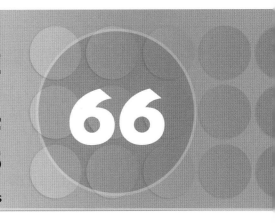

66

A 32-YEAR-OLD MAN FROM MALAWI WITH PAIN IN THE RIGHT UPPER ABDOMEN AND A FEELING OF FAINTNESS

Anthony D. Harries

Clinical Presentation

HISTORY

A 32-year-old man from Malawi presents to a local hospital with a history of pain in his right upper abdomen and a feeling of faintness, especially when standing up and walking. He was well until one month previously when he began to experience a feeling of fullness in his upper abdomen. In the week before admission he developed pain in the right upper abdomen that was particularly apparent when sleeping on his right side. He has recently started to feel breathless on lying down and feels faint, especially on standing up. His past medical history is unremarkable, except for an episode of a blistering and painful skin lesion three years previously that affected the right side of his abdomen around the level of the umbilicus – this had healed spontaneously after several weeks.

CLINICAL FINDINGS

He is thin and slightly breathless in the supine position. His pulse is regular at 130 bpm with pronounced pulsus paradoxus measured at 15 mmHg. Blood pressure in the supine position is 90/60 mmHg. The jugular venous pulse is difficult to visualize but is judged to be elevated. The apex beat is impalpable. The heart sounds are quiet but audible; no triple rhythm and no heart murmurs are heard. Auscultation of the chest is normal. There is an enlarged tender palpable liver measured at 8 cm below the right costal junction and evidence of mild peripheral oedema of the legs and sacral area.

INVESTIGATIONS

Haemoglobin 10.5 g/dL; WBC 9.8×10^9/L (reference range: 4–10). Chest radiography (see Figure 66-1) shows an enlarged globular heart with clear lung fields.

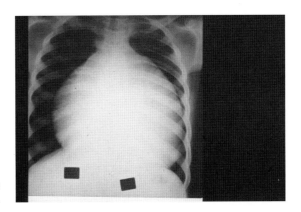

FIGURE 66-1 Chest radiograph of the patient showing an enlarged globular cardiac silhouette with clear lung fields.

1. Based on the clinical history and examination and investigations done, what is the most likely pathology to explain this man's illness and what would be the most frequent cause of the problem?
2. What other investigations should be carried out? Outline the immediate and long-term management of his condition.

Discussion

This young African man presents with a history of right upper abdominal pain, breathlessness and syncope. On physical examination, he has signs of cardiac decompensation associated with right heart failure. It is likely that his skin lesion three years previously was herpes zoster.

ANSWER TO QUESTION 1

What is the Most Likely Pathology to Explain This Man's Illness and What Would be the Most Frequent Cause of the Problem?

The history, physical examination and chest radiograph findings all point to a diagnosis of pericardial tamponade due to a large pericardial effusion. The cardiovascular manifestations of tachycardia, pulsus paradoxus, hypotension, impalpable apex beat, raised jugular venous pressure (which may be difficult to identify in pericardial effusion due to small 'a' and 'v' waves) and quiet heart sounds are indicative of pericardial effusion. The presence of syncope, pulsus paradoxus and hypotension are signs of cardiac tamponade indicating the need for a therapeutic pericardial aspiration. In Africa there are several causes of pericardial effusion that include tuberculosis, other bacterial infections, malignancy and HIV-related Kaposi's sarcoma. The presence of a previous attack of herpes zoster is a strong pointer to HIV infection, and in this case the most likely diagnosis is HIV-associated tuberculosis.

ANSWER TO QUESTION 2

What Other Investigations Should be Carried Out? Outline the Immediate and Long-Term Management of His Condition.

The most important investigation that should be carried out immediately is an ultrasound of the heart, which should show the presence of pericardial fluid and sometimes fibrous strands that are strongly suggestive of tuberculosis, especially in highly endemic areas. An electrocardiogram is useful in showing low-voltage QRS complexes and in occasional cases there may be electrical alternans. If there is pericardial fluid on ultrasound, the patient requires a therapeutic pericardial aspiration to relieve the pressure on the heart and restore cardiac output. This can be performed under local anaesthesia with a syringe and long needle being inserted just below the xiphisternal notch on the left side and directed at an angle of 40 degrees towards the left shoulder. Once fluid is aspirated and the cardiac output is restored, the patient should be started on antituberculosis treatment and corticosteroids. An HIV test should be carried out with appropriate counselling, and consideration given to starting antiretroviral therapy after several weeks if the HIV test is positive.

THE CASE CONTINUED ...

The patient underwent therapeutic pericardial aspiration and 500 mL of bloodstained pericardial fluid were aspirated. The blood pressure increased to 120/80 mmHg almost immediately. The patient was started on antituberculosis treatment with four drugs; rifampicin (R), isoniazid (H), pyrazinamide (Z) and ethambutol (E) and also on prednisolone at a dose of 60 mg daily. HIV testing was carried out and the patient was found to be HIV-positive. The patient received a full six-month course of antituberculosis treatment consisting of a two-month initial phase of four drugs given daily (2RHZE) and a four-month continuation phase of two drugs given daily (4RH), prednisolone in tapered doses for ten weeks, and antiretroviral therapy which was started at four weeks after commencing antituberculosis treatment. He made a full and uneventful recovery.

SUMMARY BOX

Pericardial Effusion

There are a number of important points that can be made about this case study.

First, hepatomegaly is a common physical sign in African patients and may be due to local hepatic pathology from cirrhosis of the liver, hepatosplenic schistosomiasis, hepatoma or amoebic liver abscess. However, hepatic congestion due to right heart failure should always be remembered as an important cause of this finding.

Second, once a diagnosis of pericardial effusion is made, it is important to determine whether tamponade is present, with the characteristic features being syncope, tachycardia, pulsus paradoxus and hypotension. The presence of tamponade is potentially life-threatening and requires prompt pericardial aspiration. Diagnostic pericardial aspiration is usually unhelpful in the district hospital setting, as the fluid is often bloodstained and acid-fast bacilli are rarely visualized in smears of the pericardial aspirate from patients who have tuberculosis.

Third, in Africa the most common cause of pericardial effusion is tuberculosis, and even if there is no confirmatory evidence of tuberculosis, patients must be treated with a full course of antituberculosis treatment.

Fourth, prednisolone during the first ten weeks of antituberculosis treatment in patients with tuberculous pericardial effusion has been shown to reduce the risk of death, the need for repeated pericardiocentesis and the need for open surgical drainage, and even if HIV infection is present this adjunctive treatment is worthwhile.

Finally, in countries in central and southern Africa there is a strong association between tuberculosis and HIV infection, with over 50 per cent of tuberculosis patients being HIV-positive. The advent of the HIV/AIDS epidemic in Africa was associated with a large increase in the number of patients being diagnosed with tuberculous pericardial effusion. Recent WHO guidelines recommend that all patients with HIV-associated tuberculosis are started on antiretroviral therapy regardless of the CD4 cell count and that antiretroviral therapy is started within 2–8 weeks of the start of anti-tuberculosis treatment. Efavirenz is the preferred non-nucleoside reverse transcriptase inhibitor. Timely antiretroviral therapy reduces mortality, is associated with excellent immunological and virological responses and reduces the risk of recurrent tuberculosis.

Further Reading

1. Thwaites G. Tuberculosis. In: Farrar J, editor. Manson's Tropical Diseases. 23rd ed. London: Elsevier; 2013 [chapter 40].
2. Mayosi BM, Wiysonge CS, Ntsekhe M, et al. Mortality in patients treated for tuberculous pericarditis in sub-Saharan Africa. S Afr Med J 2008;98:36–40.
3. Strang JIG, Kakaza HHS, Gibson DG, et al. Controlled clinical trial of complete versus open surgical drainage and of prednisolone in treatment of tuberculosis pericardial effusion in Transkei. Lancet 1988;ii:759–64.

67

A 24-YEAR-OLD WOMAN FROM THE PERUVIAN ANDES WITH FEVER AND ABDOMINAL PAIN

Fátima Concha / Eduardo Gotuzzo

Clinical Presentation

HISTORY

A 24-year-old woman from the highlands of Peru is transferred to a hospital in the capital Lima with a two-month history of upper abdominal pain, weight loss (5 kg), nausea and vomiting. She tried analgesics, which did not control the pain. She also reports intermittent fevers for the past two weeks.

Three days previously, she was seen at the emergency room of the same hospital for the above complaints. Abdominal ultrasound revealed multiple hypoechoic lesions. She was treated with ceftriaxone and metronidazole for suspected pyogenic liver abscesses but did not show any clinical improvement.

The patient reported that about 2–3 months ago she started taking over-the-counter medicines to lose weight and changed her diet to vegetarian food. She also reported the consumption of energetic hot drinks made from alfalfa and watercress. Prior to her current illness, she was healthy. She is single and has no children.

CLINICAL FINDINGS

An ill-looking patient with pale mucous membranes but no jaundice. Her blood pressure is 95/60 mmHg, pulse 105 bpm and temperature 38.5°C. On palpation of the abdomen there is right upper quadrant tenderness and the liver is slightly enlarged with a liver span of 15 cm. The rest of the physical examination is within normal limits.

LABORATORY RESULTS

Table 67-1 shows the patient's laboratory results, taken in the emergency room.

TABLE 67-1 Laboratory Results on Admission to Emergency Room		
Parameter	**Patient**	**Reference Range**
WBC (x10⁹/L)	13.94	4–10
Eosinophils (%)	43	<5
Total eosinophil count	5.97	<0.5
Haemoglobin (g/dL)	12.3	12–16
AST (U/L)	34	10–40
ALT (U/L)	55	7–40
AP (U/L)	170	20–126
Amylase (U/L)	75	3–100
Lipase (U/L)	100	10–140

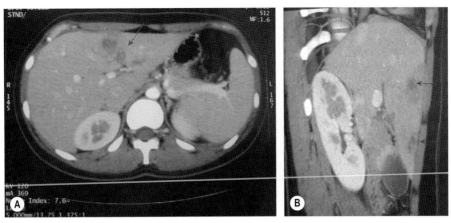

FIGURE 67-1 A contrast-enhanced CT scan showing multiple, round, clustered, hypodense lesions in left median section of liver (A, axial cross-section; B, lateral view).

IMAGING

A contrast-enhanced CT scan of her abdomen shows multiple hypodense, non-enhancing lesions in the liver (Figure 67-1).

QUESTIONS

1. What are your differential diagnoses?
2. What would be the most useful investigation to establish the diagnosis?

Discussion

A young woman from the Peruvian Andes presents with a history of fever, weight loss and abdominal pain. The blood count reveals pronounced eosinophilia. The abdominal CT scan shows hypodense non-enhancing hepatic lesions.

ANSWER TO QUESTION 1

What Are Your Differential Diagnoses?

The patient was first treated for suspected pyogenic liver abscesses based upon the presence of fever, right upper abdominal pain and hypoechoic lesions on ultrasound. However, the lack of any improvement after three days of appropriate treatment makes this diagnosis less likely.

In this patient from the Andes with high eosinophilia and a known history of alfalfa and watercress consumption, fascioliasis is the most important diagnosis to consider. Amoebic liver abscess is also part of the differential diagnosis, but eosinophilia and the presence of multiple lesions are not typical. Also, the infection should respond to metronidazole treatment.

Other endemic infections in Peru that could present with similar symptoms are brucellosis, visceral toxocariasis, or secondary infections in the context of other infections (i.e. ascariasis and hydatid disease). *Opisthorchis,* another liver fluke, could be considered if the patient had a travel history to South-east Asia, as the condition is not present in the Americas.

ANSWER TO QUESTION 2

What Would Be the Most Useful Investigation to Establish the Diagnosis?

Infection with the sheep liver fluke (*Fasciola hepatica*) is top of the list of differential diagnoses in this patient with liver lesions, eosinophilia and a history of watercress consumption.

Since ova appear in the stool only later in the course of the disease, serology is the diagnostic tool of choice. The Fas2 ELISA is a serological method with good sensitivity and specificity to diagnose the acute phase of *F. hepatica* infection.

Liver biopsy is invasive and has little benefit in this context; it could be considered if tests are negative and all treatment fails.

THE CASE CONTINUED ...

The Fas2 ELISA titre was 0.56 (normal <0.2), supporting the suspected diagnosis of fascioliasis. The patient received one single dose of triclabendazole 10 mg/kg. Her clinical symptoms rapidly improved and her laboratory parameters went back to normal. On control tomography her liver lesions were seen to be disappearing.

SUMMARY BOX

Fascioliasis

Fascioliasis is caused by the liver flukes *Fasciola hepatica* or less frequently *F. gigantica*.[1-3] Fascioliasis has the widest latitudinal, longitudinal and altitudinal distribution of any zoonotic diseases known. It is a serious public health problem, with between 2.4 million and 17 million infected people worldwide and around 90 million at risk. In South America, the infection is encountered in the Andean countries, in particular in Bolivia and Peru.[4] Egypt is another country with a very high prevalence of fascioliasis.[1]

Ova of *Fasciola* spp. are shed in the faeces of herbivores. Once they reach fresh water, miracidia hatch and infect a snail which acts as an intermediate host. Further development takes place inside the snail, then cercariae are released into the water. They develop into infective encysted metacercariae on freshwater plants. Humans acquire the disease by eating watercress (salads) or drinking water contaminated with metacercariae.

The illness includes four clinical phases: (1) incubation phase, (2) invasive or acute phase, (3) latent phase and (4) obstructive or chronic phase. The incubation phase lasts from ingestion of metacercariae to first symptoms (6–12 weeks). The invasive or acute phase begins with flukes migrating through the small intestinal wall, the peritoneal cavity, the liver capsule and the liver parenchyma.

During the acute phase, lasting 3–5 months, the patients typically present with intermittent fever, abdominal pain, malaise, weight loss, urticaria and respiratory symptoms (e.g. cough, dyspnoea and chest pain). Less common findings include changes in bowel habits, nausea, anorexia, hepatomegaly, splenomegaly, ascites, anaemia and jaundice. Eosinophilia is almost always present during the acute phase.

At the beginning of the subsequent latent phase the parasites have crossed the liver parenchyma to finally reach the common bile duct where they mature and start depositing eggs. Ova appear in the stool 3–4 months after the ingestion of infective metacercariae. The latent phase is characterized by the progressive resolution of gastrointestinal and respiratory symptoms. An unknown percentage of patients will progress to the fourth phase of the disease characterized by biliary obstruction, cholelithiasis, ascending cholangitis, cholecystitis, or liver abscess. Haemorrhage (e.g. subcapsular haematomas), hepatic fibrosis or biliary cirrhosis might also be observed.

During the acute phase, diagnosis of human fascioliasis is based on clinical and radiological findings and immunodiagnostic assays such as Fas2-ELISA. Eosinophilia is usually present.

During chronic infection, eosinophilia is rare but ova can be detected on stool microscopy. The yield can be improved using rapid sedimentation techniques. Microscopic detection of eggs is considered definitive diagnosis of fascioliasis. Eggs may also accidentally be discovered during surgery for biliary obstruction.

Typical lesions seen on CT scan are contrast-enhancement of the Glisson's capsule, multiple hypodense nodular lesions and necrotic granuloma.

Triclabendazole is the anthelmintic drug of choice. In acute cases a single dose of triclabendazole at 10 mg/kg is effective in 90% of cases and the same regimen is used in chronic disease. Triclabendazole should be taken with food to increase its bioavailability.

Further Reading

1. Sithithaworn P, Sripa B, Kaewkes S, et al. Food-borne trematodes. In: Farrar J, editor. Manson's Tropical Diseases. 23rd ed. London: Elsevier; 2013 [chapter 53].
2. Marcos LA, Tagle M, Terashima A, et al. Natural history, clinicoradiologic correlates, and response to triclabendazole in acute massive fascioliasis. Am J Trop Med Hyg 2008;78(2):222–7.
3. Cabada MM, White AC Jr. New developments in epidemiology, diagnosis, and treatment of fascioliasis. Curr Opin Infect Dis 2012;25(5):518–22.
4. Espinoza JR, Terashima A, Herrera-Velit P, et al. [Human and animal fascioliasis in Peru: impact in the economy of endemic zones]. Rev Peruana Med Exper Salud Publica 2010;27(4):604–12.

A 31-YEAR-OLD WOMAN FROM MALAWI WITH A GENERALIZED MUCOCUTANEOUS RASH

Camilla Rothe

68

Clinical Presentation

HISTORY

A 31-year-old woman presents to a hospital in Malawi with a generalized skin rash. The rash started three days before on the trunk, and then spread to the extremities and the mucosal membranes involving lips, oral mucosa, conjunctivae and genital mucosa.

There is also productive cough with whitish sputum that started one day before the rash appeared and she also reports a sore throat and dysuria for the past two days.

The patient had been found to be HIV-positive two months earlier, when she was hospitalized with cryptococcal meningitis. She was treated with high-dose oral fluconazole, since amphotericin B and flucytosine were unavailable. She improved and was discharged home on a maintenance dose of fluconazole. Antiretroviral treatment with stavudine (d4T), lamivudine (3TC) and nevirapine (NVP), as well as co-trimoxazole prophylaxis, were started one month previously.

The rest of the medical history is unremarkable and there are no known allergies.

CLINICAL FINDINGS

Her temperature is 37.7°C, blood pressure 120/68 mmHg, pulse 90 bpm and respiratory rate 24 breath cycles per minute. There is a generalized, non-itchy maculopapular rash involving the skin and mucous membranes but sparing the palms and soles. There is bilateral conjunctivitis. The eyelids and lips are covered with haemorrhagic crusts (Figure 68-1). The lips are swollen and she can hardly open her mouth; talking and eating is difficult and painful. The chest is clear.

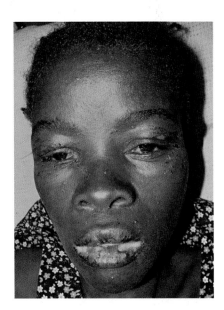

FIGURE 68-1 The face of the patient, showing bilateral swelling of the eyes with conjunctivitis and swollen lips with haemorrhagic crusts. The maculopapular rash was non-itchy and spared the scalp.

1. What is the most likely diagnosis and what is it caused by?
2. How would you approach the patient?

Discussion

A young Malawian woman presents with a generalized rash involving her skin and mucous membranes. She also complains of a productive cough of short duration, dysuria and dysphagia.

The patient is known to be HIV-positive. Within the past month she commenced treatment with co-trimoxazole and an antiretroviral triple therapy with stavudine, lamivudine and nevirapine. She has a low-grade fever, but her chest is clear.

ANSWER TO QUESTION I

What is the Most Likely Diagnosis and What is It Caused By?

The most important diagnosis to consider is Stevens–Johnson syndrome (SJS)/toxic epidermal necrolysis. This potentially life-threatening mucocutaneous hypersensitivity reaction is most commonly caused by drugs. Its incidence is much higher in HIV-positive than in HIV-negative patients. If SJS involves more than 30% of the skin surface, it is called toxic epidermal necrolysis (TEN). SJS/TEN may lead to widespread epidermal detachment and erosions of the mucous membranes. Non-specific prodromal symptoms such as cough, sore throat, fever, headache and myalgias usually precede the rash by several days and may be mistaken for a bacterial or viral infection, or for malaria in a tropical setting.

ANSWER TO QUESTION 2

How Would You Approach the Patient?

SJS/TEN is a clinical diagnosis. Once suspected, all potentially causative drugs should be immediately withdrawn. If in doubt, all drugs need to be stopped. In general, medications initiated 2–4 weeks prior to the onset of symptoms are usually responsible. In this patient's case, the major culprit drugs were nevirapine and co-trimoxazole.

This patient had only a maculopapular rash. However, patients with SJS/TEN often develop large bullous skin lesions which, once they break open, lead to considerable loss of serous fluid, similarly to a burn, and ideally should be managed in a burns unit. Topical antiseptics will reduce skin colonization. Steroid eye drops should be given in case of conjunctivitis, and early ophthalmological review should be sought to prevent conjunctival scarring and blindness. Patients need careful management of fluids and electrolytes and high caloric nutrition. A nasogastric tube is often helpful until the mucosal lesions have healed. Fever may be part of the clinical picture and there is no role for prophylactic antibiotics unless there are other signs of sepsis. Vital signs need to be checked regularly, and blood cultures and full blood count taken repeatedly.

A urinary catheter should be inserted to prevent urethral strictures. Skin and mucosal lesions in SJS/TEN are very painful. Often, opioids are necessary to control the pain.

Upon discharge, patients should clearly be warned to avoid the culprit drug and this should be clearly stated in the patient's documents.

THE CASE CONTINUED ...

Antiretroviral drugs and co-trimoxazole were stopped on admission. Since the patient was febrile, blood cultures and a rapid malaria test were taken and both came back negative. She received IV fluids and a urinary catheter. The patient and her family declined a nasogastric (NG) tube, since they had observed that patients who had an NG tube or oxygen probes were more likely to die than patients who did not have such devices.

The patient was given 0.9% normal saline as mouthwash and dexamethasone eye ointment. Fever and cough settled spontaneously. She was discharged after ten days in hospital.

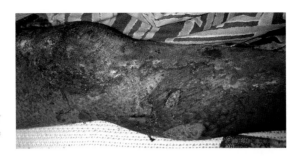

FIGURE 68-2 The right leg of another patient with SJS/TEN showing extensive epidermal sloughing and large areas of denuded dermis.

When all lesions had completely healed she was started on a new antiretroviral combination therapy and nevirapine was replaced by efavirenz. Co-trimoxazole was not replaced since there were no alternative drugs available. The new drug combination was tolerated well and no further rash occurred.

SUMMARY BOX

Stevens–Johnson Syndrome and Toxic Epidermal Necrolysis

Stevens–Johnson syndrome (SJS) is a life-threatening mucocutaneous hypersensitivity reaction. It is most commonly caused by drugs.[1–3] In SJS, less than 10% of the total body surface is involved. If more than 30% is affected, it is called toxic epidermal necrolysis (TEN). Between 10% and 30% it is classified as 'SJS/TEN overlap'. The extent of skin involvement is a major determinant for prognosis.

In Western industrialized countries, SJS/TEN is considered rare, with an estimated incidence of 1–7 per million per year. However, it is about 1000 times more prevalent in HIV-positive individuals, and clinicians working in sub-Saharan Africa and other high-prevalence settings need to be aware of this condition.

The drugs most commonly implicated in SJS/TEN are antibiotics (in particular sulfonamides, but also other classes), the antiretroviral nevirapine, anticonvulsants and allopurinol.[3]

Infectious agents (e.g. *Mycoplasma pneumoniae* and HSV) may also be responsible. Host genetic factors also seem to play a role.[2,3]

The pathophysiology is yet to be fully elucidated. Due to an unknown mechanism there is widespread apoptosis of keratinocytes and subsequent epithelial necrosis.

SJS/TEN often starts with non-specific, flu-like symptoms. After several days a morbiliform rash sets in that becomes more and more confluent. The epidermis may slough, giving rise to flaccid bullae, leaving a characteristic denuded dermis (Figure 68-2), which causes intense pain. Conjunctivitis is common and may lead to scarring and blindness.[4] Involvement of the oral mucosa and haemorrhagic crusting of the lips make it difficult for the patient to eat, drink and talk. Involvement of the urogenital mucosa is very painful and may lead to urethral strictures. The oesophagus and trachea may also be affected.

Diagnosis can often be made clinically. Skin biopsies may help rule out the major differential diagnoses such as staphylococcal scalded skin syndrome, toxic shock syndrome, exfoliative dermatitis, autoimmune bullous diseases and acute paraneoplastic pemphigus.

All potentially causative drugs need to be withdrawn immediately. Treatment is supportive and there is no clear benefit of any other disease-modifying interventions. However, data from large controlled clinical trials are lacking.

According to literature from the developed world, the case fatality rate of patients with SJS is up to 5%, in TEN on average 30%. Primary causes of death are infection and multi-organ failure.

A severity-of-illness score (SCORTEN) has been published to predict the mortality of patients with SJS/TEN.[3] Its use in resource-constrained setting is limited since it requires laboratory results (urea, bicarbonate, glucose) that may be difficult to obtain.

Further Reading

1. Hussain W, Craven NM. Toxic epidermal necrolysis and Stevens–Johnson syndrome. Clin Med 2005;5(6):555–8.
2. Hazin R, Ibrahimi OA, Hazin MI, et al. Stevens–Johnson syndrome: pathogenesis, diagnosis, and management. Ann Med 2008;40(2):129–38.
3. Gerull R, Nelle M, Schaible T. Toxic epidermal necrolysis and Stevens–Johnson syndrome: a review. Crit Care Med 2011;39(6):1521–32.
4. Schulze Schwering M, Kayange P, van Oosterhout JJ, et al. Severe eye complications from Stevens–Johnson syndrome in a human immunodeficiency virus-infected patient in Malawi. Am J Trop Med Hyg 2013;89(1):162–4.

A 22-YEAR-OLD MALE FARMER FROM RURAL ETHIOPIA WITH DIFFICULTY WALKING

Yohannes W. Woldeamanuel

Clinical Presentation

HISTORY

A 22-year-old male farmer from rural northern Ethiopia presents to a hospital in the capital with difficulty walking.

His problem started ten years ago, when he woke from sleep one morning and noticed weakness in both legs. There was no history of trauma and no prodromal symptoms; he had been in excellent health before. The weakness in his legs rapidly progressed over 4–5 days, leading to him needing a cane for mobility. He had no back pain, sensory complaints, sphincter disturbance or upper limb symptoms.

The start of his illness coincided with a period of drought and famine, when his diet almost exclusively consisted of grasspeas (*Lathyrus sativus*, local name *guaya*), which is known to be drought-resistant (Figure 69-1). Despite the monotonous diet, he had been engaged in hard physical labour on his family farm where he acted as the main breadwinner, despite his young age. He lived with his mother and three sisters, who took care of household chores; they consumed a similar diet but of overall smaller amounts of *guaya*.

During that time, several similar cases of weakness among young male farmers occurred in his village. His walking difficulty finally meant that he could not return to farm work. At the age of 20, he moved to the capital city seeking an alternative job. He migrated along with another young male farmer from his village who had suffered a similar fate; he had weakness of both legs and arms, which he had developed during the same period of drought. There was no history of cassava exposure in the region.

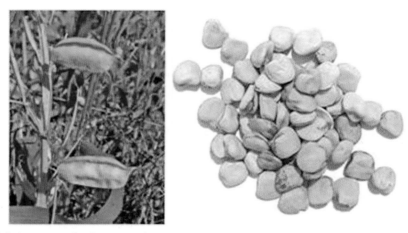

FIGURE 69-1 *Lathyrus sativus* (local name *guaya*) grasspea plant and its leguminous seeds.

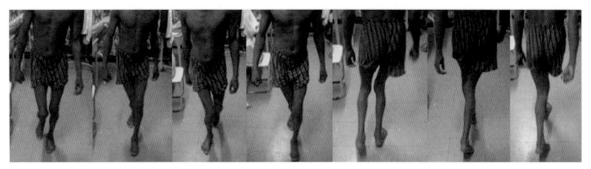

FIGURE 69-2 Images demonstrating the patient's gait: paraplegic narrow-based 'scissor gait' with foot-dragging, and toe-scraping.

CLINICAL FINDINGS

An alert young man with a normal mental state. The gait is spastic ('scissor gait'), with foot-dragging and toe-scraping (Figure 69-2). There is mild bilateral lower limb spastic weakness of pyramidal pattern, with pathological brisk deep tendon reflexes and sustained foot clonus. Extensor plantar response is elicited on the right, while equivocal on the left. Cranial nerves and upper limbs are normal. There is no sensory or bladder dysfunction.

LABORATORY RESULTS

Full blood count, liver and renal function tests, cerebrospinal fluid, nerve conduction studies and electromyography are normal. His HIV-1 serology is non-reactive. HTLV-1 and -2 serology and MRI are not available.

QUESTIONS

1. What clinical syndrome can you apply for a diagnostic approach and how do you narrow down your differential diagnoses?
2. What management and disease prevention plans can be used?

Discussion

A male teenage farmer from rural northern Ethiopia develops irreversible spastic paraparesis. The onset of symptoms coincides with a period of drought when diet mainly consists of grasspeas. There is no sensory deficit and no bladder dysfunction. Another young male farmer from the same village is similarly affected.

ANSWER TO QUESTION 1

What Clinical Syndrome Can You Apply for a Diagnostic Approach and How Do You Narrow Down Possible Differential Diagnoses?

Upper motor neuron lesion with spastic paraparesis is the clinical syndrome. Absence of radicular symptoms, sensory level, sphincter disturbance, back pain, non-progression, HIV-seronegativity and negative family history rule out most compressive, hereditary, infectious and metabolic myelopathies.

Among tropical myelopathies, HTLV-associated myelopathy (HAM) is highly unlikely. HAM has usually an insidious onset and a slowly progressive course, bladder impairment and sensory symptoms are prominent. Neurocassavism (konzo) may also present with a sudden onset spastic paraparesis but is improbable in the absence of cassava exposure. Male gender, pre-onset physical exertion, excessive prolonged *guaya* consumption and history of similarly affected village members favour a distinct form of toxiconutritional disease called neurolathyrism.

ANSWER TO QUESTION 2

What Management and Disease Prevention Plans Can be Employed?

Neurolathyrism is a preventable neurotoxic myelopathy leading to permanent disability. Treatment is symptomatic with anti-spastic drugs and physiotherapy. Tendon and muscle release surgery can be employed to lengthen contractures of calf muscles and hip adductors. Walking canes, foot braces and wheelchairs need to be provided.

Education to avoid consumption of *L. sativus* and measures to reduce toxin burden are important public health interventions. New cases of this preventable disease continue to occur. Behaviour change communication among high-risk communities can promote positive practices to reduce toxin exposure. Such practices include the use of metallic cooking utensils rather than traditional clay pots to avoid accrued toxicity from iron-induced oxidation, addition of anti-oxidant seasonings, soaking seeds in lemon-water and avoiding unripe seeds.

THE CASE CONTINUED ...

The patient received physiotherapy and muscle relaxants; however, this achieved only mild short-lasting improvement of his spasticity. A walking cane and wheelchair were provided. The patient was counselled to avoid further consumption of *L. sativus*.

SUMMARY BOX

Neurolathyrism

Neurolathyrism is a preventable toxic myelopathy caused by excessive ingestion of the *Lathyrus sativus* grasspea.[1,2] Clinical presentation is an irreversible acute to subacute spastic paraparesis or quadriparesis without prominent sensory involvement. Bladder and bowel function are maintained.

L. sativus is a hardy, high-yield pest- and insect-resistant cash crop that can endure monsoon, drought or water-logging. It has been consumed in ancient Egypt, Europe, South Asia and in the northern highlands of Ethiopia.[3] Currently more than 100 million people in drought- and monsoon-prone areas use *L. sativus* as staple crop. Being a multipurpose legume, it makes a protein-rich, filling diet. It is an 'almost perfect' crop, were it not for causing disability. *L. sativus* contains the neurotoxin β-N-oxalyl-a,b-diaminoproprionic acid (β-ODAP), a glutamate receptor agonist that results in excitotoxicity.

Toxicity is dose-dependent, and risk factors are prolonged heavy ingestion of grass peas, malnutrition, physical exertion, concurrent illness, illiteracy, male gender and young age.

Onset occurs within 3–6 months of monotonous excessive grasspea consumption. Weakness that develops suddenly or on waking from sleep is a classical presentation. Stage 1 neurolathyrism presents with spastic gait and independent mobility; Stage 2 is requiring a cane for mobility; Stage 3 is requiring a crutch; Stage 4 is characterized by the inability to bear weight with resultant contractures.

By virtue of affecting young breadwinners of rural families, neurolathyrism poses a high economic burden on poor communities in a setting where no social services or disability pensions are available.

Further Reading

1. Aronson JK. Plant poisons and traditional medicines. In: Farrar J, editor. Manson's Tropical Diseases. 23rd ed. London: Elsevier; 2013 [chapter 76].

2. Woldeamanuel YW, Hassan A, Zenebe G. Neurolathyrism: two Ethiopian case reports and review of the literature. J Neurol 2012;259(7):1263–8.

3. Tekle Haimanot R, Feleke A, Lambein F. Is lathyrism still endemic in northern Ethiopia? – The case of Legambo Woreda (district) in the South Wollo Zone, Amhara National Regional State. Ethiop J Health Dev 2005;19(3).

A 58-YEAR-OLD WOMAN FROM SRI LANKA WITH FEVER, DEAFNESS AND CONFUSION

70

Ranjan Premaratna

Clinical Presentation

HISTORY

A 58-year-old Sri Lankan woman who resides in a rural area presents to a local hospital with high-grade fever, chills, body aches, non-productive cough and progressive shortness of breath for ten days. Two days previously she developed tinnitus and hearing loss. One day prior to admission she became increasingly confused.

CLINICAL FINDINGS

On admission the patient is confused, with a Glasgow Coma Scale score of 13/15 (E4 V4 M5). Her hearing is severely impaired (WHO grade 3). Temperature 39.3°C, heart rate 120 bpm, blood pressure 90/60 mmHg. There are enlarged axillary lymph nodes on the right side. There is no rash and no neck stiffness; Kernig's and Brudzinski's signs are negative. Scattered crackles are audible on auscultation over the bases of both lungs. Her liver is enlarged to 5 cm below the right costal margin and the spleen is just palpable.

LABORATORY FINDINGS

Her basic laboratory results on admission are shown in Table 70-1; her cerebrospinal fluid results are shown in Table 70-2.

TABLE 70-1 Laboratory Results on Admission		
Parameter	Patient	Reference
WBC (x10⁹/L)	8.5	4–10
Haemoglobin (g/dL)	12.4	12–16
Platelets (x10⁹/L)	98	150–350
AST (U/L)	74	13–33
ALT (U/L)	68	3–25
ALP (U/L)	126	40–130
Total bilirubin (µmol/L)	25.7	13.7–30.8
Blood urea nitrogen (mmol/L)	6.4	2.5–6.4
Creatinine (µmol/L)	123.8	71–106
C-reactive protein (mg/L)	48	<6

TABLE 70-2 Cerebrospinal Fluid Results on Admission		
Parameter	Patient	Reference
Leukocytes (cells/µL)	35 (80% lymphocytes)	0–5/µL
Protein (g/L)	0.64	0.15–0.45
Glucose (mmol/L)	3.25*	50–75% of serum glucose

*Paired random blood glucose 7.17 mmol/L.

Her blood cultures grow no organisms; *Leptospira*- and *Salmonella*-serologies are negative. A thick film for malaria parasites is negative as well.

FURTHER INVESTIGATIONS

Chest radiography does not show any pathological changes. Her ECG shows sinus tachycardia. The EEG reveals widespread slowing; the CT scan of the brain is normal.

QUESTIONS

1. What clinical sign will you be specifically looking for?
2. What antibiotic would you include in your empirical regimen?

Discussion

A 58-year-old woman who is a rural resident of Sri Lanka presents with high-grade fever, chills, confusion and hearing loss. On examination there is a regional axillary lymphadenopathy on the right side. She looks ill and is septic on admission. FBC shows a normal white cell count but slight thrombocytopenia. The liver transaminases are slightly raised, but bilirubin and AP are normal. CSF shows slight lymphocytic pleocytosis, a mildly raised protein and a slightly decreased glucose. CT brain shows no abnormalities.

ANSWER TO QUESTION 1

What Clinical Sign Will You be Specifically Looking for?

Lymphadenopathy in the right axilla was detected on clinical examination of the patient. Her acute presentation with high fever and signs of severe sepsis make an infectious aetiology of the regional lymphadenopathy most likely. It is crucial to perform a meticulous examination in order to establish the port of entry of the microorganisms, which should be found in the skin area that drains to the enlarged regional lymph nodes.

In Asia, infection with *Orientia tsutsugamushi*, the causative pathogen of scrub typhus, is a common cause of fever, which is often associated with an eschar at the inoculation site. However, the prevalence of eschar varies in different populations and its absence does not rule out the diagnosis of scrub typhus.

ANSWER TO QUESTION 2

What Antibiotic Would You Include in Your Empirical Regimen?

In Asia, scrub typhus must be considered in every patient presenting with an undifferentiated febrile illness, regardless of the presence or absence of an eschar.

Therefore, doxycycline should be added to the empiric regimen to cover for *O. tsutsugamushi* infection. Chloramphenicol is the accepted alternative treatment if tetracyclines are contraindicated, as is the case in pregnant women, children, or patients with tetracycline hypersensitivity.

Of note, acute hearing loss or hearing impairment in a febrile patient from Asia should always arouse strong suspicion of scrub typhus. However, no single clinical sign or laboratory test can rule in or rule out scrub typhus, so empirical antirickettsial treatment is given based on clinical and epidemiological evidence. A definitive laboratory diagnosis – if at all possible in the particular setting – can be established later by demonstration of seroconversion in paired acute and convalescent serum samples.

THE CASE CONTINUED ...

On day 2 after admission she developed coarse tremors of both upper and lower limbs associated with saccadic oscillations of her eyes in all directions with further deterioration of level of consciousness (GCS 8). At this point a careful clinical examination revealed a well-demarcated crater-like lesion in the right axilla hidden within the axillary folds. Doxycycline therapy was commenced and the patient improved over the next 48 hours. She was discharged on day 6 after admission. Her hearing had returned to normal and there were no other neurological deficits.

The patient's *O. tsutsugamushi* IFA-IgG titre came back high (>1:4096), supporting the suspected diagnosis of scrub typhus.

SUMMARY BOX

Scrub Typhus

Scrub typhus is a common cause of pyrexia in large parts of Asia and northern Australia. It belongs to the tropical rickettsial infections and is caused by *Orientia tsutsugamushi*. The infection is transmitted by the bite of an infected larva (chigger) of a trombiculid mite.[1]

Infected mite larvae are found in a large variety of habitats, from scrubs and primary forests to gardens, beaches, bamboo fields and oil palm or rubber estates. Reservoirs of *O. tsutsugamushi* are rodents and the mites themselves, which can maintain the infection by vertical transmission. Humans are accidental hosts.

The incubation period is 6–10 days. A painless papule occurs at the site of the bite, which later ulcerates and transforms into a black crust or 'eschar'. Patients present with fever, severe headache and myalgia, regional or generalized lymphadenopathy and at times a macular or maculopapular rash. Conjunctival suffusions, vomiting and diarrhoea as well as constipation can also occur.

CNS involvement is common in scrub typhus, and presentations with diffuse encephalopathy or a reversible sensorineural deafness are well documented.[2] In contrast, focal neurological signs are rare. Cerebellar, brainstem and extrapyramidal manifestations have been reported, including opistosoclonus, myoclonus and Parkinsonian tremor. Further complications include myocarditis, interstitial pneumonia, ARDS and renal failure.

Immunity is short-lived and strain-specific.

Diagnosis can be challenging and in many resource-limited settings remains clinical. The diagnostic gold standard is the documentation of a significant rise in antibody titres in paired acute and convalescent serum samples. However, these serological tests are not standardized across laboratories and are usually unavailable in poor tropical areas. Rapid diagnostic tests have been developed for field use but have not yet been adequately evaluated. ELISA-based tests have a high sensitivity and specificity. PCR-based tests have been developed but await standardization and are not yet in widespread use. Culture of *O. tsutsugamushi* from the blood takes several weeks and requires a biosafety level 3 facility.

Scrub typhus is very responsive to antibiotic treatment, which should be given empirically once the diagnosis is suspected. Standard treatment is with doxycycline 100 mg bid for one week. Alternative options include tetracycline, azithromycin and chloramphenicol.

Further Reading

1. Paris DH, Day NPJ. Tropical rickettsial infections. In: Farrar J, editor. Manson's Tropical Diseases. 23rd ed. London: Elsevier; 2013 [chapter 22].
2. Premaratna R, Chandrasena TG, Dassayake AS, et al. Acute hearing loss due to scrub typhus: a forgotten complication of a reemerging disease. Clin Infect Dis 2006;42(1):e6–8.

71

A 71-YEAR-OLD MAN FROM JAPAN WITH EOSINOPHILIA AND A NODULAR LESION IN THE LUNG

Yukifumi Nawa / Haruhiko Maruyama / Masaki Tomita

Clinical Presentation

HISTORY

A 71-year-old Japanese man is referred to a local tertiary care hospital for further work-up of a nodular lesion in his right lung. He is clinically well and does not report any complaints.

The lesion was first detected two years earlier during a routine health check. Initially it was of linear shape. The patient has been regularly followed up since then. At his most recent follow-up visit it was found by chest radiography (Figure 71-1A) and CT scan (Figures 71-1B, 71-1C) that his linear lung shadow had turned into a nodular lesion of about 2 cm in diameter.

The patient was born in Kyushu district, southern Japan, where he is still living. He has no history of travelling overseas.

CLINICAL FINDINGS

The vital signs were normal. The chest was clear. The remainder of the physical examination was also normal.

INVESTIGATIONS

His full blood count and total IgE are shown in Table 71-1. Liver and renal function tests as well as electrolytes are normal. LDH and CRP are not raised.

SEROLOGIES

Cryptococcus Ag negative, *Aspergillus* Ag negative, ß-D-glucan 6.0 pg/mL (<20 pg/mL), Quantiferon-test (QFT-2G) negative.

IMAGING

Fluorodeoxyglucose-positron emission tomography (FDG-PET-CT) shows increased FDG-uptake into the lesion in the right upper lobe (Figures 71.1D–F).

QUESTIONS

1. What kind of diseases should be considered in your differential diagnosis?
2. What further information should you obtain from the patient?

Discussion

A 71-year-old Japanese man who is clinically well is worked up for a nodular lesion in his right lung. Blood tests reveal a mild eosinophilia and a slightly raised IgE. On PET scan the pulmonary lesion shows an increased FDG uptake.

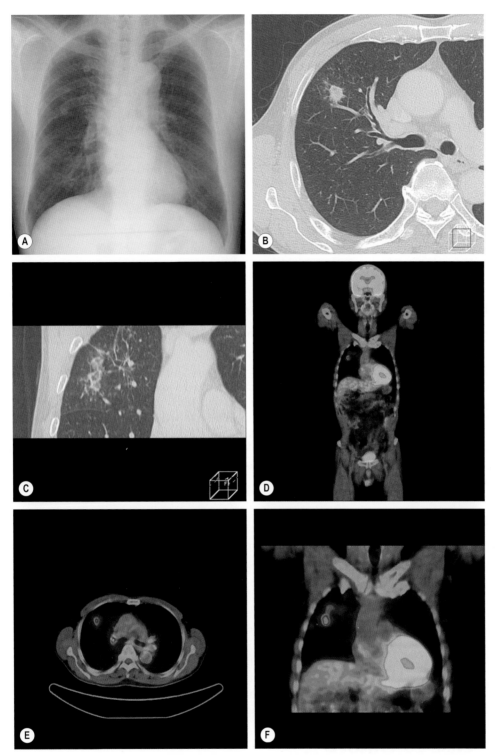

FIGURE 71-1 Chest X-ray (A) and CT scan (B,C) of the patient showing a nodular lesion in the right upper lobe. (D–F) Fluorodeoxyglucose-positron emission tomography (FDG-PET) with increased FDG uptake into the lesion in the right upper lobe.

TABLE 71-1 Full Blood Count Results at Presentation

Parameter	Patient	Reference
WBC ($\times 10^9$/L)	6.5	4–10
Haemoglobin (g/dL)	15.3	14–16
Platelets ($\times 10^9$/L)	190	150–300
Neutrophils (%)	46.1	30–80
Lymphocytes (%)	38.6	15–50
Monocytes (%)	6.4	1–12
Eosinophils (%)	8.3	0–6
Total eosinophil count ($\times 10^9$/L)	0.54	<0.45
Basophils (%)	0.6	0–2
IgE (U/mL)	185.7	<100

ANSWER TO QUESTION 1

What Kind of Diseases Should be Considered in Your Differential Diagnosis?

The most important differential diagnosis for a nodular lesion with or without cavitation in the lung is pulmonary tuberculosis or lung cancer. The PET-CT is unable to distinguish between a malignancy and an inflammatory lesion of other aetiology, e.g. an infectious process.

Systemic endemic mycoses (e.g. histoplasmosis, blastomycosis and paracoccidioidomycosis) may present with a large variety of pulmonary lesions in otherwise asymptomatic patients; however, they are not endemic in East Asia and the patient does not have a history of travelling abroad.

In addition to abnormal findings on the chest X-ray, this patient shows eosinophilia and elevated total IgE levels. One therefore needs to consider the possibility of pulmonary helminthiases, especially of lung fluke infection (paragonimiasis).

ANSWER TO QUESTION 2

What Kind of Information Should You Obtain from the Patient?

When suspecting lung fluke infection it is important to find out if the patient may at any time have been exposed to this parasite. *Paragonimus* spp. are endemic all over Asia, in West and Central Africa and parts of Latin America.

If the patient lives in an endemic area, or has a positive travel history, one should find out if s/he has ever eaten raw or undercooked freshwater crabs, which may harbour the infective stage (metacercariae) of *Paragonimus* spp. Also, consumption of raw wild boar meat is a risk, since wild boar act as paratenic hosts, harbouring juvenile worms. Traditional medicine used in some East Asian countries may contain raw crab meat and juice and potentially act as a source of infection. However, some patients have a negative exposure history and it has been suggested that even contaminated fingers and cooking utensils may act as a source of infection.

THE CASE CONTINUED ...

Bronchoscopy did not reveal any signs of malignancy. Cytology of the bronchoalveolar lavage (BAL) fluid was negative for malignant cells and acid-fast bacilli. The quantiferon-test and a wide range of tumour markers were negative.

In view of the elevated IgE levels, the patient's eosinophilia and the fact that the patient originated from Southern Japan, paragonimiasis was strongly suspected and the patient's serum was submitted for immunodiagnosis of parasitic diseases. Multiple-dot ELISA was strongly positive for *P. westermani*.

The patient was treated with oral praziquantel 25 mg/kg tds for three consecutive days. The lung lesion gradually faded and eventually disappeared. His serum antibody titre also declined.

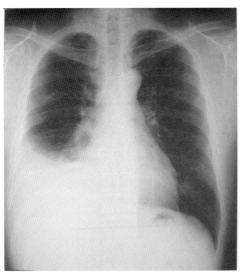

FIGURE 71-2 Chest X-ray of a patient with acute paragonimiasis, showing right-sided pleural effusion.

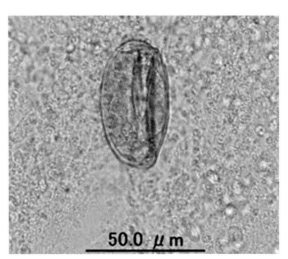

FIGURE 71-3 *Paragonimus westermani* egg in sputum.

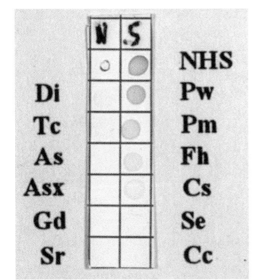

FIGURE 71-4 Multiple-dot ELISA for helminthiases showing positive reaction against *P. westermani* antigen. NHS: normal human serum for positive control; Pw: *P. westermani*; Pm: *P. miyazakii*; Fh: *Fasciola hepatica*; Cs: *Clonorchis sinensis*; Se: *Spirometra erinacei europaei*; Cc: *Cysticercus cellulosae*; Di: *Dirofilaria immitis*; Tc: *Toxocara canis*; As: *Ascaris sum*; Asx: *Anisakis simplex*; Gd: *Gnathostoma doloresi*; Sr: *Strongyloides stercoralis*.

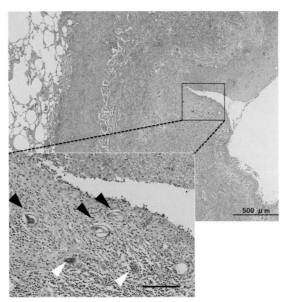

FIGURE 71-5 Histopathology of the nodular lung lesion that was surgically resected following diagnosis of lung cancer based on FDG-PET imaging. Note the chronic granulomatous lesion containing numerous *Paragonimus* eggs (black arrow). Foreign body giant cells (white arrow) are also seen in the tissue.

TABLE 71-2	Predominant *Paragonimus* spp. by Region[1]
Region	**Predominant *Paragonimus* spp.**
East Asia	*P. westermani*
	P. skrijabini[a]
South and South-east Asia	*P. heterotremus*[b]
Africa	*P. africanus*
	P. uterobilateralis
North America	*P. kelicottii*
Central and South America	*P. mexicanus*

[a]syn. *P. myazakii*.
[b]Exception: Philippines – *P. westermani*.

SUMMARY BOX

Paragonimiasis

Paragonimiasis is a subacute to chronic lung disease caused by infection with lung flukes of the genus *Paragonimus*. *Paragonimus westermani* is the most widely distributed species in Asia, but several additional species also cause disease (Table 71-2). Apart from Asia, paragonimiasis occurs in the Americas and in sub-Saharan Africa.

Adult flukes live in the lungs of a mammalian host (felines, canines, humans). Ova are coughed up and either expectorated or swallowed and passed in the faeces. When eggs reach fresh water, miracidia hatch and infect a snail (first intermediate host). After asexual multiplication, cercariae are released and infect a crab or crayfish (second intermediate host).

Human infection occurs mainly via consumption of raw or undercooked freshwater crabs or crayfish contaminated with *Paragonimus* metacercariae.[2] In addition, eating raw meat of wild boar, which is a paratenic host, is an important route of infection, especially in Japan.[2,3]

Metacercariae excyst in the small intestine and penetrate the intestinal wall. They pass through the liver and diaphragm, invade the pleural space and finally enter the lung parenchyma where they mature into adults and produce eggs. Juvenile worms sometimes migrate into subcutaneous soft tissue or the central nervous system to cause unexpected, potentially deleterious lesions.

Clinical features of the disease are similar to those of pulmonary TB or lung cancer. Patients may have chronic cough, haemoptysis, chest pain, fever, night sweats and abnormal findings on chest imaging. Pleural effusion (Figure 71-2) with marked eosinophilia in the exudate and pneumothorax without apparent nodular lesion/cavitation may occur in the early stages and/or in light infections.

Extrapulmonary paragonimiasis may present as painless, mobile subcutaneous swellings. Migration into the CNS may lead to acute eosinophilic meningoencephalitis and epilepsy.

However, about 20% of patients are asymptomatic and the disease is accidentally found on routine chest radiography, when nodules, ring shadows or cavities are typically seen.

Eosinophilia is prominent during acute and subacute infection but may be only mild or absent in chronic disease.

The definitive diagnosis is made by detection of ova in sputum, BAL fluid or faeces (Figure 71-3). However, sensitivity is below 50% in light infections. Instead, an immunodiagnostic screening test such as multiple-dot ELISA (Figure 71-4) should be used in combination with the patient's history and further laboratory results. Serological tests (e.g. ELISA) may detect early as well as chronic infections and titres decline rapidly following cure. Praziquantel is the drug of choice. A course of 25 mg/kg tds for three consecutive days is usually effective against all *Paragonimus* spp.

Even in paragonimiasis-endemic areas, physicians often do not pay much attention to this disease and misdiagnose it as pulmonary tuberculosis or lung cancer. Such diagnostic errors result in enormous socioeconomic loss, and create a mental and physical burden for the patient due to unnecessary hospitalization and laboratory investigations, surgical interventions and/or long-term medication. Figure 71-5 shows a typical example of such a case, in which postoperative histopathology revealed the presence of *Paragonimus* eggs in the resected nodular lesion, which had been diagnosed as a lung cancer by FDG-PET imaging.

Further Reading

1. Sithithaworn P, Sripa B, Kaewkes S, et al. Food-borne trematodes. In: Farrar J, editor. Manson's Tropical Diseases. 23rd ed. London: Elsevier; 2013 [chapter 53].
2. Nawa Y, Hatz C, Blum J. Sushi delights and parasites: the risk of fishborne and foodborne parasitic zoonoses in Asia. Clin Infect Dis 2005;41(9):1297–303.
3. Nakamura-Uchiyama F, Mukae H, Nawa Y. Paragonimiasis: a Japanese perspective. Clin Chest Med 2002;23(2):409–20.

A 4-YEAR-OLD BOY FROM MOZAMBIQUE WITH SEVERE OEDEMA AND SKIN LESIONS

72

Charlotte Adamczick

Clinical Presentation

HISTORY

An oedematous 4-year-old boy from Mozambique with low serum albumin is seen in the paediatric department of a central hospital in Malawi.

On admission five days earlier, the suspected diagnosis had been nephrotic syndrome and the child was started on furosemide and prednisolone; however, his oedema did not settle.

Three weeks earlier the little boy had been treated for pneumonia at a health centre. The past medical history is otherwise reported as normal. The boy is accompanied by his mother, who is visiting her sister in Malawi. The rainy season has just started.

CLINICAL FINDINGS

The patient is a miserable, apathetic boy with a puffy face and pitting oedema, most prominently on the back of his feet. The hair of the child is brittle, sparse and fair in colour. The skin is dry and hyperpigmented; it is peeling off like 'flaky paint' to reveal hypopigmented skin underneath (Figure 72-1). There are ulcerative skin lesions, most prominently in the groins (Figure 72-2). The child is refusing to eat.

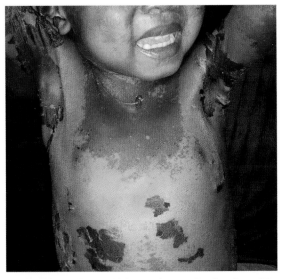

FIGURE 72-1 A 5-year-old boy with generalized oedema. The skin is hyperpigmented and dry. It is peeling off like 'flaky paint'. Underneath the skin is hypopigmented.

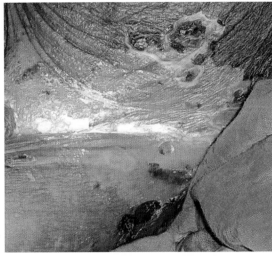

FIGURE 72-2 Ulcerative skin lesions on the lower abdomen and in both groins (where zinc ointment and GV paint has been applied).

LABORATORY RESULTS

Albumin 2.2 g/dL (reference range 3.0–5.2 g/dL), haemoglobin 7 g/dL (reference range 12–14 g/dL).

QUESTIONS

1. What is the likely diagnosis and how can it be distinguished from nephrotic syndrome?
2. How should the child be treated and what is the prognosis?

Discussion

This miserable little boy from rural Mozambique has a history of a recent infection. He developed oedema three weeks thereafter. The skin is hyperpigmented and dry, peeling off like 'flaky paint' and there is discoloration of his hair. Treatment with furosemide has no influence on the extent of the oedema. Clinically the patient is sick and refusing to eat or drink.

ANSWER TO QUESTION 1

What is the Likely Diagnosis and How Can It be Distinguished from Nephrotic Syndrome?

Generalized oedema in a child can have various causes. Nephrotic syndrome – the suspected diagnosis on admission – commonly occurs as a consequence of a recent infection. In nephrotic syndrome, serum albumin is low and there is heavy proteinuria.

However, this child is displaying further clinical features apart from his oedema that ought not be ignored, such as his skin and hair changes and his apathy. These are typical features of kwashiorkor, a form of severe acute malnutrition (see Summary Box). His low serum albumin alone is not sufficient to diagnose nephrotic syndrome, since albumin is influenced by many factors such as nutrition, liver function and intestinal resorption.

A urine dipstick test should be done to check for protein. In nephrotic syndrome, proteinuria exceeds 3.5 g per day (4+ on a urine dipstick) and the urine is often macroscopically frothy. In kwashiorkor, some proteinuria may be found but rarely exceeds 1+ on a dipstick test.

ANSWER TO QUESTION 2

How Should the Child be Treated and What is the Prognosis?

The child needs to be admitted to the high dependency area of the nutrition ward and treated according to the WHO guidelines for severe, acute malnutrition with meticulously calculated amounts of feeds. Children with kwashiorkor have a high mortality if not treated in time, correctly and monitored frequently. The risk of infection, diarrhoea, anaemia, cardiac and liver failure is high and needs to be considered. Prophylactic antibiotics, monitoring of temperature, fluid status and haemoglobin, and careful fluid replacement, are part of the initial treatment scheme.

THE CASE CONTINUED ...

The skin in the groins and armpits continued to peel off and became superinfected. The lesions could successfully be treated with Gentian violet solution (GV paint). The HIV test came back negative.

Initially the child did not tolerate three-hourly feeds and needed feeding via a nasogastric tube. On day 5 in the nutrition rehabilitation unit the child was able eat by himself and the oedema started to settle. The transition to higher caloric feeds was tolerated well.

After 15 days the child could be discharged into the community feeding programme. At this point some pedal oedema was still noticeable, but the little boy was active and his serum albumin had increased.

SUMMARY BOX

Kwashiorkor

Kwashiorkor is a form of severe, acute malnutrition characterized by hypoalbuminaemia and oedema.[1] Its aetiology and pathophysiology remain poorly understood.[2,3]

Kwashiorkor mainly occurs in areas where people live on a monotonous diet and the staple food has a low protein-to-energy ratio (e.g. maize, cassava or bananas). It is uncommon in communities where diet is supplemented by animal protein. Incidence peaks during the rainy season when staple food items and vegetables are in short supply.

However, kwashiorkor is not (just) a consequence of a diet low in protein and micronutrients. Infections often precede the onset of the disease. They lead to a fall in albumin levels in the context of acute phase reactions. Diarrhoeal diseases and capillary leak result in further loss of protein, nutrients and fluids. An imbalance between free radicals and insufficient levels of antioxidants leads to oxidative stress and damage of cell membranes. The capacity of the Na^+/K^+-pump is impaired, resulting in excess intracellular sodium concentrations and profound hypokalaemia. Production of immunoglobulins is diminished, which may lead to severe infections contributing to the high mortality associated with kwashiorkor.

The typical age at presentation is 1–3 years; boys and girls are equally affected.

Apart from oedema, children with kwashiorkor often display hair and skin changes. The hair becomes depigmented and is fair or reddish in colour. It is dry, sparse and easy to pluck. The skin is dry and hyperpigmented with pale skin underneath that is easily damaged and infected ('flaky paint' dermatosis). Ulcers may develop in flexures and around the perineum. The liver may be enlarged. Children with kwashiorkor are miserable, apathetic and often refuse to eat.

Management is challenging and involves careful feeding with increasing amounts of feeds.[1] In severe, acute malnutrition the usual signs of infection including fever may be absent, and prophylactic broad-spectrum antibiotics should be given to all patients. Diuretics are not indicated in the treatment of oedema in patients with kwashiorkor as they further deplete the intravascular volume, causing hypotension. Instead, careful rehydration is necessary, avoiding overhydration. The oedema will settle once therapeutic feeding has been installed.

Frequent monitoring of temperature is important since both fever and hypothermia commonly occur. Glucose levels, weight gain and fluid status need to be documented. Patients should also receive folic acid, anthelmintics and, once stable, measles vaccination if unvaccinated. Relapses are common and need to be recognized in time. Renal and liver function, as well as glucose levels, may be deranged well beyond the time of clinical recovery.

Case fatality rates from kwashiorkor are high, with a median of 20–30%. Additional infection with HIV further worsens the prognosis.[4]

Further Reading

1. Abrams S, Brabin BJ, Coulter JBS. Nutrition-associated disease. In: Farrar J, editor. Manson's Tropical Diseases. 23rd ed. London: Elsevier; 2013 [chapter 77].
2. Heikens GT, Manary M. 75 years of kwashiorkor in Africa. Malawi Med J 2009;21(3):96–8.
3. Golden MH. Evolution of nutritional management of acute malnutrition. Ind Pediatr 2010;47(8):667–78.
4. Heikens GT, Bunn J, Amadi B, et al. Case management of HIV-infected severely malnourished children: challenges in the area of highest prevalence. Lancet 2008;371(9620):1305–7.

73

A 38-YEAR-OLD WOMAN FROM MALAWI WITH CHRONIC ANAEMIA AND SPLENOMEGALY

Camilla Rothe

Clinical Presentation

HISTORY

A 38-year-old woman presents to a local hospital in Malawi because of general body weakness and left-sided abdominal discomfort. The symptoms have been there 'for quite some time'. There is no history of fever, night sweats or weight loss.

Her file reveals that she has presented with similar complaints many times in the past seven years. The attending clinicians repeatedly noticed a massively enlarged spleen and clinical anaemia. The patient was prescribed iron and folic acid several times.

She is a farmer residing in the lower Shire Valley in southern Malawi.

CLINICAL FINDINGS

The patient is in fair general condition. She is afebrile, with normal vital signs. She has pale conjunctivae. The spleen is visibly enlarged; on palpation it is felt about 15 cm below the left costal margin. The liver is moderately enlarged (about 4 cm below the right costal margin) with a smooth margin. There is no clinical ascites and no lymphadenopathy.

LABORATORY RESULTS

The full blood count results are: WBC 2.4×10^9/L (reference: 4–10); haemoglobin 7.2 g/dL (reference: 12–14); MVC 88 fL (reference: 80–98); platelets 115×10^9/L (reference: 150–350).

ULTRASOUND ABDOMEN

Spleen $22 \times 12 \times 7$ cm, homogeneous pattern. No abdominal lymphadenopathy. Liver 17 cm in diameter, normal echopattern.

QUESTIONS

1. What are the most important differential diagnoses in this patient?
2. How would you manage the patient?

Discussion

The patient presents with a marked splenomegaly and weight loss, moderate hepatomegaly and clinical anaemia, known for several years. She otherwise has no clinical complaints, in particular no constitutional symptoms. The full blood count shows pancytopenia with normocytic anaemia.

ANSWER TO QUESTION 1

What Are the Most Important Differential Diagnoses in This Patient?

The patient has been stable for several years without any constitutional symptoms. This makes a haematological malignancy unlikely. Visceral leishmaniasis (VL) can present with massive splenomegaly and pancytopenia, but patients usually have a history of fever and weight loss. VL furthermore is not endemic in Malawi.

The patient comes from the lower Shire Valley, a region in southern Malawi with a hot tropical climate all through the year and high levels of malaria transmission. The Shire river and other water bodies in Malawi are well known to be bilharzia-infested (*Schistosoma mansoni* and *S. haematobium*). Almost all people living in rural areas experience frequent contact with infested water during their lives when bathing, fishing, fetching water or doing laundry. Hence chronic infection with *S. mansoni* and subsequent hepatic fibrosis with portal hypertension resulting in hypersplenism is a possible differential diagnosis. The absence of the typical pattern of 'pipestem-fibrosis' on ultrasound does not rule out the diagnosis since the quality of ultrasound reports in resource-limited settings may be unreliable. Establishing the diagnosis of hepatic schistosomiasis can be difficult: serology is of no use in an endemic setting since it is nonspecific. Stool microscopy is also not helpful due to its low sensitivity; it may as well be negative in chronic infection. Liver biopsy and rectal biopsies are not commonly available. Other causes of portal hypertension leading to hypersplenism should also be considered.

The most likely differential diagnosis for this patient is hyperreactive malarial splenomegaly (HMS). HMS is the most common cause of massive splenomegaly in tropical areas with stable malaria transmission.

ANSWER TO QUESTION 2

How Would You Manage the Patient?

The patient originates from a setting where HIV prevalence is high. An HIV test should be offered to any patient. HIV infection is commonly associated with mild to moderate thrombocytopenia, leukcocytopenia and anaemia. Severe anaemia in HIV-positive patients should prompt investigation for concomitant tuberculosis. The mild leukopenia could even be interpreted as normal in the context of ethnic neutropenia, which is seen in sub-Saharan Africa.

A peripheral blood film should be done to look for abnormal blood cells. Malaria parasites should be checked, which in HMS are usually negative. If possible, a bone marrow aspirate should be done to rule out a haematological disorder.

In well-resourced settings, serological tests may demonstrate elevated serum IgM and high anti-malarial antibody titres typical for HMS.

THE CASE CONTINUED ...

HIV serology and a thick blood film for malaria parasites come back negative. The peripheral blood film does not show any further abnormalities. None of the other suggested investigations are currently available.

Under a suspected diagnosis of HMS, the patient is prescribed pragmatic once-weekly antimalarial treatment with chloroquine. She is followed up in the outpatient clinic. (Note: In Malawi, only chloroquine and sulfadoxine/pyrimethamine are available for the treatment of HMS. Other, possibly more effective drugs such as mefloquine are unavailable.)

At six months an ultrasound scan shows a significant decrease in spleen size by about 50%, making the suspected diagnosis of HMS very likely. The patient is advised to continue antimalarial chemoprophylaxis life-long.

SUMMARY BOX

Hyperreactive Malarial Splenomegaly (HMS)

Hyperreactive malarial splenomegaly (HMS), formerly known as the tropical splenomegaly syndrome, is one of the most common causes of massive splenomegaly in tropical regions with stable malaria transmission. Other important causes include lymphomas, chronic myeloid leukaemia, myelofibrosis, haemoglobinopathies, schistosomiasis and visceral leshmaniasis.

HMS is caused by an abnormal immune response to repeated infections with *Plasmodium falciparum, P. malariae* or *P. vivax* that results in an overproduction of polyclonal immunoglobulin M (IgM). IgM forms aggregates and immune complexes, which are phagocytosed by the reticuloendothelial system leading to hepatomegaly and massive splenomegaly.

Continued on following page

HMS is more common in women than in men and mainly affects the age group between 20 and 40 years. There seems to be a genetic background, with ethnic and familial clustering. HMS has also been described in expatriates residing in malaria-endemic regions.

Patients most commonly present with symptoms of anaemia and abdominal heaviness or discomfort.

Full blood count usually shows anaemia or pancytopenia reflecting hypersplenism. High antimalarial antibody titres in the absence of parasitaemia are typically seen. Patients with HMS have an increased risk of bacterial infections. There is evidence that HMS is a premalignant condition predisposing to the development of lymphoma.[1]

The clinical criteria for diagnosis of HMS include splenomegaly over 10 cm from the left costal margin and a sustained reduction of spleen size by at least 40% after 6 months of effective antimalarial treatment.

It may be difficult to differentiate HMS from splenic involvement of lymphoma when more sophisticated techniques such as bone marrow puncture are unavailable. In one study in Ghana, HMS rather than lymphoma was associated with young age below 40 years, female sex as well as an absolute lymphocyte count below 10×10^9/L.[2]

Treatment of HMS is effective with antimalarials for the duration of exposure. Proguanil 100 mg per day has been used, as well as weekly chloroquine, but high levels of resistance to both are widespread. Mefloquine is effective in nearly all high transmission settings.

Further Reading

1. White NJ. Malaria. In: Farrar J, editor. Manson's Tropical Diseases. 23rd ed. London: Elsevier; 2013 [chapter 43].
2. Bedu-Addo G, Bates I. Causes of massive tropical splenomegaly in Ghana. Lancet 2002;360(9331):449–54.

A 28-YEAR-OLD WOMAN FROM SIERRA LEONE WITH FEVER AND CONJUNCTIVITIS

74

Benjamin Jeffs

Clinical Presentation

HISTORY

A 28-year-old woman presents to a small rural hospital in Eastern Sierra Leone with a six-day history of fever, weakness, sore throat and retrosternal chest pain. She has had loose stools twice a day for the past two days. She was seen in a local health post the day before admission and given a course of artemether with amodiaquine and amoxicillin but she had continued to get worse on this. Her examination was unremarkable except some mild pharyngitis. On arrival in hospital she was treated with IV ceftriaxone and she completed the course of her antimalarial medications. Her malaria slide was negative.

She remained on this treatment for two days but continued to get worse. On the second day after admission she develops conjunctivitis. By this stage she is very unwell and is unable to walk unaided. She has developed a cough and breathlessness.

PHYSICAL EXAMINATION

Axillary temperature 38.2°C, blood pressure 80/55 mmHg, pulse rate 100 bpm. On chest auscultation she has bilateral fine crepitations.

INVESTIGATIONS

Her chest radiograph reveals diffuse bilateral infiltrates. Blood chemistry shows mild renal impairment and raised transaminases (aspartate transaminase 514 U/L (<50 U/L)).

QUESTIONS

1. What is the differential diagnosis?
2. What tests would you do and how would you manage the patient?

Discussion

A young Sierra Leonean woman has a severe febrile illness with pharyngitis, conjunctivitis and chest involvement. She deteriorates on broad-spectrum antibiotics.

ANSWER TO QUESTION I

What is the Differential Diagnosis?

Adenovirus infections can cause conjunctivitis and pharyngitis but these are normally mild. Also measles presents with fever, cough, coryza and a striking conjunctivitis. It may also cause pneumonitis, but at this stage you would expect to see a rash.

Mycoplasma pneumoniae can cause a pharyngitis and pneumonia but is rarely severe. Other forms of pneumonia are possible but do not normally cause conjunctivitis.

Leptospirosis can start with a nonspecific febrile illness. Pulmonary involvement including haemorrhages is common and it can cause renal impairment. Patients with severe leptospirosis tend to present with conjunctival suffusions than with conjunctivitis.

Typhoid can present as a nonspecific febrile illness. You would expect the patient to eventually improve on ceftriaxone, but prolonged clinical courses in typhoid are not uncommon. Pharyngitis and conjunctivitis are usually not part of the clinical picture.

Lassa fever is quite common in Eastern Sierra Leone, accounting for 16–20% of hospital admissions in some studies. All the signs and symptoms that the patient has are consistent with Lassa fever.

ANSWER TO QUESTION 2

What Tests Would You do and How Would You Manage the Patient?

Lassa fever is a serious disease. It has caused nosocomial outbreaks in which many medical staff have died. Therefore all procedures should be done with caution and the possibility of Lassa fever should always be discussed with the laboratory. All specimens should be transported in sealed plastic containers.

Serological and PCR tests are available for the diagnosis of Lassa fever, and an antigen-based rapid point-of-care test has been licensed.

PCR tests are the most sensitive but are not available in most African countries. Antigen tests demonstrate the presence of the disease but may not detect low levels of the virus, especially if taken in the first days of illness. IgM antibody tests can show a high rate of false positive tests and may be hard to interpret.

The patient needs to be isolated until the results of the Lassa fever tests are known. Since the infection spreads through contact with blood or body fluids, the patient should always be handled with gloves. If the diagnosis of Lassa fever is confirmed, use of goggles, masks, double gloves and disposable (waterproof) surgical gowns is recommended. The patient should be isolated in a side room, which

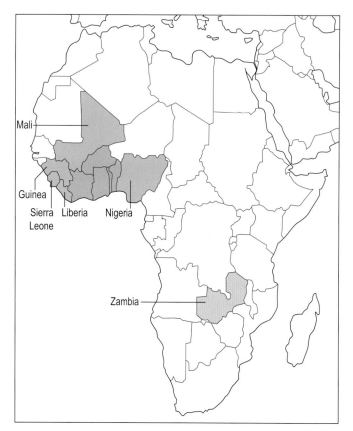

FIGURE 74-1 Endemic areas for Old World arenaviruses. Only the two arenaviruses known to cause haemorrhagic fever, Lassa and Lujo, are shown. Countries where clinical cases of Lassa fever have been confirmed are depicted in green. Indirect evidence, such as anecdotal reports or seroprevalence data, exists for most of the other countries in West Africa, shown in red. Endemic countries for Lujo virus are shown in blue. Incidence and risk of disease may vary significantly within each country. *(Reproduced from Farrar J, editor. Manson's Tropical Diseases. 23rd ed. London: Elsevier; 2013. Fig. 16.2. © Elsevier.)*

should ideally have an area outside for decontamination (i.e. removing potentially contaminated clothing). Needles and sharps should be handled with care by experienced staff. After significant occupational exposure such as a needlestick injury, post exposure prophylaxis with oral ribavirin should be considered.

The treatment for Lassa fever is with IV ribavirin, which is expensive and not commonly available. It seems to improve survival, particularly when given during the first six days of symptomatic disease.

THE CASE CONTINUED ...

The diagnosis of Lassa fever was confirmed with antigen testing and the patient received IV ribavirin in a specialist isolation unit. Unfortunately the patient was already very unwell by this stage and died two days later. All of the patient's family, close friends and medical staff were interviewed to determine whether they had had contact with the patient. All contacts were advised to monitor their temperature and seek medical help if they became unwell within 21 days of the contact.

SUMMARY BOX

Lassa Fever

Lassa fever is a severe systemic disease caused by infection with an arenavirus.[1] It is a zoonosis of rats of the genus *Mastomys* and infections in humans are likely to result from contact with infected rat urine. Lassa fever is common in Liberia, Sierra Leone, Ghana and Nigeria, although it probably occurs in a much larger area of sub-Saharan West Africa (Figure 74-1). Cases have been imported to Europe from other countries such as Mali and Côte d'Ivoire. There are up 300 000 cases estimated a year with 5000 deaths, although the confidence limits of this estimate are likely to be very broad.

Most cases are thought to be mild and patients may not even present to a health facility, but in hospitalized patients, the case fatality rate may be as high as 20%. Lassa fever is more severe in pregnant women, with a higher case fatality rate in the third trimester. It frequently results in premature labour or spontaneous abortion and about 90% of fetuses of women infected with Lassa fever die.[2]

The incubation period is 3–21 days. In individuals who are not pregnant the disease normally starts insidiously with fever, body ache and weakness. Sore throat and retrosternal chest pain are common, as are vague abdominal symptoms such as pain, diarrhoea and vomiting. Cough and breathlessness may occur in some patients. Conjunctivitis is common, especially late in the disease. Frank bleeding is rare. Raised liver transaminases are a marker of severity and are associated with a higher mortality.[3]

Serological and PCR tests are available for the diagnosis of Lassa fever, and an antigen-based rapid point-of-care test has been licensed.

As Lassa fever is common, it should be considered in anyone with a febrile condition who has visited an endemic area and appropriate infection control precautions should be implemented. It is more common in people from rural than urban areas but it does occur in towns. Treatment with IV ribavirin is likely to be beneficial if given early in the disease, but it should also be considered in patients who are diagnosed late.

Further Reading

1. Blumberg L, Enria D, Bausch DG. Viral haemorrhagic fevers. In: Farrar J, editor. Manson's Tropical Diseases. 23rd ed. London: Elsevier; 2013 [chapter 16].
2. Price ME, Fisher-Hoch SP, Craven RB, et al. A prospective study of maternal and fetal outcome in acute Lassa fever infection during pregnancy. BMJ 1988;297(6648):584–7.
3. McCormick JB, King IJ, Webb PA, et al. A case–control study of the clinical diagnosis and course of Lassa fever. J Infect Dis 1987;155(3):445–55.

A 25-YEAR-OLD WOMAN FROM ZAMBIA WITH A NEW ONSET SEIZURE

Omar Siddiqi

Clinical Presentation

HISTORY

A 23-year-old HIV-reactive Zambian woman is referred from a health centre to a local teaching hospital in Lusaka after suffering her first ever seizure. The seizure occurred out of sleep. Her son walked into her bedroom after hearing a noise and found his mother on the floor unresponsive and shaking all four limbs. This continued for 5–10 minutes.

The patient had been diagnosed with HIV infection one month earlier. She is not yet on antiretroviral therapy (ART) but has been taking co-trimoxazole prophylaxis for seven days. She was successfully treated for pulmonary tuberculosis four years ago.

The patient is unmarried with three children. She works in the hospital cafeteria. She does not drink alcohol or use any recreational drugs.

CLINICAL FINDINGS

On examination she looks well, her GCS score is 15/15, her vital signs are normal and she is afebrile. There is no meningism. The chest is clear. The neurological examination is unremarkable.

LABORATORY RESULTS

The malaria rapid diagnostic test is negative. Further blood results are shown in Table 75-1.

A lumbar puncture is done. The opening pressure is normal. The cerebrospinal fluid (CSF) is clear. CSF results are shown in Table 75-2.

IMAGING AND EEG RESULTS

A CT scan of her brain shows frontal and parietal hypodense lesions in the white matter of the right hemisphere (Figure 75-1). No contrast enhancement is present. Electroencephalography (EEG) demonstrates focal slowing in the right hemisphere (Figure 75-2).

TABLE 75-1 Blood Results on Admission

Parameter	Patient	Reference Range
WBC ($\times 10^9$/L)	5.8	4–10
Haemoglobin (g/dL)	11.0	12–14
Platelets ($\times 10^9$/L)	215	150–350
CD4 count (cells/µL)	153	500–1200
Serum sodium (mmol/L)	135	130–145
Serum glucose (mmol/L)	4.5	3.9–5.5

TABLE 75-2   CSF Results on Admission

Parameter	Patient	Reference Range
Leukocytes (cells/μL)	5	0–5
CSF protein (g/L)	0.78	0.25–0.55
CSF glucose (mmol/L)	2.9	2.25–2.97*
Cryptococcal antigen (CrAG)	Negative	Negative
India Ink stain	Negative	Negative
Gram stain	Negative	Negative
Ziehl–Neelsen stain	Negative	Negative

*½ to ⅔ of paired serum glucose sample.

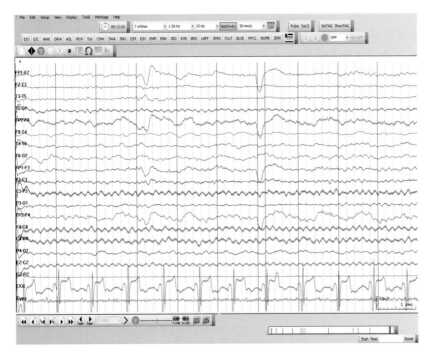

FIGURE 75-1 EEG demonstrating a slow background with superimposed delta frequency slowing of the right hemisphere.

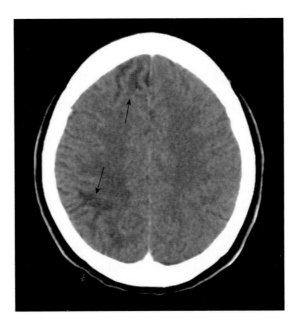

FIGURE 75-2 CT scan showing right frontal and parietal hypodensities in the subcortical white matter.

QUESTIONS

1. How would you manage this patient?
2. What is your general approach to a patient presenting with new onset seizures in sub-Saharan Africa?

Discussion

A young Zambian female presents with a new onset seizure. There are no focal neurological deficits on examination. The CSF examination is normal, apart from a slightly raised protein level. Neuroimaging reveals hypodense lesions without contrast enhancement restricted to the subcortical white matter. Electroencephalography demonstrates focal slowing in the right hemisphere. The patient is HIV-reactive, and her CD4 count is low. She is not yet on antiretroviral treatment.

ANSWER TO QUESTION 1

How Would You Manage This Patient?

The patient presents with a symptomatic seizure; there are obvious lesions in her brain and she is HIV-positive with advanced immunosuppression.

Treatment should aim at both preventing further seizures (antiepileptic treatment) and managing the underlying condition (causative treatment). The patient and her guardians should be counselled about the nature of her epileptic disorder, respecting their beliefs and attitudes.

The choice for an antiepileptic drug should take into account the local availability and costs for the patient. Phenobarbitone is the most widely available and most affordable drug in sub-Saharan Africa followed by carbamazepine. Newer drugs with fewer interactions and a better side-effect profile such as levetiracetame are not yet routinely available. Phenytoin and valproic acid are also used but their delivery might be unreliable. Reliability of supply is an important factor to consider, as the discontinuation of the antiepileptic medication might put the patient at risk of withdrawal seizures. When starting a patient on phenobarbitone or carbamazepine the effects of hepatic enzyme induction on antiretroviral therapy and hormonal contraception must be considered.

Syndromically, focal brain lesion is the underlying pathology in our patient. Differential diagnosis for focal brain lesions in an HIV patient with a new onset seizure includes tuberculoma, progressive multifocal leukoencephalopathy (PML), cerebral toxoplasmosis, cryptoccocoma, brain abscess and primary CNS lymphoma.[1,2] Neurocysticercosis, which can occur unrelated to HIV infection, also needs to be considered.

Lesions that selectively affect the white matter without contrast enhancement and without perifocal oedema are strongly suggestive of PML. There is no causative treatment available for PML. Commencing antiretrovirals is currently the only therapeutic option.

ANSWER TO QUESTION 2

What is Your General Approach to a Patient Presenting With New Onset Seizures in Sub-Saharan Africa?

The approach is influenced by (1) the high prevalence of HIV and subsequent immunosuppression; (2) the high burden of infection, including tuberculosis, bacterial meningitis and tropical diseases, e.g. cerebral malaria; and (3) lack of resources, in particular, low availability of imaging studies and antiepileptic drugs.

CNS infections are a prominent cause of epileptic seizures in sub-Saharan Africa. They can cause seizures during the acute illness (acute symptomatic seizures), as well as weeks or months after the acute episode, if the infection leaves an epileptogenic 'scar' in the brain (remote symptomatic seizures).

Three questions should be addressed when managing a patient with possible epileptic disorder:[2]

1. Is it actually an epileptic seizure/epilepsy?
2. Is there an underlying cause for the seizure disorder which can be identified and treated?
3. Does the patient require antiepileptic drug treatment and for how long should it be given?

The available diagnostic and therapeutic means dictate the clinical procedure. Mimics of epileptic seizures such as syncope and psychogenic non-epileptic attacks (so-called pseudoseizures) must be considered. Here, the history taken from the patient as well as from witnesses and guardians is decisive. Feelings of lightheadedness before the loss of consciousness, pallor and brief reorientation after the fall are typical for syncope. Psychogenic non-epileptic attacks are characterized by eye closure, long duration and bizarre motor manifestations. They often occur when the patients are subjected to emotional stress, such as during spiritual rituals and church masses.

In all patients with unknown HIV status, HIV testing should be performed. In all febrile patients, a CNS infection including cerebral malaria should be ruled out. Opportunistic CNS infections should be considered in immunosuppressed patients. In areas with high prevalence of *T. solium*, neurocysticercosis should be taken into consideration. In view of the limited resources, the diagnosis will be based on clinical and epidemiological evidence, hence, the knowledge of local distribution and prevalence of possible causes is helpful.

When initiating antiepileptic treatment, the issues of availability, including reliability of supply, affordability and interactions between antiepileptic drugs (AEDs) and patient's medication, must be taken into consideration (in particularly, antiretrovirals, antituberculous drugs and contraceptives).

Treatment of women of child-bearing age might pose some additional challenges. In all women of child-bearing age, folic acid (5 mg/day) should be added to the regimen. Antiepileptic drugs recommended for women of child-bearing age in resource-rich settings with low HIV prevalence, such as lamotrigine, are not available in sub-Saharan Africa and might have adverse interactions with ARVs, especially protease inhibitors. In those cases where several antiepileptic drugs are available, the specific drug chosen for epilepsy treatment of a woman of child-bearing age will be a trade-off between the health of the fetus and that of the mother. Here, one should consider that leaving out a drug because of its possible fetal toxicity, such as valproic acid, and using instead an enzyme-inducing drug with a better record regarding fetal malformations, might lead to a virological failure that would jeopardize both the mother and the child.

Counselling the patients and their guardians is of paramount importance. An epileptic seizure is a dramatic event. In some African communities, epileptic disorder is still attributed to supernatural causes. Patients who have experienced epileptic seizures might become socially stigmatized. Patient-tailored, non-judgemental counselling, taking into account the patient's perception of the disease, might assist in securing the patient's cooperation. Involving local health workers from the community might help overcome misconceptions and reduce stigma.

THE CASE CONTINUED ...

The patient was started on carbamazepine 200 mg bid. Valproic acid was initially requested but the patient could not afford it.

JC virus DNA was later detected in the CSF as part of a research study, further confirming the suspected diagnosis of PML. She was commenced on ART and remained on carbamazepine. After six months she remained seizure-free and carbamazepine was stopped. After one year of ART the patient's CD4 count reached 535 cells/μL and she had returned to work.

SUMMARY BOX

Seizure Management in HIV

HIV patients are at risk of developing seizures related to HIV-associated neurological diseases and metabolic disturbances.[1-4] The decision to initiate antiepileptic drugs in an HIV patient with seizures depends upon their aetiology and the duration for which the patient remains at risk of seizure activity. If the cause is readily reversible, such as hypoglycemia, there is no need to initiate antiepileptic treatment. If the patient has a seizure related to a reversible process of medium duration such as an opportunistic infection (OI), it is reasonable to initiate an antiepileptic drug (AED) and continue it for 3–6 months after treatment for the OI has been completed. If a patient develops persistent seizure activity without a reversible cause, then a diagnosis of epilepsy should be given and long-term AED will be required.

Ideally, one should select an AED that avoids hepatic metabolism due to drug–drug interactions with antiretroviral therapy. However, this may not be possible in a resource-limited setting where the only available drugs are hepatically metabolized agents such as carbamazepine, phenobarbital and valproic acid. In this case, valproic acid is the recommended agent, as it is a cytochrome P450 enzyme inhibitor as opposed to carbamazepine and phenobarbitone, which are cytochrome P450 enzyme inducers. When long-term treatment with carbamazepine or phenobarbital is the only option, the patient needs to be monitored closely for virological failure.

Further Reading

1. Modi M, Mochan A, Modi G. Management of HIV-associated focal brain lesions in developing countries. QJM 2004;97(7):413–21.

2. Radhakrishnan K. Challenges in the management of epilepsy in resource-poor countries. Nature Rev Neurol 2009;5(6):323–30.

3. Heckmann JE, Bhigjee AI. Tropical neurology. In: Farrar J, editor. Manson's Tropical Diseases. 23rd ed. London: Elsevier; 2013 [chapter 71].

4. Siddiqi O, Birbeck GL. Safe treatment of seizures in the setting of HIV/AIDS. Curr Treat Options Neurol 2013;15(4):529–43.

A 55-YEAR OLD WOMAN FROM TURKEY WITH FEVER OF UNKNOWN ORIGIN

76

Andreas J. Morguet / Thomas Schneider

Clinical Presentation

HISTORY

A 55-year-old Turkish woman presents to a hospital in Germany with remittent fever up to 39.5°C, night sweats, chest pain and abnormal fatigue. The patient had visited her relatives in Turkey several weeks before. There is a history of rheumatic fever in her childhood and mechanical mitral and aortic valve replacement at the age of 37 and 53, respectively (St Jude Medical prostheses).

CLINICAL FINDINGS

The patient's blood pressure and heart rate were within normal limits. There were unremarkable prosthetic heart sounds and a systolic grade 1 murmur over the aortic area without radiation. Liver and spleen were not enlarged. No lymph nodes were palpable. No haemorrhages or petechiae were detectable.

LABORATORY RESULTS

On admission, there was slight anaemia (Hb 11.5 g/dL [reference >12 g/dL]). White blood cell count, lymphocyte–neutrophil ratio and platelet count were within normal limits. The C-reactive protein was 15 mg/dL (reference <0.5 mg/dL). Serum creatinine and transaminases were not elevated. Blood cultures were negative. Urinary cultures yielded enterobacteriaceae.

FURTHER INVESTIGATIONS

Chest radiography showed no infiltrates. Transthoracic echocardiography demonstrated competent prosthetic valves.

The patient was diagnosed with a urinary tract infection and treated with co-trimoxazole. Body temperature dropped to normal values and the patient's condition improved, but not completely. She complained of increasing dyspnoea and eventually went into congestive heart failure.

QUESTIONS

1. What are further differential diagnoses in this patient after deterioration?
2. What are the most promising next diagnostic steps?

Discussion

The patient presented with fever of unknown origin. She had travelled to Turkey shortly before and had a history of double heart valve replacement. Treatment with co-trimoxazole resulted in some improvement, but then the patient developed signs of congestive heart failure.

ANSWER TO QUESTION 1

What Are Further Differential Diagnoses in This Patient After Deterioration?

Urosepsis could have been the underlying cause of the deterioration in this patient. However, urinary tract infection is usually easily managed with a short course of early antibiotic treatment. The patient's preceding stay in Turkey should raise the suspicion of another infection not detected so far, such as brucellosis, tuberculosis or Q-fever.

ANSWER TO QUESTION 2

What Are the Most Promising Next Diagnostic Steps?

With two prosthetic heart valves, our patient has an increased risk of infective endocarditis. Transoesophageal echocardiography is indicated to rule out cardiac involvement. Cultivation of blood cultures should be extended to up to six weeks in culture-negative endocarditis to reveal *Brucella* or *Coxiella* spp.

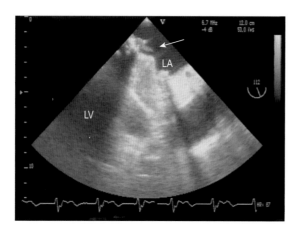

FIGURE 76-1 Transoesophageal echocardiography showing a two-cornered vegetation (arrow) measuring about 18 mm × 7 mm attached to the posterolateral left atrial side of a St Jude Medical prosthesis in mitral position (LV, left ventricle; LA, left atrium).

THE CASE CONTINUED ...

After four weeks, the blood cultures taken initially grew *Brucella melitensis biovar 2*. Transoesophageal echocardiography revealed a large vegetation attached to the prosthetic mitral valve (Figure 76-1). These findings led to the diagnosis of active *Brucella* endocarditis. Treatment with rifampicin, doxycycline 100 mg bd and gentamicin was initiated. The patient improved rapidly with defervescence within three days. C-reactive protein returned to normal after six weeks of triple therapy. Two months later, however, an annular abscess cavity around the aortic prosthesis was demonstrated on echocardiography; the patient at that time was on oral rifampicin and doxycycline. Finally, she gave her consent to a third thoracotomy, for prostheses exchange. After surgery she made a complete and sustained recovery.

SUMMARY BOX

Brucellosis

Brucellosis is one of the most common zoonotic infections worldwide.[1,2] Its true incidence is unknown as it typically affects rural communities and it is difficult to diagnose. Hot spots of the disease are Eastern Europe, the Middle East, Central and South Asia, Central and South America and Africa.[2]

The disease is caused by intracellular bacteria of the genus *Brucella*. The *Brucella* spp. most importantly involved in human disease are *B. melitensis* (goats, sheep, camels), *B. abortus* (cattle), *B. suis* (pigs) and *B. canis* (dogs).

Brucellosis is most commonly acquired by eating raw or undercooked meat and offal or untreated dairy products. Also, close contact with infected livestock poses a risk. It is an important occupational hazard amongst herdsmen, dairy-farmers, abattoir workers and laboratory technicians.

Symptoms are nonspecific, with fever, sweating, fatigue, weight loss, headache and joint pain persisting for weeks or even months.[3] Its presentation as a nonspecific febrile illness poses a differential diagnostic challenge in geographic regions where malaria and tuberculosis are highly prevalent and diagnostic resources are scarce, such as in sub-Saharan Africa. In the latter context, brucellosis is frequently missed as a major aetiology of fever, as has recently been shown from Tanzania.[4]

Brucellosis may involve nearly every organ of the body. While endocarditis is a less common manifestation of the disease,[5] cardiac valve involvement was the most frequent cause of death from brucellosis in the past.

Definitive diagnosis requires the isolation of the bacteria from the blood, body fluids or tissues. This can be challenging as culture may take several weeks. In endemic settings, serological tests are often the only available diagnostic test and their interpretation may be challenging.

Treatment of brucellosis requires combination antibiotic therapy of several weeks' duration to prevent relapses.

Doxycycline (six weeks) plus streptomycin (2–3 weeks) were considered most effective in a recent meta-analysis. Since streptomycin requires intramuscular injection, quinolones plus rifampicin for six weeks are an alternative option.[6] In children and pregnant women, a combination of co-trimoxazole and rifampicin has been used.

In the case of cardiac valve involvement, spondylitis or neurobrucellosis, extended parenteral antimicrobial therapy is recommended. Patients with *Brucella* endocarditis will frequently require valve replacement in addition to antibiotic therapy.

Further Reading

1. Beching NJ, Madkour MM. Brucellosis. In: Farrar J, editor. Manson's Tropical Diseases. 23rd ed. London: Elsevier; 2013 [chapter 28].

2. Dean AS, Crump L, Greter H, et al. Global burden of human brucellosis: a systematic review of disease frequency. PLoS Negl Trop Dis 2012;6:e1865.

3. Dean AS, Crump L, Greter H, et al. Clinical manifestations of human brucellosis: a systematic review and meta-analysis. PLoS Negl Trop Dis 2012;6:e1929.

4. Crump JA, Morrissey AB, Nicholson WL, et al. Etiology of severe non-malaria febrile illness in Northern Tanzania: a prospective cohort study. PLoS Negl Trop Dis 2013;7:e2324.

5. Agarwal SK, Rajani AR, Hussain K, et al. Brucella endocarditis: an occupational hazard! BMJ Case Reports 2013; published 22 Apr 2013.

6. Yousefi-Nooraie R, Mortaz-Hejri S, Mehrani M, et al. Antibiotics for treating human brucellosis. Cochrane Database Syst Rev 2012;10:CD007179.

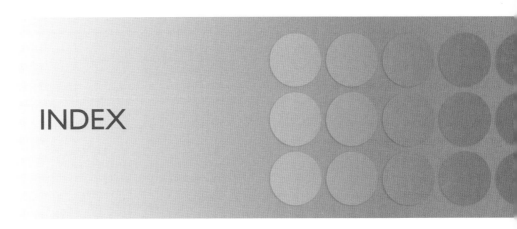

INDEX

Page numbers followed by 'f' indicate figures, 't' indicate tables, and 'b' indicate boxes.